Just Care

In the series *Dis/color*, edited by Cynthia Wu, Julie Avril Minich, and Nirmala Erevelles

James Kyung-Jin Lee, *Pedagogies of Woundedness: Illness, Memoir, and the Ends of the Model Minority*
Milo W. Obourn, *Disabled Futures: A Framework for Radical Inclusion*

Akemi Nishida

JUST CARE

Messy Entanglements of Disability,

Dependency, and Desire

TEMPLE UNIVERSITY PRESS
Philadelphia • *Rome* • *Tokyo*

TEMPLE UNIVERSITY PRESS
Philadelphia, Pennsylvania 19122
tupress.temple.edu

Portions of Chapter 3 are reprinted by permission from Springer Nature: Palgrave
Macmillan, *Subjectivity*, "Relating through differences: disability, affective relationality,
and the U.S. public healthcare assemblage," Akemi Nishida, © 2017 Springer Nature.

Library of Congress Cataloging-in-Publication Data

Names: Nishida, Akemi, author.
Title: Just care : messy entanglements of disability, dependency, and desire /
   Akemi Nishida.
Description: Philadelphia : Temple University Press, 2022. | Series: Dis/color |
   Includes bibliographical references and index. | Summary: "Just Care examines
   care as a site where the somatic, the political economy, and intersectional social
   oppressions manifest and materialize interactively, while it is also a vision and
   praxis for radically collective and affectionate ways to live and transform society"—
   Provided by publisher.
Identifiers: LCCN 2021059336 (print) | LCCN 2021059337 (ebook) | ISBN 9781439919897
   (cloth) | ISBN 9781439919903 (paperback) | ISBN 9781439919910 (pdf)
Subjects: LCSH: Health services accessibility—United States. | People with disabilities—
   Home care—United States. | Home care services—United States. | Community health
   services—United States. | Social justice—Health aspects. | Caring—Political aspects. |
   Caring—Moral and ethical aspects.
Classification: LCC RA418.3.U6 N56 2022 (print) | LCC RA418.3.U6 (ebook) |
   DDC 362.2/40973—dc23/eng/20220318
LC record available at https://lccn.loc.gov/2021059336
LC ebook record available at https://lccn.loc.gov/2021059337

♾ The paper used in this publication meets the requirements of the
American National Standard for Information Sciences—Permanence
of Paper for Printed Library Materials, ANSI Z39.48-1992

Printed in the United States of America

9 8 7 6 5 4 3 2 1

Contents

Notes to Readers

Image Description of the Cover

In the center of the cover, the title, *Just Care*, appears in all capital letters, large-sized font, and in black color. At the top of the cover, the author's name, Akemi Nishida, appears in medium-sized font and in black color. At the bottom, the book's subtitle, *Messy Entanglements of Disability, Dependency, and Desire*, appears in medium-sized font and in black color. The background is a close-up of a mural that may remind people of walls at schools or parks. It is made up with multiple colors and many overlapping abstract shapes that are painted on a concrete surface. Orange, blue, turquoise, red, black, cream, purple, and yellow paints fill in shapes including circles, squares, and other abstract shapes involving many curvy lines.

Notes on Content Warnings

This book in general includes mentions and depiction of ableism and intersecting social oppressions taking place during care routines such as daily personal assistance. This includes interlocking systems of oppression, experienced by those who are situated as care receivers and workers, and expands to not only ableism but also sexism, racism, xenophobia, queer-phobia and transphobia, and (settler) colonialism. In different chapters, there are mentions of slavery, colonialism, eugenics, various forms of confinement, forced medical treatment, and police brutality as well. These depictions at large do not entail vivid, detailed, and visual descriptions of such violence. Please refer to the first endnote in each chapter for further content warnings specific to the chapter. Please prioritize your self- and collective-care as you read this book.

Acknowledgments

この本を始めるにあたってまず日本とアメリカの家族にお礼を言いたい。日本でケアまたは世話といえば家族中心というのが当たり前な中、それを無視して渡米し自分の学業を優先したことで日本の家族には色々と迷惑をかけたと思う。そうすることで得られた家族の形もあるのだろうけど地球の反対側で生活をしていくことで心配や面倒をかけてしまったことは否めない。そんな中で私のことを遠くから見守り、自分勝手させてくれた両親、弟、祖父母、叔父叔母、従兄弟たち、そして近所の方達には感謝しかない。

　そしてアメリカでの家族。この本を執筆するにあたってサポートし続けてくれたパートナー、ジョーと子供の譲生は常にケアという題材を実際の生活の中で体現してくれた。ありがとう。この本は日本とアメリカの家族の助力なしには存在しなかったということは断言できる。I begin this book with the preceding special thanks to Itsuko, Akira, Akifumi, Joe, and Yuzuki.

I have never said "I love you" and I have rarely used the word *love*, because the word to me is so *U.S.*, or more accurately it does not align with the cultural norms and customs I grew up with. I never heard people around me say "I love you," as I grew up in the countryside of Japan. Once, I saw a seemingly Southeast Asian teenager reading a book titled *I Love Yous Are for White People: A Memoir* (by Lac Su) on the New York City subway. I almost jumped and screamed "YES!" Love is certainly not only for or used particularly by white people, but it captured my sentiment. And yet I catch myself repeatedly saying "I love you" back to my closest friends nowadays. Maybe that's a sign that I am more Americanized. Or it is because I am now in long-lasting relationships with many of the people whose names I write in the following. And I do not know a better word to express the magnitude of appreciation and fondness I have for these people. Thank you all. I love you all.

In addition to the families in Japan and the United States whom I thanked earlier, I would like to thank my crip family and communities. It is they who shaped my understanding of the world and taught me what is dreamable and visionable that I would have never been able to realize without them. Those who mentored me since the early days after I migrated to the United States include Leroy F. Moore Jr., Sebastian Margaret, Patty Berne, Eli Clare, Charone Pagett, Jane Dunhamn, and Gykyira. Other crip family, friends, and comrades include Alejandra Ospina, Park McArthur, Nick Dupree, Michelle Mantione, Leslie Freeman, Julie Murray, Tina Zavitsanos, Amalle Dublon, Trina Rose, Stacey P. Milbern, Dwayne Bibb, Bhuttu Mathews, Collette Carter, Nadia, Aaron Ambrose, Kay Ulanday Barrett, Stephanie Infante, Jay Toole, Vandana Chaudhry, Liberte Locke, Dynah Haubert, Sandie Yi, Carolyn Lazard, Alice Sheppard, Lezlie Frye, Angel L. Miles, Liat Ben-Moshe, Candace Coleman, Timotheus Gordon Jr., Kim The, other members of AYLP in Chicago, Rahnee Patrick, Carrie Kaufman, Ting-Ting Grace, Jenny Charlton, Esther Lee, Yi Ping Lin, Kennedy Healy, Dean Adams, Olivia McAdams, Euree Kim, Leah Lakshmi Piepzna-Samarasinha, Lydia X. Z. Brown, Abia Akram, Walei Sabry, Pater Trojić, Lawrence Carter-Long, Matthew Clark, Margot Cole, Nadina LaSpina, Harilyn Rousso, Adrienne Asch, the people at CUNY Coalition for Students with Disabilities (special thanks to Charmaine Townsell and Chris Rosa), Toby MacNutt, Marjorie McGee, various care collectives I was part of, and many more people whose paths crossed with mine and those who are with me in this world and in whatever world comes next.

The generous support of my academic mentors and dissertation committee helped me to articulate and communicate what I was feeling and thinking: Michelle Fine, Nirmala Erevelles, Dan Goodley, Wendy Luttrell, and Josh Clegg. Such support continued at my current job at the Racialized Body cluster at University of Illinois Chicago with Cynthia Blair, Rod Ferguson, and Lorenzo Perillo.

I was fortunate to be surrounded by people who shared a core belief that academic and scholarly work must happen for social justice and must be done collectively by resisting the individualism engraved in academia and elsewhere. I thank Michelle Billies, Kendra Brewster, Rachel Liebert, Puleng Segalo, Ali Lara, Wen Liu, Colin Ashley, Duquann Hinton, Caro Muñoz-Proto, Steph Anderson, David Caicedo, Adeola Enigbokan, Vicky Barrios, Isabella Elisha, Sonia Sanchez, Sabrica Barnett, Shawndel Fraser, Bill Cross, Judith Kubran, Suzanne Oullette, Mariette Bates, Lauri Hyers, Pam Block,

Rachel O'Connell, Ronak K. Kapadia, Aly Patsavas, Zhiying Ma, LaWanda
Cook, Juliann Anesi, Sami Schalk, Jina Kim, Alison Kafer, Eunjung Kim,
Margaret Price, Jess Waggoner, Ally Day, Carrie Sandahl, Michele Friedner,
Joan Ostrove, Michelle Nario-Redmond, and Karen Nakamura. Special
thanks to Patrisia Macías-Rojas for our daily check-ins to sustain each other
beyond university walls. Many whose names are listed here have read different versions of chapters in this book and not only gave me tremendous
feedback but also modeled how to engage in feminist peer reviewing.

Thank you for many collective writing, workshopping, reading, and
chatting spaces including Free Space (organized by Michelle Fine), NYC Disability Studies Group (organized by Lezlie Frye and Rachel O'Connell),
Anti-Oedipus Happy Hour Group and Affect Theory Reading Group (both
organized by Ali Lara), Write on Site (organized by Marisha Humphries and
Lorena Garcia), Team Chiya Chai (organized by Ronak K. Kapadia), Writing Our Ass Off, while Wiping Yuzu's Ass Up (with Angel L. Miles and
Sandie Yi), Chicago Feminist Disability Studies Workshop Group (with Liat
Ben-Moshe, Aly Patsavas, Zhiying Ma, and Michele Friedner), Summer
Writing Retreat (organized by Sami Schalk), and UIC Institute for Research
on Race and Public Policy (IRRPP) Writing Retreat. Thank you, Jill Petty, for
coaching me at the IRRPP writing retreat.

Thank you, Timotheus Gordon Jr. and Ashley Volion, for the brilliant
insights you shared with me as research assistants. Thank you to students,
staff, and faculty members in the Critical Psychology program at the Graduate Center and Disability Studies program at the School of Professional
Studies (both at City University of New York) as well as the Disability and
Human Development and Gender and Women's Studies Departments at
University of Illinois Chicago.

Thank you, Shaun Vigil, Cindy Wu, Julie Avril Minich, and Nirmala
Erevelles for creating and nurturing a platform, the Dis/Color series, to discuss race and disability in depth. I am proud to be part of the endeavor.
Appreciation also goes to the people at Temple University Press who have
been very accommodating and supportive.

Thank you for all your care and labor to nurture and expand disability
studies and inviting me to share my ideas when they were not quite in shape
yet—School of Professional Studies at the City University of New York (special thanks to Mariette Bates); Second Life (thanks to Gentle Heron/Alice
Krueger), Western Massachusetts Disability Studies Conference (thanks to
Sarah Orsak); Chicago Disability Studies Student Council Conference
(thanks to Disability and Human Development, Student Association); University at Buffalo (thanks to Cindy Wu and Michael Rembis), University of
Chicago (thanks to Michelle Friedner and Zhiying Ma), Japanese American
Service Committee (thanks to Ryan Yokota), University of Kansas (thanks

to Ray Mizumura-Pence and Sherrie Tucker), University of Wisconsin–Madison (thanks to Sami Schalk and Ellen Samuels), University of Connecticut (thanks to Laura Mauldin and Nancy Naples), Arika, Performance Space New York, and Whitney Museum (thanks to Amalle Dublon, Jerron Herman, Carolyn Lazard, Park McArthur, Alice Sheppard, and Constantina Zavitsanos), University of Minnesota (thanks to Angela Carter), Sawyer Seminar at UIC (thanks to Jennifer Brier and Stacey Sutton), Newbery Library Gender and Sexuality Seminar (thanks to Francesca Morgan, Elizabeth W. Son, and Ronak K. Kapadia), University of Texas at Austin (thanks to Alison Kafer, Grayson Hunt, and Lisa Moore), Williams College (thanks to Emily Mitchell-Eaton), and Bard Graduate Center (thanks to Therí A. Pickens and Nadia Rivers).

Speaking of care and labor, Oliver Fugler of Queer Edit is the one who read every word in this book and helped me with developmental and copy editing over the years. Thank you, Oliver, for how you practice editing in very genuine and social-justice-oriented ways.

Thank you, Bella Chen, Jennifer Sowell, Duygu Durmus, Hiro Namba, Linh Le, and Terria Brown for our long-term friendships that sustained me since the time of the ESL class at Delaware County Community College. Finally, credit for the book title goes to Joe Martello. Thank you for your talent for coming up with silly puns.

Just Care

Introduction

Needing Care and Caring Needs

All living creatures have needs. To need is to be alive. Still, we often let ableism classify some needs as socially accepted and others as not. Instead of receiving support, people [with] intellectual disabilities often lose their autonomy if they need help making decisions. Cities send police officers [with] guns if a person needs psychiatric support. People who need daily assistance are called "drains" on the state. Capitalism is most exploitative when it focuses us to ignore limitations or needs. *How can we hold need as sacred?* [emphasis added]
—Disability Justice Culture Club, "All living creatures"

I

Needing You

On the late afternoon of October 28, 2012, I was needed by and simultaneously needing my friends.[1] Texts from a number of friends from disability communities flooded my cell phone. They were all desperately looking for emergency care supports for our friends Michael and Sonia, as Superstorm Sandy was approaching New York City.[2] Although they direct their own long-term care routines—twenty-four-hour home nursing care for Michael and several hours of care a day for Sonia—they urgently needed someone to come over and carry out care tasks that they direct during the hurricane.

The urgency was palpable as the sky got darker and the wind caught speed—all signaling that the storm was about to land on New York City. City officials had announced the closure of the subways, bridges, and tunnels that connect Manhattan with other boroughs and New Jersey. It meant that nobody—including the care worker who was supposed to take the next shift—was entering or leaving the island. I immediately hopped onto one of the last subway trains from Brooklyn to Manhattan. The subway cars as well as the streets leading to their apartment were almost desolate—occupied only by people who were experiencing housing insecurity, wearing layers of clothes, sitting with shopping carts full of their belongings to prepare for the hurricane. Acknowledging their presence from the corner of my eyes and feeling the chill in my backbone as the city's lack of care for certain people was more alarming than the hurricane itself, but I continued rushing to my friends, who were my priority that afternoon. Finally, I arrived at the tall residential building where they lived in lower Manhattan. Many apartments in the building seemed vacant as the occupants had left to seek safety and comfort, while building managers hurried to get ready for the hurricane.

As I walked into Sonia and Michael's familiar and warm apartment, I was immediately embraced and competed for space with power chairs, beds, complex connections of wires, computers, and other communication and entertainment devices, as well as the tall towers filled with medical devices, including Michael's ventilator. These devices filled the room with the rhythms of different and constant sounds signaling that they were functioning just fine. This is their living room/bedroom/community gathering space, which was covered by the decorations from the last birthday the room had witnessed. The room acts as activism strategy office, movie-watching social space, and home-away-from-home for disabled wanderers from all over the world. Michael and Sonia are, after all, a power couple and the keystones of disability communities both virtually and in real life, and they do not hold back support for anyone who comes their way. They are activists and cultural workers who are friends and crip family to me and so many others. They took care of me, as they fed me emotionally, physically, intellectually, financially and much more in this room, just as they did for anyone who comes their way.

That afternoon, the apartment was a cave, protecting its inhabitants from the anxious rush on the other side of the door. Sonia and Michael welcomed me with a smile just like any other day—Sonia from her power chair, sitting between her and Michael's beds, and Michael from his bed. Michael's care worker and friend, Jason, was engaging in tasks as usual, and just like any other day he was leaving after his shift in the early evening (instead of extending his stay and care shift) in order to take care of his own and his family's needs, which meant leaving Lower Manhattan before all the transportation got shut down. There was no sign of other care workers coming to take the next shift, or any shift in the near future, because of the emergency situation—hence Michael and Sonia had reached out. They had prepared several gallon jugs of water and their fridge was filled with just the usual amount of food. After all, we were not sure how big the hurricane would actually be, and we also were facing the limits of what we could prepare as disabled people leading the life of the financially poor (but rich with community love).

Going to a shelter or hospital was not an option, they told me early on. The shelters and even hospitals were not accessible enough or ready to provide the particular care they needed. Electricity is key to providing Michael with air, nutrients, and medicine as he lies on his bed and to enable Sonia's power chair and their reclining beds to do their work. Hundreds of tiny pieces of plastic, metal, and fabric must be assembled and work together perfectly for them to live. In these circumstances, anywhere but home felt precarious. Any hiccup with hospital generators; a lack of time, energy, or will of nurses to learn specific and individualized ways to provide care to Michael (particularly his tracheostomy care); lack of wheelchair-accessible space for Sonia to be near Michael to direct his care; or even a tiny dislodge of Michael's oxygen bag, which provides him with air, while he was transferred to a hospital could end my friend/family's life. Michael had endured the trauma of institutionalization in his earlier life and was determined not to go back. Based on how disability services and programs are set up and budgets are allocated, it was easy to imagine, and pretty much guaranteed, that evacuating to a hospital would automatically lead to Michael's being reinstitutionalized without any promise of getting out.[3]

We lost electricity the second night after I got there, and then water, and eventually cell service. Lower Manhattan never gets dark—ever. It is home to Wall Street, city hall, and the heart of this nation's economy. And yet that night, it was weirdly dark—except for the construction site of Freedom Tower, which was intensely lighting up nothing but concrete and metal.

The sudden cutoff of electricity acutely showed why I was needed. Electricity enabled them to live. Without electricity, the battery of Michael's ventilator would run out in a few hours and stop assisting Michael to breathe. Here my needs kicked in too—I needed my friends to survive the hurricane and continue allowing me to be embedded in their lives. I was the only one in the household—consisting of three disabled people (since Jason had left already)—mobile enough to take the stairs to go to the nearby fire station to use their generator to charge a spare ventilator battery. The game plan was this: I would go there every few hours to charge the spare battery, the ventilator would keep working, and my friend would keep breathing and living. A straightforward and simple task—except that it is not. To do so throughout a night without adequate sleep, go down and up staircases in absolute darkness for at least a dozen floors which were occasionally occupied by strangers, seemed nothing compared with the alternative—Michael wouldn't get to breathe. And yet, it was hard in its own right—to be beyond exhausted, walking up and down staircases with a body not used to such exercise in the middle of the night, passing strangers who were way bigger than me and intoxicated, in the complete darkness, and knowing that most of the apartments in the building were vacant, so no one could hear me or come to help. But the hardest part, which still gives me chills today, was the sense that my friend's life literally depended on me. My head told me to stay calm and rational, yet my body and imagination exploded with anxiety and panic. Every nightmare from the past occupied my head, and all the anxiety of the future thrummed in my skin. My friend's life depended on me, in an acute and direct way, as much as my safety also felt precarious in a different way, as a Northeast Asian disabled cis woman living in a world filled with race-based gender violence—but again, I repeated to myself, this was nothing compared with the anxiety Michael and Sonia must be feeling to put all their eggs in one basket—me.

By the third day, the sun was shining, the hurricane was gone, and we sat and lay in the sunlit room together, alive but still desperate with no water or electricity, not much food, and dying phone batteries with no cell signal. Our phones had been our lifeline connecting us with the outside world, so losing them activated another level of devastation.

It was then that an unexpected knock on the apartment door vibrated the air of the quiet apartment. Surprised, we looked at each other exhaustedly, and when I opened the door, there were two strange men. They were holding a box of food, water, and other supplies and quickly told us that our friend and local disability rights activist had sent them, and they were in the middle of delivering more supplies to other people.

Right before we lost our phone signal, I posted on Facebook: "Day 2, no power. Which means Ive [sic] been running up and down of 10+ stories stairs every few hours to charge batteries. Which means no food. While the city offers a car to pick up nurses, no nurse since Sunday night. HELP." What we did not know in that small New York City apartment was that the disability community had gotten together online, collecting supplies needed to keep us alive and connecting with local strangers or disability community members who were mobile enough to send supplies our way.

Using Google Docs, a virtual network was ever-expanding with friends and strangers signed up to take turns making the battery run for Michael's ventilator, to provide ad hoc care for Michael and Sonia, and to coordinate people to collect gas and drive to pick up and drop off their home care workers. People all over the United States sent marine and car batteries so that Michael and Sonia could have electricity at their own home eventually without running to the fire station every few hours. A community-based care and support structure was established, and it lasted for months. So many connections were forged and many new friends were made. In particular, queer communities came first by bike to Manhattan to support Michael and Sonia—strangers to them.

Weeks later, still in the middle of my own recovery from what had happened, I sat down with participant observation assignments submitted by the students in my disability studies qualitative research method class at a continuing education college. The class was filled mainly with those who worked as care workers at group homes for people with intellectual and developmental disabilities. They were almost all Black and Brown migrant women.[4] Given that the hurricane happened in the middle of the semester, many documented their experiences during the hurricane. What filled their participant observation papers was how they had to work day after day—even a week and more—nonstop during the hurricane and its aftermath. There was nobody to come and release them from shifts, as transportation, bridges, and tunnels were still shut down or operating in a very limited capacity. Some care workers were forced to go back to work while their own disabled elderly parents sat in flooded homes without electricity. Many of those care workers, in other words, had to make hard and yet familiar choices of work or family—which is ultimately about whose care needs to be prioritized.

New York City's recovery was not done equitably. While the business district of Manhattan recovered in a blink of an eye, people living in the periphery of New York City lived without gas and electricity or among debris for months to come.[5] A documented 106 lives were lost during this deadliest hurricane of 2012.[6] This includes a death caused by failure of an oxygen machine due to the electricity shortage.[7] Furthermore, countless people lost their wheelchairs and other assistive devices in floods and during the mess of evacuation.

My need to keep my friends alive was met, and I gained new friends and assurance of community support during the ad hoc care shifts; however, it took me a while to regain a calm mind, however temporary. Questions from those days still occupy me: How can government meet people's needs and where are their limits? What are the possibilities of community-based and grassroots care and what are its limitations? What happened to other disabled people (and their needs) who did not have the kind of social capital and resources that Michael, Sonia, and I had? Whose needs are highlighted and whose are put aside? Why are we trained to prioritize people's needs: Are the needs of disabled people in group homes more urgent than the needs of disabled elderly parents whose children who are the primary family care providers and also work as care workers for wage have no choice but to leave them behind to go back to their work to attend to other disabled people?

Are some people's needs more sacred and urgent? How are their lives more precarious than others'? How do we measure people's needs and determine priorities regarding whose needs will be attended to first? Whose and what needs can wait? How do we know whether needs are met or not? How do we meet the needs of those who are unaware or taught to ignore that they have needs? Who is allowed to need? Whose needs are met with care? Reflecting on the opening quote from Disability Justice Culture Club, how can we shift society and our ideologies to "hold need as sacred?" What would our daily lives be like, and how would it feel to embrace and center our needs and dependencies as our principal values?

Care often emerges from needs, while needs are not always met with care. The preceding story, at a glance, seems an extreme case of care—caring during the superstorm. And yet it is not. It is a mere extension and continuation of the precariousness and challenges of everyday care that people negotiate whether they are situated as care givers, care receivers, or both. Exploitative labor conditions for care workers and of the difficulties that disabled people and others with long-term care needs face in securing ad hoc care have been a chronic issue, as the care crisis has become a regular occurrence in the United States.[8] How to decrease expenditures by public healthcare programs (e.g., Medicaid) while the number of people who need daily care and support only increases, and how to find care workers who will work under unjustifiably difficult conditions (i.e., low wages with meager benefits) have been the challenge politicians are tackling—but this problem also shows how poorly they understand and imagine the structure of care and people's needs for care.[9] On the ground, though, those who perform care work have always had to decide every day whose care needs to prioritize (e.g., their clients', their children's, their aging parents', or their own). People who are situated as care recipients, including people who are disabled, have always had to improvise when care is lacking by being carers for one another, as much as they cry, complain, and advocate together to end the low-quality care (aka ableist abuse) that they are subjected to.

In *Just Care*, I investigate the multiplicity of care—how it is turned into a mechanism of social oppression and control while simultaneously being a tool with which marginalized communities activate, engage in, and sustain social justice fights. Care has been turned into a business opportunity for care industries, especially under the current neoliberal political economy.[10] Care offered by the U.S. public healthcare system represents the line the nation draws to divide protected citizens (those who are cared for) from the unprotected ones (those left without care), while there is no guarantee that the care it provides is of high quality or is not used for surveillance and control of welfare beneficiaries.[11] The structure of care is deeply embedded in and embodies the cruel social order (e.g., racism, cisheteropatriarchy, ableism, neocolonialism).[12] All of these elements determine who is made to survive and thrive with and through care in the current political climate and who is made to deteriorate under the name of care. However, care also consists of everyday support systems woven together by everyday people and is embedded in each breath of our lives. Care at the micro level can facilitate connecting or gluing people and thus entails the potential to foster solidarity and mobilize mass.[13] Care is inherently collective and can activate and enable more sustainable relationships, and care is a necessary foundation for the more-just world that social justice activists fight for. Additionally, many social justice movements are undergirded by care, no matter how invisible an act of care is made to be.[14] It is community-based care or care for one another that lets marginalized communities survive and thrive, when they have been deprived of structural and public care, which I call state violence.[15] Care is the foundation and necessity for inclusivity, accessibility, and from-the-ground-up social transformation. It is a life-making and world-changing practice, while it is simultaneously used for money making—or worse, life sucking and sometimes life taking. Given this contradiction, I begin this book by thinking of care broadly as a site where bodymind, political economy, and historically formed social oppressions and social justice struggles intersect and interact. It is thus a way to envision and practice alternative, radically collective, and affectionate ways to live.[16]

In short, I examine *care injustice* where people—whether they are situated as care workers, care receivers, and others—deteriorate under the name of care when care is used as a mechanism to enhance political economy and neglect the well-being of those situated as care workers and care recipients. I also examine *care justice*, or *just care*, which occurs when people feel cared for affirmatively, whether they are situated as care workers, care receivers, or both, and when care is used to improve the well-being of people, the community, and the surrounding (i.e., natural and built) environment, and for more-just world building. The first half of the book looks into lives unfolding in the assemblage of Medicaid long-term-care programs taking place in people's own homes (instead of residential facilities like group homes). We assume (and hope) that governments guarantee a safety net when we are or become disabled and lower-income (including poor and working-class people)—but do they? Who is granted U.S. public healthcare support, and how? Who is made to assume responsibility for care under such programs, and how? I examine how the circumstances of those who are situated as Medicaid enrollees and care workers are different, overlap, and are interwoven, and whether they are cared for as care recipients and as workers in the U.S. public healthcare sector. The neoliberal status quo has been intensifying the social injustices that are directed toward those who are situated as care workers and care receivers and within which their lives unfold while their everyday lives are profoundly embedded in each other's. In this context, what kind of resistance can they (and others) activate and nurture in the middle of care-based structural oppressions? What visions for better care practice are dreamed of, shared, and enacted by those who are situated as care workers and care receivers?

The second half of the book explores how care justice is imagined and enacted as well as how care undergirds and expands social justice activism. To do so is also to tap into various marginalized communities' tactics to survive and thrive by caring for one another when government fails (or actively neglects) to meet people's care needs. My particular focus is on care collectives (community-based mutual-aid groups) formed by disabled and queer people to meet each other's care needs and to actively practice interdependence—a principle that disability justice activism advocates for. What is it like to practice such social justice vision—interdependency—in their everyday lives, when the surrounding world operates the opposite way: enforcing individualist independence? As members of the collective desire to be entangled in each other's messy dependency, what does such desire activate and how does it enable different ways to be with each other? What are the implications of yearning to reclaim their dependencies, when dependency has been used as a key tactic to justify ableism inflicted on disability communities?

Finally, this quest to unfold the multiplying and contradicting layers of care lands on *bed activism*—resistance and visioning that are happening in bed space. Sick and disabled people of color (among others) have put forward *crip wisdom* from their bed spaces. Crip wisdom emerges from the everyday lives of disabled, neurodivergent, Deaf, Mad, sick, injured, and debilitated people.[17] What and how do critiques of the status quo and normalization of activist works, as well as unique resistance and visions, emerge from bed space? What do moments of enduring pain, fatigue, depression, and other bodymind conditions in our beds activate and animate? What becomes dreamable as we take seriously the resistance and visions bubbling out and embodied in sick and disabled people's beds? What possibilities, wisdoms, and even struggles does a bed space hold, offer, and teach us and the world?

Caring

Care is present throughout the opening story of Superstorm Sandy. For example, the government determined what care was offered (or was not offered) to those who were experiencing housing insecurity and/or disabled people like Michael and Sonia who rely on Medicaid and whose complex care needs are hard to meet at evacuation sites—all of which dictate their well-being, vitality, and ability to stay alive. Or what the building managers may have thought of as care by calling 911 to send firefighters to check on us during an electricity outage can also be read as their concerns about liability, in which we are turned into their risk. It was simultaneously care from friends and strangers that enabled us to continue living under desperate circumstances. Care is transient, malleable, and subjective. Multiplying meanings, intentions, and impacts are contained in and enacted by a gesture of caring.

What care does is the focus of this book. My curiosity is about care as a modality of power dynamics. Care is used to enforce top-down dominant power as much as care is exercised at the grassroots level to enable resistance against such dominant power and enact transformative power for a more-just world and way of living. Care is structured and institutionalized in the interlocking system of racist, cisheteropatriarchal (i.e., sexist, transphobic, and queer-phobic dominance), neocolonial, and disability economies. It is commodified by care industries or turned into a way for governments to manage and control people, particularly those who are involved in public healthcare programs. And yet care has also been an everyday tool of everyday people to survive, thrive, and transform the violent status quo. In short, our lives are enabled and hindered by care (and the lack thereof) as much as we enact care.

I begin this book by thinking about and understanding care as the energy and time we spend in intention to contribute to others' well-being, vitality, and lives. Care is a way to orient ourselves and direct our energy toward something or someone. I begin with such a broad definition to avoid prescribing the notion of who can care or normalizing and hierarchizing different forms of care that are evident in the narrow way care is structured and set up in the larger society. Specifying care as a particular action (e.g., the physical care of feeding someone), for example, can obscure care by disabled people who may not be able to perform the particular action. Standardization of care offered by the care industrial complex often values physical care over emotional and spiritual care. It also dictates who can care and which people are exclusively considered as receivers of care. My understanding of care has profoundly grown from the work of disability justice activism and the writings of Patty Berne, among many others who advocate for interdependency, which illuminates that we all are capable of care, need care, and are worthy of being cared for.[18] In other words, the act of sending positive vibes to others from one's bed is care, just like the physical act of care (e.g., cooking for others) that is built into long-term-care support services. Additionally, care is highly subjective, and one's intention to care may not be always met with observable outcomes such as a change in vitality and well-being, or it may not be received as care by the person the care was intended for.

Care is a name we give to our experiences—what we do, sense and feel, or think. Care is inherently relational, whether it actually ties together humans and other living and nonliving entities, or even our inner self (i.e., self-care).[19] It can touch (physically and metaphorically) lives to various depths. Care manifests in various modes: physical, material and financial, emotional, cognitive, and spiritual care, to name a few. Care transgresses time and space—words from an elder may touch a youth decades later, for example. It is subjective as much as it is susceptible to and embedded within the forces of political economy as well as the intersecting social oppressions. This means that what one person thinks of as caring can be experienced by others as violence, control, pity, love, debt, a life saver, and so on. The practice of care is deeply cultural, sociopolitical, and historically situated—which I further explain later. My understanding of care is further shaped by how it is defined by theorists including Christina Sharpe, who describes care as "a way to feel and to feel for and with, a way to tend to the living and the dying,"[20] or Berenice Fisher and Joan Tronto, who define care as "species activity . . . to maintain, continue, and repair our 'world' [which includes] our bodies, our selves, and our environment."[21] Additionally, the teachings of disability justice activism illuminate how care *circulates* among people, although it is often arranged to be given from a provider to a recipient.[22] People are simultaneously care recipients (who, after all, can live without care?) and care providers in varying degrees, though not everyone is equally provided with care or subjected to care-providing. To address this multiplicity of care, I use the term *care practice* in this book to portray the expansive layers and forms of care—care as provided, received, and circulated—as they are often indistinguishable and noncompartmentalizable.

Thinking of care as open-ended and circulating is my intervention on how care has been often compartmentalized in the field of care studies. Defining care often entails and prescribes dichotomization of people as either carer or cared—"Care is conventionally defined as the activities and relations involved in caring for the ill, elderly, handicapped [*sic*] and dependent youth."[23] This example definition used in labor studies of care not only restricts care solely as an action but also prescribes the *subjects* and *objects* of such actions. It also simultaneously indicates who needs care and who does not, or who is capable of caring and who is not. Different schools of care studies—including feminist, labor, and disability studies of care—have highlighted and prioritized studying circumstances of different constituencies who were embedded in the care structure.[24] Paying attention to how the term *care* is scrutinized and described with different synonyms and adjectives, alone, gives us a glimpse of various approaches one can take to studying care. *Burden* and *responsibility*, for instance, are commonly used synonyms to describe care, particularly in feminist and labor studies of care.

Those words explain that the care consists of daunting yet unavoidable work often tasked to women and gender-nonconforming femme people who are situated as care providers. Another commonly used term, *dirty work*, illustrates that care is work that involves feces, sweat, vomit, mucus, and other bodily discharge that is considered dirty.[25] Those terms shed light on how care is taxing *labor* and how people are disproportionately situated to that labor under the intersecting forces of cisheteropatriarchy, white supremacy, neocolonialism, and more that shape labor stratifications. Such an approach to care illuminates and problematizes the inequality bubbling on one side of the care equation—care giving. What is rarely mentioned in such analysis is the other side of equation—care receiving and the stories of those who are exclusively situated as objects and roots of such burden and responsibilities or dischargers of the "dirt." Thus, the care needs of those who are situated as care workers are rarely acknowledged.

The term *assistance*, rather than *care*, has been advocated in U.S. disability communities and studies, particularly following the Independent Living Movement, which emerged in the 1970s in the United States and elsewhere.[26] Disability communities and studies have problematized the ways disabled people are exclusively considered care recipients and dependent. This is true especially because their dependencies on others are constructed, amplified, and considered as a *social burden,* which is thus used to justify to deprive them of their agency to exercise self-determination. Care is, therefore, understood as a modality of patronizing power dynamics where disabled people are inherently made powerless. The term *personal assistantship* is put forward to avoid association of disability communities with the idea of care, which is thought specifically for "children, sick people, and older people, and [instead the term assistantship is believed to] highlight the empowering nature of consumer-directed models of support."[27] It is, in other words, a part of fight to end objectification of disabled people enacted within and through the practice of care. Here, too, what is rarely touched on is the other side of the equation—care giving—as disability communities advocate to establish employer-employee power dynamics with care workers, where disabled people are the ones with the authority of an employer. Also, it is often assumed that care workers do not have a disability.

Different approaches to studying care within these fields tease out how various oppressions are disguised and exercised through care; how cisheteropatriarchy shapes oppressions care providers experience, and ableism is interwoven in the experiences of care receivers.[28] Such focused approaches in these fields enable more in-depth analysis and understanding of care-based injustices. They also provide a way not to erase different degrees and unique needs of disabled people, as well as idiosyncratic ways that care workers experience exploitation. We can also observe how such distinct approaches and specific focuses traditionally taken in disability and feminist studies of care separately mean that the creative resistance and interventions of those who are situated as care workers and care recipients are often recognized separately, and so justice and liberation for those populations are often fought disjointly.[29] These distinct approaches can also be interpreted as the hidden assumptions in these fields that care workers do not experience ableism, and that cisheteropatriarchy does not shape the care experiences of those who are situated as care recipients.

To bridge these discrete analyses and to approach studies of care in radically different ways, feminist disability studies scholars have been exploring ways to study care more holistically. Feminist disability studies philosopher Eve Kittay's classic work, *Love's Labor*, for instance, inserts dependency critiques to the theory of justice by writing about her caring relationship with her disabled daughter.[30] Critical feminist disability theorist Nirmala Erevelles brings transnational feminist analysis into her examination of the care-based injustice disabled people are subjected to in the United States by engaging in historical material analysis.[31] By learning from and joining (intersectional) feminist disability studies, what I am putting forward is the overlap, intersection, and interaction between the circumstances granted to those who are situated as care workers and care recipients. Such analysis shows that it is marginalized populations who are pulled into the assemblage of care structure (whether as care workers or care recipients), particularly within U.S. public healthcare programs, which further marginalizes them. In reality, those who are situated as care workers and care recipients spend most of their waking time together and co-experience each other's day-to-day occurrences. This reality means that care workers' and care recipients' oppressions are experienced together and through one another, witnessed by one another, and thus entangled. Structurally, disabled people and their need for care are situated in the middle of and interwoven with the exploitation of care workers, and care workers are situated as the direct deliverers of care that many disabled people describe as ableist violence. This is to say that their daily care encounters are where macro-level care injustices trickle down and crystallize, and care justice cannot be achieved without justice for both those who are situated as care workers and care receivers.

Specifically, I analyze care by using what I call relational analysis. This analysis embodies and further expands what feminist disability studies scholars have been working on—exploring both care worker and care receiver roles and their relationships to develop a more holistic understanding of care formation.[32] To engage in relational analysis in this book is not only to center how the circumstances and oppressions of those who are situated as care workers and care recipients are interwoven and interactive but also to investigate and untangle the inherent dichotomization in our understanding of care. Such dichotomy can quickly trick us into thinking that care workers do not experience disabling conditions, that disabled people who are situated as care receivers are incapable of providing care, that ableism does not impact care workers, or that care recipients are immune from cisheteropatriarchal exploitation. It also obscures the mutually implicated genealogies of how care worker and receiver populations are shaped historically. Certain populations come to be constructed and considered solely as laborers who are dispensable in the public care setup, while other populations are exclusively considered as needing care since their dependencies on one another and public services are amplified as peculiar and burdensome. The profound devaluation of care thus accelerates further marginalization of those who come to be situated as care workers and care recipients in public healthcare programs. And most importantly, I use relational analysis to illuminate and (re)activate the many times when care is used to forge solidarity to reassure and reaffirm marginalized communities' worth and fundamental power. Dichotomized understanding of care also hinders the framework used to recognize how those who are situated as care providers and care receivers can come and are already coming together by co-engaging in nurturing care to lift one another. What kinds of dreams for care justice become imaginable with such an analysis?

Recognizing the historical development of care scholarship in feminist and disability studies as well as feminist disability studies and further inserting relational analysis, I use the term *care*, instead of *assistance* and *attendant*. Although these terms may not absolutely meet the demands of the disability rights community and disability studies, I am using the term to address how care is turned into a vehicle of oppression that disability and other communities face by calling it what it is (i.e., many disabled people are abused under the structure of care), in order to untangle such care-based oppressions. Similarly, I use the terms *Medicaid enrollees* or *those who are situated as care recipients* as well as *care workers* and *those who are situated as care workers* in this book. I do so, although they signal the dichotomy, in order to have the framework to articulate and make visible and denaturalize the energy and time that women and gender-nonconforming femme people devote to caring for others.[33] In other words, dissolving the role of care workers contains the risk of erasing the unequal ways that people's needs for care are made into the responsibilities of largely women and gender-nonconforming femme people. It also risks overlooking the reality that people do embody different kinds and degrees of capacities and care needs, while such capacities and needs are amplified or overlooked by ableism and other interlocking systems of oppression in this society. Also, by repeating the unwieldy phrase *those who are situated as* care workers and care recipients, instead of automatically designating care workers as nondisabled and care receivers as disabled, I resist the widespread assumption that care workers are nondisabled or immune to pain, fatigue, and other disabling conditions, and disabled people are not agents of care giving.

Controlling Care

Care is a racialized, gendered, trans, and queer matter, as well as entangled in power dynamics rooted in the matter of (neo)colonialism, transnationalism and migration, disability, age, and class. In other words, it is mutually structured in the racial and cisheteropatriarchal capitalism as well as the neocolonial and ableist economy. In those multiplying forces, ideas are formed about who needs or does not need care, who is suited or not suited to care, or who is worthy or unworthy of publicly funded care; these ideas simultaneously dictate and determine care worker and public healthcare enrollee (i.e., care receiver) populations.[34] Enabling and further enforcing those notions are the dichotomous understanding of care and devaluation of care practices, particularly when it involves caring for lower-income people, which is distanced from the care that more affluent people purchase for themselves and their family members.[35]

Unfolding care injustices helps to explain how people's capacities and debilities or disabilities are constructed, amplified, and differently valued. It is to trace the historical roots of how mainstream society came to dictate whose needs for care supports will be recognized or unrecognized and deemed worthy or unworthy of public supports. Race, for example, has been a crucial element that is used to construct and dictate people's capacities to take up labor and particularly physically taxing and low-paying jobs. The fundamental categorization of disability has been developed based on people's incapacities and inabilities to enter the capitalist labor force—which is how the state legitimates and grants the status of disability and associated public supports to its people—and sets it up as if disability and labor capacity are mutually exclusive; people are either disabled or workers.[36] A ripple effect of this categorization includes the oppressive and reductive understanding of racialized populations solely as workers, which leads to extra complexity in order for them to be recognized, legitimated, and identify as disabled and hence needing and deserving of the public services and supports. In the realm of care structure, women of color have historically and structurally been often primarily situated as care workers as their capacities to engage in domestic and care labor are amplified. This came with systemic ignorance of the reality that they have care needs too. This fundamental categorization and stereotyping of women of color as workers thus paved more complex paths for them to claim and be legitimated with disability status and considered deserving of public supports.[37] This setup is said to manifest in the welfare program for single mothers and families in need, for instance, that shapes today's care worker population among other elements—which I untangle more in Chapter 1.[38]

This is all to say that the construction of care labor capacities and incapacities and notions of being deserving or undeserving of public supports are inherently formed in intersecting social oppressions. Gender and sexuality are deeply influential to determine care giver-receiver dynamics too. Care is, for example, forged as family-based unpaid labor that is provided by mothers, daughters, and other female family members (and at a time gender-nonconforming femme members if they are not disintegrated from their families) to their biological family members.[39] This structure has simultaneously excluded many queer people from the familiar care circle, when they are pushed out of or run away from their biological families who enforce cisheterosexual ideology. Patriarchal and cisheteronormative family ties, in this case, draw lines between those who are cared for and those who are not, as well as delineating who performs care tasks in the family sphere.[40] I use the term *cisheteropatriarchy* to signal the intricate ways that forces of transphobia and queer-phobia, sexism, and heterosexism undergirds family-based and other care formation.

Additionally, behind each U.S. citizen who needs long-term care are often migrant women of color providing lower-wage care labor.[41] This is the case despite the fact that these women have next to no margin to become disabled and claim disability status themselves or receive any public care supports, as their legal residency in the U.S. often hinges on their capacity to work and any sign of them needing public supports can deter them from obtaining legal status (e.g., a green card).[42] The history of colonialism dovetails with global neoliberalism and neocolonialism to determine who will receive care and who will provide care on the global front.[43] Additionally, feminist philosopher Uma Narayan explains how exploitation and dehumanization under colonization have often been justified by discursively flipping this violence into a discourse of care—care provided by colonizers to "civilize" the colonized: "care discourse can sometimes function ideologically, to justify or conceal relationships of power and domination . . . 'paternalistic caring' of the sort found in colonial discourse can also be wielded as a form of control and domination by the powerful and privileged."[44]

These factors also mean that not everyone who is experiencing disabling conditions (i.e., impairments and debilities) is granted disability status from the governments that determine their rights to receive public supports (e.g., Medicaid) or recognized as needing and deserving care. Even when people are bureaucratically legitimated as having a disability and successfully enrolled in long-term-care programs funded by governments, however, this does not guarantee that they are inherently cared for. Their care needs, in particular, are woven into the fabric of ableism and interacting social injustices.[45] What is given as care is, therefore, often experienced as paternalistic violence and abuse to control and manage disabled people situated as care recipients.[46] Their dependency on and need for long-term care are, for example, amplified and framed as a *social burden*, whereas nondisabled people's dependency on others (e.g., domestic workers to clean their houses) is naturalized. In a society where independence is enforced as a virtue, their dependencies are turned into justification for ableist violence against them and thus locate them exclusively as care recipients and incapable of care—overlooking their contributions to others' well-being and to society.

Furthermore, this making of divisions—care giver and care receiver—in interlocking social injustices does not mean that marginalized communities and people passively experience care as a form of oppression or as care manifest only through such mechanisms of control. I tease out different structures of care that they invent and exercise in the next section. Also, this division does not reductively mean that disabled women of color who are situated as care recipients do not exist, simply because care labor is often reserved for (or forced on) women of color under the racialized, gendered, and migration-based occupational divide enforced by the care industrial complex. I will further complicate and challenge this dichotomy to assert that such a divide, if anything, indicates how the lives of disabled women of color are constantly pushed deeper into the shadows and ignored (though those women fight back—which I will examine further as well).[47]

The ways in which care is turned into and functions as a mechanism of control and oppression is only intensified and further enforced in the climate of the neoliberal political economy: "Neoliberalism is a political, economical, and ideological system that privileges the market as the most efficient platform for distributing social goods, minimizes the role of government responsibility in assuring collective well-being and highlights instead personal responsibility for assuring individual well-being."[48] Not merely an economic structure, neoliberalism is an ideology that shapes popular beliefs, thoughts, opinions, attitudes, and behaviors as well as implementing the new social order that organizes society in an economy- and market-centered way.[49] In political philosopher Steven Shaviro's words, the emergence of neoliberalism is the rise of "*new*, flexible forms of social organization [that] have their own traps, their own mechanisms of oppression, their own devices of exploitation and subordination" through which the rich get richer and the poor get poorer.[50] This new social order builds itself on and further intensifies already existing social injustices and social orders. Since the 1970s, this political economy and form of governing principle have spread across the world, though its manifestation varies from region to region.[51]

Neoliberalism further accelerates individualism and already existing social injustices and stratification that shape various ways that care is structured and exercised. Disability studies scholars Dan Goodley, Rebecca Lawthom, and Katherine Runswick-Cole, for example, have described neoliberalism as an incubator for ableism by addressing the reality that shrinkage of public supports and expansion of the privatized free market mean that austerity measures are constantly enforced to reduce or terminate public disability services that are lifelines to many disabled people.[52] In geographer David Harvey's words, "each individual is held responsible and accountable for his or her own actions and *well-being*. This principle extends into the realms of welfare . . . [and] health care."[53] Not doing well or thriving in the free market is then turned into an individual responsibility. Thus, the long-term-care needs of disabled people are increasingly pushed out of the purview of state responsibility with shrinking welfare programs, and instead made into an individual or family responsibility. Simultaneously, care industries have been flourishing by taking advantage of this responsibility as a business opportunity to develop care provision services. Public governmental responsibility is increasingly transferred to the private sphere (if these are indeed distinguishable). In such a context, inequality expands between those who can purchase care (e.g., quality healthcare insurance for medical care to keep well and thriving) and those who cannot, which leads to the gap between those who can fit the prototype of the ideal citizen and succeed in the free market and those who cannot. Discrimination between these two is not only a matter of individual financial wealth. It is also a matter of intricate social formations that determine who is deemed worthy of social supports and whose lives matter, as well as the values attached to people's (assumed) labor capacities or lack thereof. Not only is care formation in the status quo a *result* of neoliberalism, but such care formation simultaneously functions to further enforce the value system put forth by the neoliberal political economy.

Resistive and Visionary Care

As much as care is deployed as a mechanism of control and oppression, it has also been a tool for people to resist oppression and engage in alternative and collective ways of living. Such a way of living thus not only makes one's life more sustainable, but also gives them the power to distract the flow of the status quo and enable another kind of world making. I put forth those nurturing aspects of care to show that care is the foundation of and undergirds various social change activisms and practices, a notion that is often

made invisible.[54] Many marginalized communities have relied on care offered within them to survive and thrive, particularly when such care is
needed to tend the damage of social oppressions or to counter the lack of
public care supports (which is part of discriminatory state violence).

The Black Panther Party came up with a revolutionary health justice
practice, for example, when white supremacist policies and climate violently prevented members of Black communities from accessing quality
and comprehensive institutional medical care.[55] They created an alternative structure of healthcare provision for communities, including supply-
ing free meals for children, offering health education and free health
checkups in the community, and accompanying elders to doctor visits.
Their approach to healthcare as a basic human right and the foundation of
community living was visionary and revolutionary, particularly against
the backdrop of the rising industrialization (and hence commodification)
of healthcare and care in general. Another example of community based
care is observable in queer communities forging chosen families to take
over the care granted and limited within family of origin. Specifically, during the rise of the HIV/AIDS epidemic, such chosen families and queer kins
attended to those who were ill by caring for them at every level (providing
food, physical and emotional care, and more).[56] Preceding this, the Street
Transvestite Action Revolutionaries (STAR), founded by trans activists of
color Marsha P. Johnson and Sylvia Rivera, created community-based care
circles to provide home and nurture for trans and queer youth of color who
needed them.[57] When care has been and still is often located in the unit of
family of origin and deeply shaped by cisheteropatriarchal ideologies,
trans and queer communities have transgressed this foundation by engaging in peer intimate care for one another without blood-based and law-
based family boundaries and restrictions. Migrant communities, particularly those who are not U.S. citizens and do not have legal documents, are
also left to forge their own care structures because of the lack of healthcare
supports from the state.[58] Houston Health Action (a pseudonym), for example, is a grassroots group of undocumented uninsured migrant people
who have become disabled during the physically taxing labor to which
migrant populations are often subjected. In the absence of affordable
health insurance and limited access to hospital medical care, they raise
money on their own to buy devices such as catheters and visit one another
to exchange care.[59] Finally, disabled people too have come to forge alternative and community-based care structures, as public healthcare programs
are unavailable to or underserving them or as such structure has been
described as functioning as surveillance and control than nurturing care.[60]
They have followed the call from the disability justice movement, for

instance, to create alternative ways to meet one another's care needs by transgressing the boundary that situates disabled people exclusively as care recipients. Instead, many disabled people work together collectively to provide care needed by their community members as much as they also receive care.

Although I laid out snapshots of collective care that have emerged from different communities in the preceding paragraph, they certainly overlap and influence one another, as people occupy intersecting identities and communities. The rise of care needs within a community thus indicate the manifestation of disability (i.e., impairments), signaling the impossibility of clearly drawing a line to divide those communities.[61] Further, these examples also demonstrate how care and relationalities forged through care enabled and sustained those communities to thrive and engage in social changes.

Beyond the care structured by the state, family, or communities, care circulates, sustains, and affirms people in our everyday lives and at the micro level. Seeing #BlackLivesMatter chalked on streets, for example, to affirm the value of Black lives and existences can be crucial in a political climate that constantly gives the opposite message.[62] When a queer youth runs away from their family, meeting a senior queer person and receiving mentorship are forms of care that can change the future trajectory of the youth.[63] What would it mean for an undocumented migrant person to receive hundreds and thousands of signatures from strangers on a petition demanding that they be given safe and legal space in the United States?[64] Finally, the magnitude of emotion that disabled people may feel as their care to others is recognized and appreciated—in an atmosphere that automatically turns them into social burdens—is incalculable.[65] The magnitude of the sensations that I call *care* here are hard to capture, but they can entail transient moments that inherently integrate the power to affect people and activate changes in their well-being. In this book, I aim to capture these life-altering and life-affirming moments of care justice or just care that are buried under the layers of care injustices inflicted by industries and the state. When care is used to trivialize or even dispose of many people's well-being and lives—through exploitation in the care labor force, being subjected to abuse under the name of care, or being left without care supports—people dare to continue caring for one another. They engage in care simultaneously as a way to survive and thrive, as a modality to show love, and to form a radical collectivism that interweaves people's lives beyond the individualist boundary enforced in the United States and under the neoliberal climate. Throughout *Just Care*, I illuminate these contradictory and multiplying realities of care to understand the life-making that is happening in disability and other marginalized communities in the middle of a debilitating socio-political climate.

Grounding

So much of the care that was experienced during and after Superstorm Sandy was invisible or existed only between lines of what I could observe and articulate. I will not know the experiences of caring and being cared for that Sonia or Michael felt. Yet those invisible, inarticulable, between-the-lines feelings, senses, and actions undoubtedly add color and vitality to our lives.

In the broadest sense, how I understand care as being embedded in the larger sociopolitical forces and nurturing a vision for a more-just society was founded on the teachings of disability justice activism, affect theories, and critical feminist, race, and disability theories. Disability justice activism, in particular, illuminates different ways to engage in care in order to live in more sustainable and interdependent ways and also how care is the bedrock of marginalized communities and their social change fights. Developed and nurtured by disabled gender-nonconforming, trans, queer, Black, Indigenous, activists of color as they weave together their community and cultural wisdom, this activism centers on ten principles: intersectional analysis, leadership of those most impacted, anticapitalist politics, building cross-movement solidarity, recognizing wholeness of people, prioritizing sustainability in social justice fights, commitment to cross-disability solidarity, investing in interdependent relationships, working for collective access, and collective liberation.[66] Although these principles emerged to reimagine or reactivate radically inclusive and accessible social justice movements, they also guide us in how to conduct our everyday lives in more-just ways, which simultaneously allows us to build and embody a different world. The care justice or justice enabled through care that I write about here, therefore, is an attempt to reflect this activism, while I write this book with a hope to further contribute to the deepening of this movement. In other words, disability justice activism teaches me how to dream collectively while it also equips me with the sharpest analysis to detangle the violence we witness and experience in the status quo under the name of care. In this way, I am thankful for leading disability justice activists such as Patty Berne, Mia Mingus, Leroy F. Moore Jr., Sebastian Margaret, and Eli Clare as well as Stacey Park Milbern, Leah Lakshmi Piepzna-Samarasinha, Lydia X. Z. Brown, and more and more people who developed and nurtured the disability justice activism since the early 2000s and who are, thus, cited heavily in this book.[67] Disability justice—which I often describe as a mash-up of race-based, trans-specific, queer, feminist, migrant, decolonial, and cross-disability (i.e., Deaf, neurodiverse, Mad, and anti-psychiatry) social justice work—is the prism through which I understand the status quo of care and visions of what care can be and do.

With disability justice as a foundation, I also examine care through critical theories—mainly critical disability, race, (transnational) feminist, and also queer and migration studies. Building from these frameworks, therefore, I untangle an aspect of care as an oppressive mechanism that relies on white supremacist, cisheteropatriarchal, neocolonial, xenophobic, and ableist logics—the logics that critical theorists have articulated. Critical theories also help me uncover the overlapping yet distinct histories of how care and the needs of people have been the center of community building and resistance in the marginalized communities mentioned.[68] Writing this book on the foundation on the teachings of disability justice activism and critical theory also involved attending the emergence and development of theory happening in the everyday life of everyday people, regardless of their affiliation with academic entities.[69] Boricua Ashkenazi disability justice artist and activist Aurora Levins Morales uses the term *homemade theory* to describe the theories emerging from people's everyday lives and to bring theory out of academic walls: "we create [homemade theories] out of our shared lives, [and it] really help[s] us to make sense of everything that we are and all that we find to love."[70] She transgresses the inaccessible and exclusionary ways that theory is written within academia and instead reclaims and engages in theory building, which is rooted in shared lives of people regardless of their academic training and affiliations. Learning from her and other like-minded feminists, I bring together theories primarily emerging from academic spaces with theories that emerged and developed from and during my conversations with Medicaid care workers and enrollees, members of community-based care collectives (mutual-aid groups developed by disabled people), and those who engage in bed activism together to better understand the status quo through the analysis of care and needs.[71] The critical theories (which are mainly emerging from academia) that I unfold in this book include differential inclusion (conceptualized by Yến Lê Espiritu) in Chapter 1, necro-theories (developed and written by Achille Mbembe, Lauren Berlant, and Jasbir Puar) in Chapter 2, affective body (theorized by Audre Lorde) as well as hapticality and undercommons (written by Stephano Harney and Fred Moten) in Chapter 3, critical analysis of interdependency (woven by Baggs) and messiness (explored by Martin F. Manalansan VI) in Chapter 4, and dreaming from bed (put forward by Aurora Levins Morales, Leah Lakshmi Piepzna-Samarasinha, and Johanna Hedva) in Chapter 5—all of which I further describe throughout the book.[72]

These ideas and thoughts are further enhanced by homemade theories of those whose lives are intimately embedded in public healthcare programs and community care collectives.

Affecting Care

I situate care directly in relation with life: shaping the vitality and well-being of people. To recognize and write the relationality, I rely on the concept of *affect* together with the aforementioned activist, critical, and homemade theories. I use the idea of affect to describe the invisible, inarticulable, between-the-lines feelings and senses that care activates. As much as care can be thought of as a concrete action, it can also be understood as what circulates among and through us and transforms us (for better or worse). It is the invisible force or energy that impacts us as much as we emanate it and influence others. Affect becomes feelable as we are evoked and recognizable as we attach emotion to name the affect—excited, tired, depressed, anxious, and angered, for example.[73] Therefore, to talk about affect is also to pay attention to the transient and ever-changing energy level of our bodyminds: capacitation and debilitation.[74] In the context of care, I explore how care becomes a site or modality of this transition. This idea put forward as affect, I argue, is familiar to disability communities. Indeed, it is an integral part of community knowledge, as people constantly communicate their fluctuating energy levels with or without the metaphor of spoons, which I bring up in the following.[75]

Political philosopher Gilles Deleuze has described affect as follows (in his interpretation of Dutch philosopher Baruch Spinoza's work):

> The affections (*affection*) are the modes themselves. The modes are the affections of substance or of its attributes. . . . These affections are necessarily active. . . . The *affection* refers to a state of the affected body and implies the presence of the affecting body, whereas the *affectus* refers to the passage from one state to another, taking into account the correlative variation of the affecting bodies. . . . "By affect I understand affections of the body by which the body's power of acting is increased or diminished, aided or restrained."[76]

Affect theorists Melissa Gregg and Gregory Seigworth have described affect as a synonym for the *force* emanating from people and manifesting at the site of encounters by connecting us with our surroundings (i.e., other people and environments) that can draw us toward or repel us from one another.[77] Also, affect can be a flow of energy that influences—enhances or decreases—one's vibrancy and vitality.[78] It escapes the comb of empirical measurement while moving people and shaping lives, or it is interpreted (i.e., cognitively registered) as a certain emotion. To apply affect theory is to pay attention to experiences and phenomena as being felt in the gut and sensed through the skin.

Viewing girls with muscular dystrophy on TV telethon programs, for example, moved many viewers to open their wallets and donate—this force or affect might be named as a feeling of pity or fear that is deeply rooted within ableism in society. Images of disabled people, including disabled children, abandoning their wheelchairs to crawl and drag themselves up the staircases of the Capitol to advocate for the Americans with Disabilities Act in 1990 pushed many disabled people to join the movement—such an affect can be registered as empowerment. In affect theorist Brian Massumi's words, affect is "a prepersonal intensity" and "govern[s] a *transition* where a body passes from one state of capacitation to a diminished or augmented state of capacitation," and thus "every transition is accompanied by a feeling of the change in capacity."[79] To encounter others, surrounding environments, and political atmospheres entails the potential to be influenced in how we feel, act, think, and dream. The encounter, therefore, activates an increase or decrease in a bodymind's capacity and vitality.

Affect theory informs this book in multiple ways. My primary understandings of care as modality, transient encounter, or what circulates among and through us are all shaped as I conceptualize care through this theory. My use of the terms *capacitation* and *debilitation* to illustrate the fluctuations in a person's capacity (i.e., increased or decreased vitality or energy) through care is another way. On one hand, these fluctuations are part of *every bodymind's* daily and transient experiences, corresponding to the ever-changing energy level or vitality of the bodymind. I use the terms, therefore, regardless of a subject's status as a disabled or nondisabled person. On the other hand, I also use the terms *capacitation* and *debilitation* to describe the prolonged status of a bodymind. Disability and race theorists (among others) have deployed this latter use of these terms largely to depict a more permanent status of a bodymind as debilitated—whether it is recognized or identified as disability or not—which has been caused by social injustices (e.g., armed conflict, police brutality, labor exploitation, lack of quality healthcare).[80] Accordingly, I use the term *care* to entail the sense of a modality that shapes people and their well-being and vitality. To use affect as a theoretical framework for this book is, therefore, to pay attention to (1) the realm of sensual experiences, (2) people's fluctuating energy as well as states of bodymind, and (3) what circulates *between* people, other (non)living entities, institutions, and surrounding environments, which is to set a unit of analysis as connections and relationships among elements rather than the element itself.

I engage with affect theory through and with the aforementioned critical and homemade theories and under the prism of disability justice teachings. This includes taking critiques against the theory seriously by making efforts to decenter who is considered as knowers of affect and by integrating its diverse developments before and since the theory's initial popularity in the 1990s (e.g., the field's initial overlook of Indigenous wisdom and knowledge on *felt theory*).[81] In particular, many people have pointed out the field's initial lack in recognizing how social power dynamics are present in experiences of affect.[82] Mad studies theorist and artist Rachel da Silveira Gorman points out that "[Queer of color theorists assert] affect as a product of repetition and sedimentation of ideology, rather than of 'preindividual bodily capacities' in which the diversifying complexes mediating social relations vanish into the appearance of unmediated essence."[83] As this quote demonstrates, there have been developments of affect theory that insert or follow the tradition of critical theory. Building on this, using affect theory for my analysis and understanding of care does not mean letting go of sociopolitical and cultural power dynamics that are profoundly present in care—but bringing them together and centering them. Also, it is to recognize, for example, Audre Lorde's writings about the erotic as seminal text theorizing about the affective capacity of bodyminds, without relying solely on those mainstream affect theorists (on which I further elaborate in Chapter 4).

Affect studies' focus on the body, its sensation, or its capacity and debility as an area of exploration, I argue, is compatible with and useful for disability studies. Affect theory has shifted the paradigm of studying a body away from an investigation of representation or meaning attached to bodies (which was popular prior to the affective turn in the 1990s) and toward a body itself.[84] It explores what a body can do or how a body affects or is affected by its surroundings. To refocus on bodies in affect studies terms is not equal to solely measuring bodies based on the functionality and values attached to them, a measurement that disability studies has wrestled to dismantle over decades. Although I engage in the capacity- and debility-based commodification and exploitation that people are subjected to in the current political climate, this refocusing on bodies expands on more than that. One principle of affect theory is to illuminate the vitality and capacity emanating from the *existence* of a living body (and bodymind) itself by paying close attention to subtle ways that a bodymind affects others—the heat it releases, the rhythm it beats, the odor it radiates, the touch sensed by others and with which it saturates others.[85] What are the aspects of care practice that such illumination and attention make feelable and recognizable? This theory, in other words, allows us to acknowledge the power of a bodymind and the power that it emanates on a very micro and subtle level and its shaping of care. This overlaps with disability studies' call to understand disability as part of diversity without pathologization and criminalization.[86]

What does it mean to recognize and value people based on their bare existence, which emanates energy, instead of evaluating them solely on their functionality and its usefulness to the political economy? Using such an affect studies approach to bodymind is also to ask how to recognize the power of existence beyond and against the neoliberal extraction of debilitated bodyminds and oppressed status (e.g., how the toxic-waste-management business flourishes by discarding trash to marginalized neighborhoods and the Global South, and how their marginalized status itself forms the foundation of this business as it uses that status to justify this form of social oppression manifesting through environmental injustices and enacted under the political economy). It also means grasping care as being more than physical actions (and also happening emotionally and spiritually, among other ways). Cognitive function is often deployed as the foundation upon which to define, standardize, and value people, for instance.[87] People's experiences, agency, and ultimately human-ness are overwhelmingly recognized in the ways they assert themselves verbally and through exercising certain functionality, for example.[88] Disability studies as a field has been critiquing this bias and grappling to make a shift by analyzing and problematizing the overt focus on *mind* (e.g., the deployment of IQ to measure, categorize, and value human beings, which simultaneously has led to discrimination against and devaluing of those with intellectual and developmental disabilities).[89] Indeed, there has been a move within disability studies to prioritize a body or blur the division between body and mind, instead of exclusively prioritizing or privileging minds.[90] Mad activist-scholar Margaret Price, for instance, questions the fundamental divide between mind and body by describing how both elements interactively shape our experiences and existences by putting forward the term *bodymind*.[91] Focusing on how disability studies along with affect theory can further assert different understanding and valuing of bodyminds does not neglect the reality that ableism is rooted in the function-based valuing of disabled people and dictates our desires (e.g., overt emphases on enhancing one's abilities through rehabilitation to be part of the political economy). Or this highlighting of existence (i.e., ontology) is not the same as saying that disabled people cannot function or have no function in this society. Instead, I am following the insights and knowledge of disability studies and communities as well as neurodiverse communities who fight against the pathologization of certain ways our minds work and to acknowledge and value the diverse ways people's bodyminds operate.[92] Further, such focus can make visible multiple ways that we care and experience care, while physical care is considered as default and the basis for paid care labor formation.

This idea that bodyminds are dynamic as their energies fluctuate is wisdom that is always and already nurtured in disability communities. Describing and communicating such fluctuations of energy and capacity have been crucial for disabled people to articulate what kind of care and supports we need and to illustrate the state and needs of our bodyminds, which are not necessarily visible to others. In particular, those with chronic fatigue and pain have developed *spoon theory* to explain their energy level and how it changes across the day in a visualized and quantified way that is easily comprehensible to others. When Christine Miserandino, who lives with Lupus, wanted to explain what it is like to live with such chronic illness and fatigue and how her energy is drained or regained differently than that of her nondisabled friends, she grabbed spoons to use them as a metaphor for the energy she had for a given day.[93] The number of spoons she has and how quickly she loses a spoon is a dynamic combination of her disabled bodymind and internal and external influences. Weather and temperature (external factors) or the amount of sleep one gets the night before (an internal factor) can cause one to lose spoons quickly, and different tasks can cost a different number of spoons as well. Community members may tell their friends, "My spoons are low this evening due to the cold weather, and I cannot go out anymore," to explain the need for last-minute cancellation of plans. Having care or a personal assistant, in this context, allows disabled people to reserve their spoons and have more choices on where to spend their spoons (while their care worker can assist them with daily activity without losing too many spoons). Although spoon theory has been developed based on the needs of those with chronic fatigue and illness (that are often invisible) in particular, to communicate and make visible their changing stamina or bodymind conditions, affect theory illustrates such fluctuations of energy as happening to any body in various degrees. The theory offers language to discuss the dynamic nature of the degree or speed of how fast we debilitate (i.e., losing spoons), how much innate energy we embody (i.e., the number of spoons we have), how fast we can recover our energies (i.e., regaining spoons), and how care shapes or dictates these transitions. The community-born wisdom of spoon theory embodies what I am trying to put forward in this book by bringing together affect theory and critical studies and by relying on terms like *debility* and *capacity*. It illuminates and introduces language to capture the dynamic materialization of the political economy and social injustices in and through bodyminds. Now, what does it mean to recognize disability in this theoretical framework, which conceptualizes lives—vitality and well-being—as constantly evolving or *becoming* instead of *being*?

Affecting Disability

When I'm writing about bodies it pulls me back to the lived experience
of bodies, reminding me that bodies are not metaphors and symbols but
visceral, lived experiences of bones, muscle, blood, and shit.
—Eli Clare, "Resisting Easy Answers"[94]

I highlight in this book how disability is assembled in multiplying intersecting power dynamics as much as disabled bodyminds inherently transgress the restrictive framework of the disability-normalcy binary by leading
unexpectable and rich lives that are woven with resistance and crip (also
Deaf, Mad, neurodiverse, sick, and debilitated) wisdom in the middle of
ableist oppressions. Disability is a name given to particular bodyminds,
their conditions, and their visceral and sensual experiences in a dynamic
assemblage of political and economic forces, the medical industrial complex, legal recognition, capitalist investment or divestment, interlocking
systems of social injustices, cultural setup, and disability community formation, among others. Who comes to be recognized as disabled, identifies
as disabled, or acquires disabling conditions, and how they experience disability are deeply interwoven with forms of privilege and oppressions associated with race, gender, sexuality, geopolitical origin and indigeneity,
migration status, class background, age, and so on. I investigate how care
and care structure (assembled with federal and state governments, the care
industrial complex, domestic workers' rights and disability rights communities, and so on) interactively shape the notion of disability through the
mutual construction of care worker and care receiver populations and how
people break through such prescribed roles by engaging in interdependent
care for one another.

Intersectional reading of disability illuminates various ways that people
relate to disability and how discourses of disability and ableism are deployed
to shape their everyday lives.[95] The label of disability is constructed and attached to particular bodyminds (including their behaviors, attitudes, and
expressions) in a mixture of forces including examination, diagnosis, and
pathologization by the medical industrial complex; bureaucratic recognition and classification (i.e., eligibility for disability-related public services)
by local and federal governing institutions; inclusion and exclusion from
legal protections; capitalist industrial investment and divestment (e.g., commodification of disabilities through the care and rehabilitation industrial
complex and other forms of disability economy); cultural ideas about which
bodyminds are to be disgusted, feared, pitied, paternalized, inspiring, or
sacred; and U.S. disability communities' soliciting of disability as individual and collective identity and a source of pride. Interlocking systems of

oppressions and privileges are fundamentally present in these constructions and attachment of disability onto particular bodyminds.

Additionally, at the level of bodymind itself, disabling conditions (i.e., impairments) do not occur for everyone equally. Recent works in critical transnational, disability, and race studies articulate that disability occurs for many as a result or process of social oppressions including slow and acute violence that is the materialization of interlocking social oppressions, and thus the majority of disabled people are concentrated in the Global South.[96] "Becoming disabled" is a term that critical disability studies theorist Nirmala Erevelles conceptualizes and critical race and queer studies scholar Jasbir Puar expands on. As Puar explains, "bodily experiences . . . can be capacitated through a reorganization of resources, of white privilege and class and economic mobility. For others, disability is a product . . . of exploitative labor conditions, racist incarceration and policing practices, militarization, and other modes of community disenfranchisement."[97] Whether we recognize disability as a label or an identity or a bodymind condition, it does not occur for people randomly, equally, or neutrally but is unevenly distributed "across bodies, identities, and experiences."[98] This includes different access to notions of disability as identity, community, and a source of pride, which I further discuss shortly.

Further, interwoven with this notion of being attached to a disability label and becoming disabled is how disabled bodyminds are met with various degrees of pathologization, criminalization, and dehumanization as well as state protection, community supports, and more.[99] Whether one self-identifies as disabled or is labeled or perceived as such, disabled bodyminds elicit a diverse range of reactions from the world at the intersection of various forms of social oppressions and privileges. Such reaction can be state and public supports for some disabled people, for example, since disability recognition is deeply connected to eligibility for supplemental income, Medicaid supports, and on, while such *protection* certainly does not guarantee quality supports or comes with the state surveillance and control.[100] Disability can be turned into an area where police and state violence are mobilized, such as when police violently engage in ableist readings of people's behaviors and attitudes as deviant and threatening, which leads to criminalization and police brutality against some disabled people.[101]

In other words, interlocking social oppressions profoundly shape and are shaped by ableism, which is the making and maintaining of the hierarchies and values attached to different bodyminds that determine which people are disposable and which people are worthy to the society, to cite critical race and disability activists Talila A. Lewis and Azza Altiraifi.[102] It means that people of different communities, backgrounds, and intersecting identities have different relationships to disability.[103] Not identifying as proud disabled people is, therefore, not necessarily and exclusively a sign of internalized ableism, as disability rights communities (overwhelmingly led by white, cisheterosexual, physically disabled U.S. citizens) have quickly assumed. It can be a sign that different cultures and communities have developed unique ways to define and relate to the matter of disability.[104] Our relationships to our bodyminds, disabling conditions, and disability labels and identity are deeply mediated by those intersecting social forces. It is care that I examine to see how the mechanism and practice of care mutually construct a disability-nondisability binary. Which people experiencing disabling conditions are legitimated as disabled by the state to receive Medicaid long-term-care supports? How does the denial of such public supports further disable them? Which people are considered not disabled enough and hence situated to conduct care labor? Which people are debilitated or becoming disabled under the mechanism of care (e.g., Medicaid public healthcare supports)? How do the interlocking systems of oppression (i.e., intersecting racism, cisheteropatriarchy, ableism, settler colonialism, and so on) determine the answers to these questions?

Simultaneously, though, I highlight that disability is more than a label and diagnosis, and thus, disabled people and our lives are more than that of victimhood under ableism and the intersecting social forces that made us (further) disabled. Disability is inherently transgressive, and disabled lives are way more nuanced and richer and full of crip wisdom. In his book *Brilliant Imperfection*, disability justice activist and writer Eli Clare repeatedly uses the phrase "a multitude of visceral differences" to describe disability and experiences through disabled bodyminds.[105] With this phrase and the opening quote of this section, Clare has recognized disability first and foremost as a bodily experience or a bodymind itself (i.e., "bones, muscle, blood") and thus expanded and included the sensual aspect of bodyminds (i.e., visceral) to understand disability. Situating disability in the sensual and ontological realm rather than cognitive or epistemological (as if fully knowable), he highlights the expansive nature of disability beyond the expectation of disability to be neatly categorized and framed. In other words, disability is unpredictable and messily transgressive of what is medically reportable, categorizable, and diagnosable as well as bureaucratically measurable, legitimatable, and archivable. It is more than frameworks (e.g., category, status, the disability model) can contain, label, and comprehend.

Further, I insist that this transgressive nature be the very bedrock of disability as a concept. Disability is used to draw the line of what is considered normal or deviant as much as such dichotomization constructs disability. That is, disability is a catch-all for whoever does not neatly fit into the notion of normal, while such a notion is also sociopolitically constructed in the web of white supremacy, cisheteropatriarchy, settler colonialism and neocolonialism, and on. It means that not *every* inability we experience is made into the category of disability, as women's inability or resistance against following sexist submissive expectation has been historically pathologized, for instance, while their inability to be financially independent was not only normalized but expected.[106] In a way, disability is inherently outcast.[107] Essentially, disabled people are simultaneously the target of stigmatization and discrimination, as we do not fit into the social expectations of "normal," and also embody the potential to live outside the narrow restriction by defying the exclusionary normative life that is enforced. While such restriction limits the general population's imagination regarding what humans are and can be, disabled people have been always and already forced to creatively reimagine our day-to-day lives and redefine who we are and what we can become while negotiating ableism inflicted on us.

This is so even when disability is inflicted by violence or used to justify further violence. I contend that rich, nuanced, and complex lives continue for those who become disabled, sick, maddened, debilitated, and injured even in the wake of extreme ableist harm that causes such conditions of the bodymind, and that is never containable in a simplified notion of *victimhood*.[108] While disability and debility theorists rightly articulate that we live in a society that is oppressive and hence debilitating and disabling to members of marginalized communities, it is crucial to also widen our perspective to recognize people's resistance, resilience, and other-world-making practices in the middle of these oppressive forces. Where there is a disabled life, there is always crip wisdom, whether it is recognizable and squarely aligns with disability politics put forward by disability activists or not.[109]

Intersectional analysis not only points out these multiplying oppressions but searches for and illuminates the visions that are only dreamable at the intersection and nurtures cross-community solidarity.[110] To state that ableism happens in interaction with other forms of -isms is to say that disability justice and liberation can be achieved only by eradicating all forms of social domination, through solidarity with other marginalized communities and recognition that people are always and already part of multiple communities. I make these connections not simply to juxtapose the dichotomy of violence and hope but to demonstrate the complex realities of disability experiences that reflect the intricacy of violence and hope and much more. In the chapters to follow, I investigate how practices of care can be the mechanism of disability- and debility-making while, simultaneously, disabled people engage in care to envision different and radically collective ways to live. What does caring among those who are marginalized and oppressed under U.S. public healthcare programs, for instance, activate and enable? How do the unique insights of care by disabled people allow them to envision and guide care-based justice and social change with and through care?

Finally, recognizing disability in its multiple layers is crucial in this book to avoid setting an exclusionary boundary to define who or what is considered disabled and disability and who or what is not—a boundary that leads to the stark dichotomization of people as either disabled or nondisabled.[111] When I speak of disability in this book, therefore, it entails much more than psychiatric disability or Madness; chronic fatigue and illness; and intellectual, developmental, learning, emotional, sensory, and physical disabilities, or the bearing of stigmatized marks (e.g., burn scars, birthmarks). By *disabled people*, I mean anyone who actively identifies as disabled, those who do not identify as disabled but experience disabling conditions, and those who are assumed to be and labeled as disabled. Ableism, as well, is dynamically experienced and constantly evolving in relation with interacting social oppressions and privileges that impact people not only acutely but also longitudinally. This is to note that ableist oppressions can accumulate within us to deteriorate our bodyminds slowly or change the trajectory of our future by psychologically dictating to us about what we can(not) do and what we can(not) become.[112] Additionally, the term *ableism* is used to encompass sanism, audism, and healthism—all of which pathologize and devalue particular bodyminds.[113]

II

Researching Needs

The first thread that became this book was woven during a conversation I had with a bunch of my crip families and disability activists, when I asked them, "How can research be used for the justice of disabled people?" A friend and disability rights activist, Nick Dupree, responded that my research should (1) reveal how Medicaid became profit-centered, while it should be people-centered; and (2) challenge the medical model of care, which is normalized and institutionalized in state-sponsored care he received.

This provocation called together many scenes of how care and disability were integral in my own life, having been born with a disability and growing up within a mélange of care, ableist bullies, and medical interventions; engaging in care labor in order to survive after I migrated to the U.S.; being an instructor of disability studies for a continuing education school that largely served a student body that consisted of care worker populations who are largely (migrant) women of color. Further, years of working for disability rights and then disability justice activism, participating in activist meetings and conversations with domestic worker activists under the national campaign Caring Across Generations, and finding a home with my crip families—chosen families formed with people in the disability community and their allies—all laid the foundation to this book as well. The crip family-dom, to me, was formed by centering our love, care, and needs, as well as a pinch of cynicism, rudeness, tears, and laughter. This means that crip family-dom was possible only because we all took roles of both the cared for and the caring. It did not matter what disability we had or how incapable society thought we were, we all had to chip in in order to be together. It was through those many moments of me occupying both caring and cared-for subjectivities that this book emerged.

Also woven in to shape this book are the many testimonies on care and needs that people have shared with me. Whether they identify their primary roles as care worker and/or receiver, or as being part of disability and/or domestic worker activist communities, I bring up perspectives that they shared with me as expert testimonies and (homemade) theories.[114] I integrate those testimonials-cum-theories in a similar vein to how I use theories that emerged from that academic sphere throughout this book. Therefore, while I used traditional research methods (as laid out shortly) to listen to, observe, and understand those testimonies, how I engage with them does not follow typical positivist research analysis to capture the statistical significance per se. Testimonies that shape this book were shared as unique personal stories, and yet as those people shared their *personal* stories, it became quickly clear that they were profoundly overlapping, interactive, and interwoven (while there are still some degrees of uniqueness to them) across the given roles of care worker and receiver. These conversations unfolding in focus groups were often filled with energetic exclamations of "yeah!," "um-hum," and "Amen" directed at each other with big nods and enthusiastic agreements. It was as if these individual stories were reaching out their synopses to one another to become a collective story. What I do in this book is, then, connecting those dots of homemade and academically driven theories to offer one way to understand the structure and everyday practice of care, care activism, and visions emerging in the sites of care.

In the fall of 2013, I hosted two focus groups (i.e., expert discussions) with disabled people who receive their long-term care via Medicaid community- and home-based service and support programs in a U.S. northeastern state. They echoed each other that perspectives and testimonies they shared were deeply impacted by their backgrounds, including their race, gender, migration, and other identities. Out of twelve disabled people who joined the focus groups, the majority identified as African or Black American—six in total; three identified as Hispanic or Latino/a; and three as white or Caucasian.¹¹⁵ Most of them told me that they have physical disabilities, while two of them identified as having intellectual and developmental disabilities as well as learning disabilities (a few of them had multiple disabilities). A majority of them (eight people) identified as cis women, and the rest (four people) as cis men. The number of years they have been receiving Medicaid long-term services and supports varied from eight to forty, while their ages varied from thirties to sixties at the time of the focus groups. And a few mentioned during the focus group that they or their parents are migrants to the United States. They gathered to teach me how Medicaid works and how they navigate it.¹¹⁶ Some of them invited their care workers to the focus group so that I could have a more comprehensive view of care practices. While *focus group* is a dry term used for this research method, what I witnessed was more like a disability community hangout where support systems were forged and crip wisdom was shared. They all took this opportunity to compare notes on how they are treated by their care agencies and exchange tips on how to navigate the system. We discussed how they came to the role they are in today (Medicaid enrollees and care recipients); what care means to them; positive and negative care relationships they had with care workers; critiques of the care industrial complex; how they and their care partners engage in just care; and their care-related dreams. Those focus-group-turned-informal-gatherings were followed by homemade Japanese lunches that we enjoyed together, which further offered a space for us to come together to socialize. We gathered to talk about care, while care was simultaneously embodied in the group. Here is an example of such moments as I noted right after one of the focus groups.

As disabled experts began to fill the conference room and gathered around a big white table, it became clear that this focus group was quickly turning into a multigenerational disability community gathering. As many used power chairs, others moved chairs that were already in the room to create a space for them. We took turns opening the door when people moved in and out of the room. As almost all of us identify as part of the disability community, interdependence was our way to share a space together. People worked together to interpret and help pass messages across the table, when some participants' speech was shaped by their disabilities and when I had a hard time understanding people as English is my second language. We took turns filling out demography questionnaires with each other's consent, as some of us read and others do not; some of us write and others do not. Some read and write in English and others in a mixture of English and Spanish. After the focus group and during our group lunch, we took turns feeding each other, so everyone's stomach was filled. We were seasoned experts in creating a warm, supportive, and affirmative space to welcome anyone and everyone regardless of our intellectual and/or physical disabilities, including those who were super vocal and friendly as well as those who were shy and needed some time to warm up. It was particularly memorable when an elderly man who identified as intellectually disabled answered my question, "In what ways do you (as being situated as care recipient) provide care to others," by telling us, "No, I am a care recipient and not giver." A number of other participants immediately disagreed with him by telling the group how he taught them—younger advocates of disability communities— how to work in this complex disability service system. We were all helping and helped by each other, as we transgressed the care recipient-provider binary where disabled people are often situated exclusively as recipients of care.

I pictured myself going through a similar research process with care workers, though my plan did not come through. Care workers constantly work overtime with minimal to no days off. They do so in order to make a living with the minimum wage they receive. Additionally, the fact that their work schedule is contingent on the needs and schedules of their care partners (Medicaid enrollees) means that last-minute changes and cancellations were part of this research. One care worker told me, "Look, I have only one day off. And I have been running around with laundry and grocery shopping all day already. I usually don't have time for something like this [research interview]. But you seemed nice. That's the only reason I came here. Because you looked like a nice person at the karaoke party [offered by a care agency where you volunteered]." Responding to that reality, I conducted individual interviews with care workers, instead of focus groups, in order to meet their availability. In total, I interviewed ten people who have been working as care workers from seven to fourteen years (or possibly more, as a majority of them skipped this demographic question). Other than one white man, the rest of them identified as either Black or Latina women (seven Black women and two Latinas), and about half said that they are either migrant themselves or children of migrants. Ages varied from thirties to fifties, while many of them skipped this question. We discussed similar topics to the ones that I discussed with those who are situated as care recipients—how they came to the role they are in today (care workers); what care means to them; positive and negative care relationships they had with their care partners (i.e., recipients of care); critiques of the care industrial complex; how they and their care partners engage in just care; and their care-related dreams. I brought home-cooked foods to some meetings or offered coffee and snacks—all depending on where we met and how much time they had with me.

Participant observation of care practices entailed me participating and hanging out as care workers and Medicaid enrollees engaged in care practices. I tagged along with them at their convenience. Two pairs of care workers and Medicaid enrollees generously invited me into their daily care practices. This included engaging in morning routines—using the bathroom (during which I stayed outside), applying skin cream, braiding hair—and a cake baking session or preparing and hosting music classes that one Medicaid enrollee organized. Respecting privacy and staying out of their way were my priority as I shadowed, hung out, and chipped in to assist with their care tasks (for two three-hour blocks with one pair of care partners and two hours with another pair). All of these events took place in the fall of 2013.[117]

My writing on community-based care collectives (i.e., mutual-aid groups) is based on my own experiences in two care collectives I was part of as well as individual interviews or conversations with those who were involved in care collectives across North America. I was in formally organized care collectives between 2011 and 2015, though such collective and mutual care is inherently part of crip hangouts regardless of the formal scheduling and formation of such collectives. During the summer of 2017, I talked to six disabled people and one ally who were part of care collectives and shared their wisdom and knowledge on care collectives with me. All of them, except for one ally, identified as disabled (physical disabilities, psychiatric disabilities, and a mixture of these). A majority of them were cis women, while two identified as gender nonconforming; almost all of them (except one) identified as queer. This information is significant in that their knowledge is also rooted in the wisdom of queer community as well as migrant and racialized communities in some extent, as two of them identified as children of migrant families and one of them as a person of color. Three of the interviewees received some form of public care supports (i.e., Medicaid long-term care), while five of them used long-term care. All of them, thus, lived in their own home and not a group home.[118] Our conversations were open-ended; I asked them to share about their experiences in care collectives they were part of, what they enjoyed, what they found challenging, and everything else they thought was important to share in order to depict their experiences in the collectives. I used pseudonyms for everyone I talked to and hung out with for this research, given the nature of conversations we had on care (which covered intimate, private, and often shamed topics in the larger society) and their critiques of the care industrial complex they profoundly rely on.

Finally, the writing on bed activism was deeply shaped by my own time spent in bed enduring migraine-related pain, fatigue, and nausea as much as my reading and being in imaginative conversation with writings by sick and disabled activists, artists, and thinkers of color who makes magic from their bed spaces and in dreams. Artists whose work I engaged closely in the chapter include Aurora Levins Morales, Leah Lakshmi Piepzna-Samarasinha, and Johanna Hedva, while so many others have influenced me and this chapter (whose names I list in the chapter). I came to read their writings in books and web articles and blogs throughout the 2010s. Given my training in social science research method and not literature analysis, I read these pieces in a similar way to how I read focus group and interview transcripts. It is by paying attention to overlapping and stand-out themes across writings by these activist-artists that we can capture the peculiar characteristics of bed activism.

Needs and care, when they are written about within the academic rules of logic and rationales, may sound logical and rational—even rosy. In reality, they are the opposite of that. Respecting privacy and staying out of the way of the care workers and Medicaid enrollees, for example, was not simple and was also based on my own assessment; those I interviewed and interacted with may disagree. Like the everyday reality of care practice and activists working toward care justice, research is messy even with the approval of a university ethics board. Conducting and writing about care is always a balancing act, because care can and does entail the most intimate, private, and hidden parts of our lives. I am forever in debt to those who opened up their daily lives to invite me in and educate me on how care is practiced.

Mapping the Book

Chapter 1: Differential Debilitation and Capacitation: Neoliberalization of the U.S. Public Healthcare Assemblage

By teasing out the neoliberalization of U.S. public healthcare programs, I trace the political economy of care with particular attention to the making of care recipients, or Medicaid enrollees, and care workers. Care has historically been deployed for sociopolitical control and management and deeply embedded within the racial, gendered, disability, and (neo)colonial economies that construct and amplify certain people's capacities and debilities to categorize them into care worker and care recipient roles. It is on this ground that the neoliberal U.S. public healthcare assemblage flourishes to commodify and exploit marginalized populations based on their capacities and debilities. Those arguments are built into this chapter as I lay out the neoliberal turns of Medicaid with the implementation of its managed-care program and of welfare for single mothers (and families in need) as well as the flourishment of transnational care migration (and related industries)—all of which positions or at the same time forces certain populations to become care workers and care recipients and shapes today's care formation within U.S. public healthcare programs. I end this chapter by addressing global and domestic *chains of care* to understand how U.S. citizens' care needs are nested within the chain and not unconnected to that of disabled people in the Global South and other locales, and how some people's care needs come to be prioritized over others'.

Chapter 2: My Body Pays the Price: Necropolitics of Care

The everyday care practices that care workers and Medicaid enrollees co-conduct are unfolded to trace how they are situated and treated in the neoliberal U.S. public healthcare assemblage. As both populations are evaluated and exploited based primarily on the financial values attached to their care labor capacities and degrees of debility or care needs, their well-being is overlooked and their actual bodyminds are treated as if they are disposable. By using a relational analysis, I theorize such realities to argue that *both* care workers and Medicaid enrollees are exploited and deteriorating under distinct and yet also mutually implicative mechanisms shaped within the current political economy. This analysis complicates the concept of biopolitical labor, which is widely used in care studies to explain how it is those who are situated as either care workers or care recipients who deteriorate under the name of care, while the other flourishes. Instead, I conclude by describing that the care circulated in today's public long-term care assemblage is necropolitical: care workers and Medicaid enrollees are structurally set up for mutual debilitation, while the U.S. public healthcare assemblage thrives.

Chapter 3: Affective Collectivity: Beyond Slow Death and toward Haptic Relationality

The main focus of this chapter is that the lives of those who are situated as care workers and Medicaid enrollees contain more than victimhood under necropolitical care. I develop the notion of affective collectivity to depict the unique haptic tie that some care partners (i.e., workers and Medicaid enrollees) develop as they co-conduct care tasks over and over. Affective collectivity is an ontological and sensual connection that is nurtured as care partners co-experience one another's differently shaped bodies, movements, rhythms, heat, and odors, among other sensory information through recursive care tasks or as they go, side by side, through every up and down of each other's daily lives. I illuminate such collectivity to invoke nuances in the rich lives they continue to lead and possibly co-capacitative relationships they weave in the middle of the exploitative macro care setup. Also, I highlight the notion of affective collectivity to diversify and transgress the ways people's connections are normalized and primarily theorized as happening in a cognition-centered way. At the end, I explore affective collectivity as a foundation of collective resistance happening within the neoliberal public healthcare assemblage.

Chapter 4: Living Interdependency: Desiring Entanglement in Messy Dependency

Shifting the focus from public healthcare programs to community-based care collectives, I explore the idea of interdependency with particular attention to how this idea is actualized in community settings of care collectives. Specifically, my curiosity was piqued when the care collective members I interviewed shared their desire to reclaim their dependency (instead of interdependency or independency) and be entangled in each other's messy dependencies. Enacting the social justice ideology of interdependency in disabled and queer people's everyday lives by developing care collectives turned out to be full of challenges and messiness that led them to the desire. Analyzing such challenges as manifesting in material and affective modes, I theorize them not necessarily as collective members' dismissal of interdependency but as a critique of capitalist and neoliberal care formations—how certain modes of care practice are normalized and standardized and interdependency has come to be translated as reciprocation of care (in as equal a manner as possible) in the care collectives I looked into. Desiring messy dependency was a way for members to reclaim their dependency as far messier, unruly, and wild and to view it as their crip wisdom—instead of something to be ashamed of. I end this chapter, then, by contemplating what it means for collective members to desire dependencies, when individualism and independence are enforced as requirements to successfully navigate and survive in the neoliberal political economy.

Chapter 5: Bed Activism: When People of Color Are Sick, Disabled, and Incapable

Bed activism addresses resistance and visioning emerging from bed space. It entails not only the conventional activism that disabled and sick people engage in from their beds (e.g., joining protests via the internet), but also bed-born wisdom and dreams emerging in the middle of bed dwellers' moments of enduring pain, fatigue, depression, and other bodymind conditions. By putting forward writings on bed lives woven by three sick and disabled queer activist-artists of color, I explore some characteristics of bed activism, including its assertion of ontological resistance ("our existence is resistance"), its inherent collectivist pulse, whether the connection is happening by writing to each other or meeting one another in their dreams, and its radical reimagination of the paradigm on how activism and protests are defined and formed. Bed activism shows how rich lives continue for injured, disabled, sickened, and maddened people even in the middle of constant debilitation. It also illuminates how marginalized populations always carve a space to revalue themselves and refuse the neoliberal values attached to their constructed capacities and debilities. I weave those features of bed activism with key theorizations I develop in this book. Through writing about bed activism, additionally, I explore how we can engage in a kind of disability studies which helps us, disabled people, to live.

Postscript: What about COVID?

While this book was written before the COVID outbreak, I end this book with some notes on the COVID pandemic and care. Using care as an analytical tool, I write about various ways that different disabled people are impacted by this pandemic, questions of needs and desires, disposability of *essential* workers, and silver lining of crip wisdom. To write this postscript was also to insert the disabled-life-realness on how exhausting it can be to survive and how impossible it is to form a cohesive thought on the pandemic in the middle of a pandemic.

1

Differential Debilitation and Capacitation

Neoliberalization of the U.S. Public Healthcare Assemblage

How a social order organizes care . . . is a matter of social justice.
—Eva Kittay, *Love's Labor*

Neoliberal discourses of care are increasingly used as a technology of *control*, to both reify normative constructions of the heterosexual middle-class family and to morally, socially and culturally regulate poor people with care responsibilities, for themselves and others, under workfare structures and programmes. [emphasis added]
—**Karen Soldatic and Helen Meekosha, "The Place of Disgust"**

On the morning of June 6, 2017, a corner in downtown Chicago became crowded as it witnessed the "Don't Cap Our Care!" Rally (#NoCapsNoCuts #SaveMedicaid) to oppose the attempt to cut Medicaid funding by the Trump administration.[1] As the noise and smells of the busy traffic swallowed the corner, people gathered slowly. Some were using power wheelchairs; others were using manual wheelchairs or white canes or were accompanied by service animals. They were people of different ages and genders, and the majority were people of color. They carried colorful signs—in their hands, attached to their wheelchairs, or held together by multiple people—"Disability Rights = Human Rights," "Medicaid = my life," "Medicaid cuts kill," "Medicaid <3 saves," "Don't cap kids' futures," "Save the people." A few dozen meters away, the corner was also surrounded by police observing the Medicaid rally unfold.

At a glance, it was strikingly clear that the rally was largely occupied by people from various marginalized communities—indicating that not everyone was equally affected or agitated by the proposed downsizing of Medicaid; instead, mostly marginalized communities are negatively affected by the shrinkage of public healthcare programs. People wore T-shirts representing Planned Parenthood, Metropolitan Chicago Breast Cancer Task Force, Therapists for Children, AIDS Foundation of Chicago, and Access Living (an independent living center for disabled people in the Chicago area), among many others. The rally was put together by disability rights communities with the help of queer communities, feminist communities, senior communities, communities of working-class people, multiple race-, ethnicity-, and migration-based communities, workers' organizations (e.g., the care worker community, or therapists for children relying on Medicaid), and many more. They shared concerns, fears, anger, and a commitment to fight side by side. They chanted that Medicaid was lifesaving and ultimately *life itself* for them, their loved ones, and clients.

"NO CUTS, NO CAPS!"

"WHAT DO WE WANT, REALLY WANT?"—"HEALTH CARE!"

"WHAT DO WE NEED, REALLY NEED?"—"MEDICAID!"

"HOW DO WE GET IT?"—"PEOPLE POWER!"

"PEOPLE POWER!"—"PEOPLE POWER!"

While the Chicago protest was taking place, the United States at large was witnessing nationwide uprisings of disability and other communities in coalitions for the "Don't Cap Our Care!" rally against the Trump administration's push to downsize U.S. public healthcare programs.[2] Care = Life. During this series of rallies, protesters repeatedly brought up the language of life and death such as "Kill the Bill. Don't Kill Us" to signal care as directly a matter of life. In disability activist Alice Wong's words, Medicaid is "more than a health care program. It is a life-giving program."[3] Care or the lack thereof is profoundly interwoven with people's well-being, vitality, and ultimately lives. Additionally, what this rally crystallized and illuminated is how the government and subcontracted care industrial complex directly affects and shapes people's well-being—and particularly that of lower-income people (including working-class and poor people), and whether they are assigned to be care workers or recipients under publicly funded care programs.

In this chapter and the one that follows, I unfold how care is used as a mechanism to control and manage people, and not all people but *certain* people. The opening quotes by Eva Kittay, Karen Soldatic, and Helen Meekosha highlight such points that I build on in the following. Care is a response to needs that emerge in every living being in varying degrees and manners. And therefore, while who receives care or not is primarily based on the degrees of complex care needs that one embodies and whether they require long-term care supports, it is also indicative of whose lives are prioritized and whose are not. Also, which people are tasked to meet other's care needs and which people are not, along with the devaluation of care practice (including needing, receiving, and providing care) at large, all show how care dictates lives unequally. To trace the history of care is, therefore, to trace the history of racialized, gendered, migrant, (neo)colonial, and disability economies within which care is constructed and different lives are taken up. I assert that the line drawn between those who are cared for in the United States (and particularly in public healthcare programs) and those who are not is profoundly intertwined with these economies, while the economies also dictate the quality and quantity of care that those who are cared for receive (which many disabled people describe as abuse, and I will trace it further in the following). It is also the case in terms of which people are situated to labor as care workers and how it is determined in the web of these economies. By referring to racial, gendered, migrant and (neo)colonial, and disability economies, I am pointing out how the capitalist system is profoundly and inherently developed and implemented with racist, cis-heteropatriarchal, ableist, colonial forces and formations. It is a way to acknowledge how the economy is used to deploy and further engrave those oppressions for some and privilege for others, whether through exploitation, dispossession, and downward mobility or accumulation of wealth and upward mobility. This is so as much as these interlocking systems of oppressions enable capitalist assemblage.[4] This web of sociopolitical regulations, or control and exploitation, particularly in the context of U.S. public healthcare programs, highlights that care is not only a mechanism to divide who matters and who does not. It is also a mechanism to further enforce the marginalization of already marginalized populations by pushing them to perform economically undervalued (and underpaying) care labor or by subjugating them into low-quality and sporadic care provided under U.S. public healthcare. In such a mechanism, the upward mobility or improvement in well-being through caring labor and care itself is not necessarily guaranteed for those who are situated as care workers and receivers in the system.[5]

To untangle an aspect of care as a mechanism of control, I build on the concept of *differential inclusion*. A critical ethnic studies scholar, Yến Lê Espiritu, examines the lives of migrants from the Philippines, in relation to the United States under neocolonial global migration, to describe how they were not totally excluded from U.S. society but were put into the "process whereby a group of marginalized people is deemed integral to the nation's economy, culture, identity, and power—but integral only or precisely because of their designated subordinate standing."[6] I expand the definition by thinking about how people are included in the U.S. public healthcare assemblage because of their designated exploitable standing. Thus, such exploitation is based on the financial value attached to their capacities and debilities under the mechanism of *differential capacitation* and *debilitation*.

I argue that people's inclusion, exclusion, or pressured placement in the U.S. public healthcare assemblage, whether as care recipients or as care workers, is based on the evaluation, categorization, and commodification of their degree of debilities and capacities. Thus, such placement further engraves the divide between care worker and care receiver positions and dictates the making of these populations.

Care is more than an attitude or behavior, I argue. It can be a site of care injustice, which is how social stratification manifests and materializes through its unequal making of care receiver and care provider populations as well as devaluing them through and under the structure of care. The opening illustration of the Medicaid rally and the fact that it was attended and advocated by those who are situated as care recipients and as care providers under Medicaid exemplifies impacts of care formation for both of them. Public healthcare programs, and particularly Medicaid, is a site where I engage and examine the notion of care as political in this chapter.

Despite the popular belief that Medicaid and other public healthcare programs (such as Medicare) are readily available safety nets for people in need in the United States, I contend that such assessment needs further examination.[7] Tracing the neoliberalization of U.S. public healthcare programs in this chapter demonstrates the careful calculus of people's debilities and capacities that is used to determine who is granted publicly funded care and who is not, as well as who is assigned to care labor and who is not. Medicaid and other U.S. public healthcare programs, therefore, can be understood at a glance as a measurement of how people's care needs or capacities to care and ultimately lives are de/valued—decisions that are left to the discretion of governments and the care industrial complex. It is so while services provided by them do not necessarily mean quality and life-making care for recipients of publicly funded care. Not everyone is equally tasked to provide care under Medicaid, and the fact that Medicaid workers' wages and benefits were not historically protected by the U.S. Department of Labor also shows whose labor capacity is regarded as exploitable and hence whose lives are placed at the periphery of governmental concerns and protections.[8]

Medicaid is increasingly becoming a profit-centered, multi-industrial, and governmental project in the current neoliberal political economy. In this context, it is based on the commodification of one's degree of capacity or debility wherein the roles of care worker and care receiver are constructed, and certain populations are assigned to these roles. On the frontier of U.S. public healthcare programs, such capacity is about caring labor capacity and debility as reflected in the needs for care assistance. These capacities and debilities are commodified in exchange for funding from federal to state governments and then to the subcontracting care industries, for instance. I describe how the neoliberalization of public healthcare programs have intensified the ways in which people are recognized, reconfigured, and revalued based on their changing degrees of capacity and debility within the system. As different degrees of capacities and debilities are amplified or attached to certain populations, they become the basis for the populations' differential inclusion in the U.S. public healthcare assemblage. Additionally, this analysis equally portrays how the stark division between care giving and care receiving roles and attached stereotypes are sociopolitically reinstated in this neoliberalization of public healthcare programs. In what follows, I review newspaper articles of current times (since the 2000s) and feminist and disability studies scholarship on care formation and bring them together to illustrate how the making of care recipients (theorized largely within disability studies) is deeply intertwined and mutually shapes the making of care workers (theorized mainly in feminist studies) and vice versa.

Finally, I end this chapter by illuminating and speculating on how the effects of U.S. public healthcare as a mechanism of control and management extends beyond those who are directly made into care workers and care recipients under the programs. My particular attention is about speculatively connecting U.S. Medicaid enrollees with others whose care needs are also met by the same set of care givers. Much of the literature on the migrant care labor force, for example, discusses the drastic changes and adjustments that families of migrant care workers are forced to deal with. In other words, disabled U.S. citizens' demands for the right to receive care are deeply nested within the global, racialized, and feminized economies that create care providers for them. With the speculative connection between disabled people needing care in the Global North and Global South or Medicaid enrollees and their care workers' family members who also rely on the same *worker* who is also a carer for her family members, I seek to reimagine and rethink U.S. disability activism for healthcare in a more holistic and global way.[9]

Dichotomy in Care Studies

Disability and feminist theorists have had similar goals. Both are concerned with the elimination of the exploitation and oppression of their respective constituencies. The notion of care has been a focus of debate for both movements but the approach has been very different. [In feminist movements,] the focus of attention has been the carer rather than the "cared for." In contrast, for the disability movement, notions of care have been addressed predominantly in instrumental terms since care has been conceived as a practice that contributes significantly to the marginalization and confinement of people who are "cared for."[10] . . . [T]here is significant scope for a clash of standpoint between the emancipatory goals of the two movements.

—Nick Watson et al., "(Inter)Dependence, Needs and Care"

The scholarship of care has often been premised on an assumed divide between those who are cared for and those who provide care. Nick Watson and his colleagues exemplified this foundational divide in the opening quote, although an increasing number of scholars (and especially feminist disability studies scholars) are bridging together the two analyses that I hope to join with this book.[11] What is rarely analyzed in this divide and not yet mainstreamed within studies of care is the overlap or mutual construction of care worker and care receiver populations. Every life entails a need for care and is thus capable of contributing to the well-being of others, though the degree of such needs and capability varies. And yet the process of setting up the positions of care worker and care recipient often exclusively highlights and amplifies one aspect of an individual or group and simultaneously shadows the other side. A care worker's need for care is often overlooked or actively neglected, as much as the contributions of those who are situated as care recipients are unrecognized. In other words, the making of care workers simultaneously determines who is granted the position of care receiver and who is solely situated as a care giver and vice versa. Tracing the making of care worker and care receiver populations is, therefore, equally about tracing how care comes to be solely understood and divided into giving and receiving—the dichotomized and linear one-way action—as if care is neatly packageable, givable, and receivable and does not leak out and circulate.

Further, what is implied in this dichotomy of how care is studied and theorized is the homogeneity of *disabled care recipient* and *female care provider* populations, suggesting that *all* disabled people with lower incomes receive quality long-term care through public healthcare programs and are guaranteed state protection with such a safety net. Also suggested is that *all* women are equally subjected to care tasks, while such "woman-ness" is exclusively thought about as cisgender and in a gender- and heteronormative manner and overlooks gender-nonconforming and trans femme people who are also pushed into or take up care responsibilities.[12] And how about the fundamental assumptions that care recipients are cared by receiving quality supports, or that care workers are receiving wages, benefits, and other support from their employers that meet the depth of care work they engage in? Are care workers not disabled and not in need of care supports, and can't those who are situated as care receivers care? Where are disabled women and gender-nonconforming femme people situated in the dichotomy of disability and feminist care studies and activism? I complicate this implied dichotomy and homogeneity of either population by asking which people are granted public supports and which people are assigned to care labor.

Within feminist studies, care work has been theorized and constructed as women's work. While the diverse standpoints of women who take up the care laborer role have begun to be articulated in more recent years, the intersectional analysis of care work is historically not mainstream or the norm.[13] A common explanation of the U.S. care crisis within mainstream feminist care studies, for example, often begins with the era of second-wave feminism, when women were said to have begun entering the job market (or public sphere) and their families experienced the loss of their primary care provider. This phenomenon is attributed as one of the causes of the U.S. care crisis in many feminist care scholarships.[14] What underlies this common explanation is an assumption that women were historically able to (and allowed to) stay home to attend to their family members' care needs for free, because their husbands (i.e., the breadwinners) brought in enough income for the household on their own. In other words, the explanation is centering and reflecting largely a white, middle- and upper-class cisheterosexual lifestyle of U.S. citizens. Invisible and excluded in this narrative are those who always worked (or were forced to work) for wages, for various reasons, or those who do not or cannot fit into such a lifestyle.[15] For instance, single parents assume both breadwinner and caring responsibilities; queer people were historically denied institutional and legal access to the marriage-based household-dom; single mothers of color were denied access to welfare supports and forced into the labor forces in various points in history; and migrant people left their families in their nations of origin to bring income. This also means that these groups of people have invented and engaged in new and creative ways to conduct their households, which simultaneously resists and interrupts the standardization of family-based care formation.[16] Tracing the historical making of the care provider population, indeed, shows that certain women—migrant and nonmigrant women of color from lower-income backgrounds—were always and already working as carers for more affluent families before the U.S. second-wave feminist movement began to focus on women's right to work.[17] In other words, different women have been differently capacitated and tasked to take up care responsibilities in the United States. Additionally, it is crucial to note that the foundational absence of men and masculine-presenting people in care analyses and studies speaks clearly of the profoundly gendered nature of caring tasks.[18]

Furthermore, it is not only capacity to work that is commodified and exploited under the capitalist economy, but debility and disability are also commodified, which has been particularly intensified under the neoliberal political economy, as many disability studies scholars have articulated. Critical theorist Jasbir Puar has explained that people have come to be measured and financialized "in relation to their success or *failure* in terms of health, wealth, progressive productivity, upward mobility, enhanced capacity."[19] Disability studies scholars David Mitchell and Sharon Snyder have symbolized the shift from disciplinary society to neoliberal and control society by highlighting the deployment of disabled bodyminds: "The historical shift from liberalism's carceral restraints on deviant bodies to neoliberalism's referencing of deficiencies across all bodies provides a key transition in historically distinct approaches to body management. . . . [T]he era of biopolitics turns the corner and proliferates pathologies as *opportunities* for new product dissemination opportunities."[20] In other words, people's debility, disability, or inability to work is turned into an opportunity for industries to build new markets to supply capacitative and normalizing means to them (e.g., insurance companies, pharmaceutical industries, and the medical and care industrial complex). Such industries proliferate without necessarily promising capacitation and normalization, which may not in fact be ultimate goals for the industries, or without ameliorating the notion of their debility and dependency as burdensome.[21] Disabled people's actual, amplified, and constructed debilities or needs for care lay one of the foundations for the emergence of public healthcare and the care industrial complex. While debility-based business flourishes in the neoliberal world, as theorized by Puar, Mitchell, and Snyder, I further complicate theorization of debility commodification by contemplating that it is based on people's *different degrees* of debility; they are further siphoned into the care structure, which functions as a mechanism of commodification and exploitation.[22]

Neoliberalization of the U.S. Public Healthcare Assemblage

When you are disabled and rely on public services and programs [such as Medicaid], you face vulnerability every day. This vulnerability is felt in my bones and in my relationship with the state. . . . The fragility and weakness of my body, I can handle. The fragility of the safety net is something I fear and worry about constantly.

—Alice Wong, "My Medicaid, My Life"

Government totally sucks. They can determine when you can live and how you can live. They give you that assistance and it determines your lifestyle . . . your weight and your health and all those things.

—A man experiencing house insecurity interviewed on his experience in Medicaid by Jamila Michener, *Fragmented Democracy*

A quick glance at one aspect of U.S. public healthcare, Medicaid, demonstrates how care has been historically turned into the realm of rights and governmental responsibility as well as being commodified and turned into business opportunities for the care industrial complex.[23] Medicaid is the single largest source of health coverage in the United States, or "government insurance," which has made health and medical care services available to its citizens and denizens since 1965.[24] It has been described as the safety net for those who are considered vulnerable in the nation's perspective, and those who are eligible include children, disabled people, pregnant people, senior people, and parents/caretakers who live with lower income (between 100 percent and 200 percent [depending on states and programs] of the federal poverty line).[25] The expansion of its eligibility criteria pushed through under the Patient Protection and Affordable Care Act (also known as Obamacare) means that Medicaid covers the care needs of nondisabled and non-caretaker adults with lower income in selective states, as precarious as this expansion may be, which was demonstrated and protested at the Medicaid rally that opened this chapter.[26] This means that 66 million U.S. citizens (more than 1 in 5 people) received Medicaid supports as of 2019, and its budget is the third biggest portion of U.S. federal mandatory spending after the Social Security and Medicare budgets.[27] Thus, the Medicaid budget makes up the largest revenue that flows from the federal government to state governments.[28] Medicaid represents 1 dollar out of every 6 dollars spent on healthcare in the United States at large, or 1 dollar out of every 2 dollars in terms of long-term care.[29] One in 3 disabled U.S. citizens are said to be receiving their healthcare under Medicaid (as of 2019).[30] Additionally, although elderly and disabled people account for only 23 percent of Medicaid enrollees, expenditures on their care occupy almost two thirds of its entire spending (61 percent).[31] Although Medicaid is jointly funded by federal and state governments, it has traditionally been administered by state governments within the boundary set by the federal law.[32] This administrative authority has been changing in recent years, though. The care industrial complex is passed down with increasing administrative authority by the state governments and aggressively taking over Medicaid and other public healthcare arrangements and provisions, which demonstrates the privatization of public welfare programs and exacerbates the blurring border between government and business industries. These changes in administrative authority and hence more involvement of industries in the public sphere demonstrate the neoliberalization of Medicaid. I use the term *care industrial complex*, therefore, to refer to a variety of for-profit and nonprofit care organizations that carry out subcontracted tasks to manage publicly funded care with the revenue from government entities.[33] Medicaid, in sum, is a major force mobilizing a large portion of the U.S. federal and state budgets and bulldozing administrative authority previously directly regulated by state governments to open up market space for the care industrial complex. It is directly shaping the health and life trajectories of lower-income people in the United States.[34]

The lifesaving significance of U.S. public healthcare programs can never be overstated. The nationwide protest to save Medicaid and the constant fight to expand Medicare for all demonstrate this point; so does the opening quote of this section by disability activist Alice Wong. It is as crucial, though, to critically examine public healthcare programs too. In reality and up close, it becomes clear that unfortunately Medicaid has never been a stable safety net or a net that has lifted the needs of *all* lower-income people who require such supports. At the macro level, non–U.S. citizens are fundamentally excluded from the majority of governmental supports. It is so no matter how integral they are to U.S. history and its day-to-day operation, not only by contributing to the U.S. economy but also by being crucial builders and nurturers of U.S. social and cultural life.[35] The continuous threats against the Affordable Care Act and its Medicaid expansion policy under the Trump administration also illuminate the complexity and precariousness of drawing a line of who is (not) eligible for supports. The fact that state governments have historically been the primary managers of Medicaid means that who receives what kind of care dramatically differs from state to state.[36] Additionally, at a more micro level, which people's healthcare needs are legitimated and thus which people are considered vulnerable enough and deserving enough to be eligible for Medicaid is negotiated and determined in the complex web of medical professionals and government officials, among others, who are all given authority to examine and dictate such decisions. These decisions regarding deservingness, however, should not be considered separately from these authorities' subjectivities and internalized stereotypes of who is considered deserving of medical welfare such as Medicaid.[37] Dictating who can enroll and receive public healthcare supports is, therefore, more subjective, ambiguous, political, and even business-related. In political scientist Jamila Michener's words:

> A study of the history of poverty in the United States shows that there is no escaping the enduring distinction between the "deserving" and the "undeserving."[38] The inclination to classify people living in poverty according to desert is the most critical component of American poverty governance [including Medicaid].[39]

Finally, it is argued that Medicaid functions not only as a gatekeeper to draw the line of who is worthy of public supports or not, or whose lives and well-being matter and whose do not, but also as a mechanism to exercise governmental surveillance and control that further exacerbate the inequitable status quo. Michener summarized this in the opening quote of this section and in the following statement: "[Medicaid] beneficiaries are overwhelmingly poor, disproportionately people of color, and unduly prone to health troubles. As such, Medicaid policy brings government directly into the lives of the most marginal citizens."[40] Indeed, Medicaid recipients in general are disproportionately those who are lower-income, have attained a high school diploma or less, and come from racialized communities, while long-term-care programs tend to have relatively more white, formerly middle-class enrollees in comparison to other programs under Medicaid.[41] Medicaid, in general, is still an area where intersecting social oppressions (e.g., classism, racism) manifest and materialize, because such oppressions determine not only who has to rely on such medical welfare but also who is excluded or included in such healthcare programs.

Not only are the lives and well-being of Medicaid enrollees profoundly shaped within Medicaid programs, but so are those who are situated as care workers. In this globalizing neoliberal era, for example, U.S. public healthcare programs are not merely a matter between the U.S. government and its citizens. What enables U.S. public healthcare programs includes an ever-expanding transnational labor migration force and the transnational care industries that facilitate this migration.[42] On the global front, transnational industries and many governments of Global South nations facilitate and broker the migration of their citizens as care workers to nations of the Global North, including the United States.[43] Simultaneously, U.S. governments and care industries also intervene in this migration in terms of where workers land and how they are treated.[44] Because the U.S. capitalist economy (and thus neoliberalism) was built on the history of its settler colonialism, imperialism, and slavery, the care labor force as we know it today is deeply embedded in this historical context.[45] I survey the genealogy of care worker making in this chapter and its interwovenness with the genealogy of care recipient making. With it, I point out how historically constructed roles and divides between care workers and care receivers are mutually constitutive.

I describe and tease out these complex forces that shape and enable U.S. public healthcare programs in this neoliberal political context with the word *assemblage*. The term—initially conceptualized in French, *agencement*—signifies the notion of connection or being in connection with something, and the "design, layout, organization, arrangement, and relations—the focus being not on content but on relations, relations of patterns."[46] It illustrates and highlights the dynamic nature of a social structure—in this case Medicaid. Medicaid is constructed and animated through a network of multiple moving elements and relationships. These elements include federal Medicaid policies, state and local administrative guidelines, the care industries that directly coordinate care, those who are situated as care recipients and care workers, transnational care industries, labor migration policies in both sending and receiving nations, and the histories (e.g., colonialism, slavery, and more) that laid the foundation for the care formation among other evolving parts. Each element, with its own force, assemblage, and networks, enables and functions within the neoliberal U.S. public healthcare assemblage as much as some of those elements are enabled, impacted, and sustained by the U.S. public healthcare assemblage. Thus, between and within each element are financial circulations and exchanges, including Medicaid funding, wages for care labor, subsidies to care industries, revenues for transnational care industries, and taxation of remittances sent to families of care labor migrants, for instance.[47] I would like to add the capacities and debilities of individuals to this list of elements circulated and exchanged within the assemblage and simultaneously shaping it. I chose to work primarily with the term *assemblage*, instead of *institution* or *structure*, in order to acknowledge the dynamic and ever-changing or unstable and precarious natures of Medicaid. This term also signifies that the daily lives of those who are sucked into the assemblage (i.e., care workers and Medicaid enrollees) are dynamically influenced and shaped by the changing nature of Medicaid.

Differential Debilitation: The Making of Medicaid Enrollee Care Recipients

It is of compelling public importance that the State conduct a fundamental restructuring of its Medicaid program to achieve measurable improvement in health outcomes, *sustainable cost control and a more efficient administrative structure*. [emphasis added]

—Former New York State governor Andrew Cuomo in New York State Department of Health, "Redesigning New York's Medicaid"

One of the dynamic events I examine in this chapter is the transition of Medicaid to managed care, which I describe as a neoliberal turn of Medicaid. It is under this turn that the disabled care recipient population was reconfigured and further divided based on their degree of debilities or needs for care. The managed-care program has been widely and quickly implemented into public healthcare programs across states in the 1990s and onward, with the hope of suppressing ever-growing Medicaid expenses.[48] Since the original implementation of Medicaid, its expenses have grown from $1 billion in 1966 to $639.4 billion in 2019, or, an increase of nearly 170 percent in the last decade (from $378.6 billion to $639.4 billion).[49] This trend in increasing national health expenditures is expected to continue.[50] Given the ever-expanding need for Medicaid long-term care and ever-growing expenses, states across the nation rapidly began implementing the managed-care program.[51] Replacing the former "fee for service" system, managed care is "a health care delivery system . . . which provides for the delivery of Medicaid benefits through contracted arrangements between state Medicaid agencies and *managed-care organizations* that accept *a set per member per month payment* [or capitation] for these services." Thus, within this system, "patients [*sic*] agree to visit only certain doctors and hospitals, and [. . .] the cost of treatment is monitored by a managing company."[52] It is, in sum, characterized by (1) transfer of administrative authority from state governments to the care industrial complex (i.e., managed-care organizations and agencies), which now "determines the level and intensity of services" for each enrollee; and (2) a transition to a per-capita funding model where the government pays a standardized fee per Medicaid enrollee to the care industrial complex or agencies that handle Medicaid-funded care (regardless of detailed differences in individual specific care needs).[53] This can be also read as the "privatization of public issue," or the neoliberal turn of Medicaid.

Since managed care has been promoted as "[improving] access and [reducing] costs by eliminating inappropriate and unnecessary services," the federal government strongly endorsed its implementation by passing various waivers that allow equally eager states to *mandate* managed-care enrollment.[54] As states began to mandate managed-care enrollment for beneficiaries, enrollment in managed care increased more than seven times in a decade (from 2.7 million enrollees in 1991 to 18.8 million in 2000), which grew to over 54 million people as of 2017—almost 72 percent of all Medicaid enrollees are receiving benefits through managed-care programs.[55] Finally, close to half (45 percent) of national Medicaid spending is directed toward managed-care organizations, which is a major portion of spending, especially since the second-highest amount of Medicaid spending amounts to only 12 percent.[56] Originally, the transition to managed care was promoted more for acute and non-long-term-care plans that are used more by nondisabled Medicaid enrollees. Long-term care for disabled adults and senior citizens was only slowly pushed to managed care. Slowly but surely, the trend is to keep moving long-term care to managed-care programs; as of 2019, twenty-three states provide their Medicaid long-term care under managed-care programs and via care industries that handle managed care (including New York State).[57] Managed-care programs and accompanying drastic changes in care services have become reality for the majority of Medicaid enrollees at this point, regardless of critiques and suspicions over their effectiveness.[58] Their increased authority has been a major game-changer for care industries, as well as for Medicaid enrollees and care workers in terms of their daily lives.

I further illustrate this process of transition as it occurs in New York State, whose Medicaid program is often viewed favorably in contrast to those of other states, since it is reported that New York's state Medicaid program spends the most dollars for its lower-income population, and its quality is ranked second after that of Massachusetts.[59] Managed care was strongly endorsed by former governor Andrew Cuomo as soon as he took office in 2011, as is shown in the quote that opened this section. He convened a Medicaid Redesign Team to conduct a major reform of the state's Medicaid programs, in order to end corruption under the previous fee-for-service structure to control its cost.[60] The Medicaid Redesign Team thus began to overhaul New York's state Medicaid program with the implementation of managed care, a new assessment system for prospective enrollees, and the Medicaid Global Cap, which limits the state's Medicaid budget. This set of profound reforms proceeded against the backdrop of an ever-increasing population who needed Medicaid supports.[61] This clear imbalance between the move to cap its budget and the ever-increasing population that required public healthcare supports becomes even more problematic once attention is shifted to the role and force of the care industries that are now granted Medicaid administrative authority and to whom more than half of the state's Medicaid spending goes.[62]

New York Times healthcare journalist Nina Bernstein summarized the new mechanism of care under managed care as "the new system's calculus: the more enrollees, and the less spent on services, the more money the companies [the care industrial complex] can keep."[63] She and her colleagues have reported repeatedly that a new "per capita" payment mechanism means that if agencies aim to recruit those with fewer care needs, the agencies' costs of providing care can stay low, and what is left from the per-capita funding will stay with the agencies.[64] In other words, it portrays how people's degree of debility is commodified based on the amount and kind of care they need and its cost. Determinations of who is supported by U.S. public healthcare programs and how become deeply impacted by commodification of debility. New York's state Medicaid program is generally known as a very generous and *better one* within disability communities, though a close look at it may spike concerns regarding how meager the Medicaid programs in other states could be.[65]

As the managed-care program was implemented, care industries flourished at the national level. Although only 7 percent of Medicaid-certified home care agencies were for-profit in 1980, the number had jumped to 70 percent in 2007 and was close to 80 percent in 2010.[66] One study shows that the Medicaid budget, paid from federal and state (and in some areas local) governments to care industries, makes up almost half (49 percent) of these industries' revenues. In terms of New York State's Medicaid expenditures, spending on managed-care programs increased 178.7 percent within six years between 2008 and 2014 and was expected to increase 429.4 percent within the decade between 2008 and 2018 ($8.5 billion in 2008, $23.7 billion in 2013, and $45 billion in 2018)—certain parts of which go to the care industrial complex.[67] Funding, in other words, circulates within the U.S. public healthcare assemblage from the government to industries, enabling the care industrial complex.

In the transition to the neoliberal state, it is not only people's labor capacity that is commodified but also people's need for care, making debility and disability into capital.[68] Against this backdrop of managed care becoming a new business opportunity, there have been reports of the reconfiguration—and even pushout—of Medicaid long-term-care enrollees. *Mismanaged Care*, a report published by Medicaid Matters New York and the New York chapter of Elder Law Attorneys in 2016, for example, documents the alarming increase in service deductions and terminations under the managed long-term-care program (managed-care programs for long-term care).[69] Degrees of service deduction and termination are correlated to enrollees' degrees of debility or hours of long-term-care services they previously received. Researching all fair hearing decisions that were made between June and December 2015 and are archived by the Office of Temporary and Disability Assistance, authors of the report identified 1,042 decisions on care reduction under managed long-term-care plans and unfolded them. They recognized, first of all, that the steep increase in the numbers of such appeals mirrors the increase in changes to long-term-care services. Upon closer examination, they found that those who received longer care hours (sixty hours or more a week, and hence with more complex care needs) had their long-term-care hours dramatically cut down. On average, close to 50 percent of long-term-care hours were cut down among this set of enrollees who appealed. The normal bell curve that once represented the distribution of New York State's Medicaid enrollees across the hours of long-term care they received is now skewed to the left. These statistics signify that the majority of people are receiving shorter hours of care (one to twenty hours per week) and the number of those who receive longer hours of care is drastically cut down.[70] Additionally, those who made the appeals reported that they did not receive any notification of or reasoning for the change and, therefore, such dramatic changes in care hours often hit them abruptly. It is crucial to note that most of those appeals (90 percent) ended up in favor of the demands of the appealing enrollees and their families to keep their service hours as they had been. These successes occurred partially because the care industries that reduced or terminated the long-term care did not show up to the hearing, or they were unable to provide appropriate justification for the care cut.[71]

The *New York Times* follow-up reports also indicate that the issue of debility-based service changes are not uncommon. Reporting personal stories of Medicaid enrollees and their family members who faced sudden service decreases, Bernstein noted, "The flat rate [per-capita funding given to the care industries] creates a perverse incentive. . . . The less care they provide to each [enrollee,] the more [the industries] earn."[72] She further reported that the profit-based service changes those enrollees once faced and fought did not end when they won their appeals. An elderly disabled woman who relied on both a paid care worker and her daughters for her long-term care, for example, testified that she was subjected to another set of service reductions even after she and her daughters won the original appeal reported under *Mis-managed Care*. During the second appeal, the agency's lawyer justified the service cut by arguing that she "could urinate or defecate in a 'pull-up' diaper and wait in a chair for two or three hours until a family member could leave work and come to change her." This quote exemplifies that the mechanism of drastic service cuts is built upon the profound disregard for Medicaid enrollees' comfort, safety, humanity, and dignity.[73] Also overlooked is the secondary impact on her family members to witness their loved ones being mistreated and this lack of care supports from the state being turned into their full responsibility. It is increasingly left to disabled people themselves and their family members (if they have any) to deal with the lack of government care supports. Such experiences vary as well based on the degrees of debilities and of care needs one embodies.

It all boils down to what these reports echo in each other:

> [Legal advocates for disabled Medicaid managed-care enrollees] said representatives of [care] agencies [the care industrial complex] running the managed-care plans deterred people who were bed-bound [sic] or affected by dementia from enrolling in a plan, often by refusing to do an assessment at all, or by falsely saying that the plan's budget or policies did not allow as much care as the person needed. . . . While high-needs cases were shed, the race was on for cheap ones. . . . [Built on the assumption that] one low-paid aide can serve many people, some of the same players who exploited the old Medicaid system found the [Medicaid enrollees under managed care] were still a *valuable commodity*.[74]

These reports reveal the ways that disabled enrollees are further divided based on the degree of their debilities and needs for care and circulated and embedded within the profit-focused assemblages of public healthcare. Those who require longer service hours are, for example, considered *too disabled*, as their care is more costly to be provided at their own homes because of the extensive hours and more complex medical care requirements that can be met only by certified nurses. They are then pushed out or deterred from applying for home- and community-based care or put into residential facilities such as nursing homes, because the cost of providing extensive medical care is cheaper when it is done en masse.[75] While many have faced drastic service cuts and have been left without care, more reports are coming out detailing that those who do not necessarily need day-to-day long-term-care supports are recruited or at times forced to sign up for managed-care programs so that the industries can receive more subsidies from the state while the cost of care remains minimal.[76]

In an era where the numbers of those who require long-term care are skyrocketing, Medicaid enrollees are further reexamined, rerecognized, and at the same time pushed out or placed in different programs within the assemblage of public healthcare programs where their different degrees of debilities are most marketable. Testimonies shared in the preceding reports make it clear that Medicaid enrollees' actual circumstances are grossly ignored, and their debilities are amplified and reconstructed in order to fit into the profit-making formula under managed care. They are thus recognized and taken up in these assemblages as mere debilities, while their personhoods as a whole, their actual needs, as well as other aspects of their lives that shape their care needs are ignored in the shadow of commodification of their debilitation. It is as if disabled people's debility and care needs become tokens for which industries receive funding from the government.

As an increasing portion of the healthcare budget becomes allocated to Medicaid managed care, and as New York State is, for example, projected to save more than $200 million annually with the initiation of managed-care programs, these numbers and testimonies from enrollees raise the question: Who bears the inconveniences—or even the life-threatening consequences— as some money is saved and other flows from the state to care industries and as profit takes center stage in the U.S. public healthcare assemblage?[77] What does it mean to live in a society where suppression of the public healthcare budget is prioritized over people's care needs and lives?

Finally, I end this section by noting the eerie absence of critical race and gender analyses in this discussion on debility commodification in managed care. Medicaid at large is occupied disproportionately by those with lower income and people of color, whereas Medicaid long-term-care programs are often seen as unique with their relatively large presence of white, formerly middle-class enrollees compared to other Medicaid programs.[78] The high costs of long-term care and its long-lasting nature often suck up savings and put even those with class privilege near the poverty line and eligible for public healthcare supports.[79] Thus, this unique characteristic of long-term care also means that many of those white enrollees' families often become powerful lobbyists and major advocates for keeping long-term-care programs' eligibility criteria more open and protecting the programs from further scrutiny or reforms.[80]

Nonetheless, the more I have looked into this phenomenon of differential debilitation or the pushout and deduction of care hours for some Medicaid enrollees, the more I have noticed and been filled with questions about the lack of demographic information on Medicaid enrollees who went through these reconfigurations. This absence became even more prominent when I requested that the New York State Department of Health (DoH) share demographic information and rationales for pushouts of Medicaid long-term-care enrollees during the transition to managed care. Although the DoH released the report on how many people were pushed out from each care agency during the transition to managed-care, detailed information about those people (e.g., demographic information) and the reasons for termination of their services were not mentioned.[81] The response I received from the DoH included that (1) they do not keep demographic records on those who were pushed out, and (2) they reasoned that the push-out was not due to the implementation of managed care but to implementation of the new function assessment measurement used to determine who can enroll in Medicare programs. This was despite the fact that the time frame of this new measurement's implementation and the DoH web report on those who were pushed out rarely overlapped. One thing this unsatisfactory response illustrates is a difficulty or incompetency regarding documenting and following up on who experienced the drastic service cuts or terminations at the time of transition to managed care, particularly when this reconfiguration was managed at the level of care industries (i.e., agencies) with their newly gained authority. This unsatisfactory response also illuminates the gap between what is traced by the state and what is actually going on at the agency and individual level. When one has no choice but to rely on court cases of those who appealed the pushout or reduction of long-term-care hours, detailed demographic information is often omitted. This suggests that these pushouts and the reconfiguration of the enrollee population were purely constructed based on their care hours, and this may be so in the cases I have laid out. Nevertheless, I cannot dismiss entirely how the evaluation and placement of people on the spectrum of capacity-debility (hence needing Medicaid services or not) is profoundly constructed in relation to stereotypes based on race, gender, class, migration, and disability. For example, even though the measurement of functionality, to some extent, is self-reported, it is also examined by medical institutions where people's capacities, debilities, and other bodymind conditions are constructed in relation to the representation of their intersecting identities.[82]

Medicaid at large, for example, is occupied with children and adults of color, signifying who has access to private insurance and who has access only to public health insurance.[83] The photos used in the *New York Times* reports I brought up in this section, indeed, include images largely of Black and Brown women.[84] They pose alone or with their daughters, sitting in small, crowded, New York City apartments wearing expressions of despair. The absence of (or extreme difficulty in finding any) demographics in official documents of those who were pushed out or whose services were reduced gets more and more suspicious next to the disproportionate racial makeup of Medicaid enrollees at large and the newspaper images used over and over to represent this case. Further, this lack of critical race and gender analyses of the Medicaid managed-care transition becomes even more obvious as analyses of how care workers are constructed show the deep history where gender, race, migration status, and class are crucial factors in care worker making and deeply tied to notions of their capacity to labor.

Differential Capacitation: The Making of Care Workers

[The area of care] is where the lives of privileged women intersected with poor women and women of color, who were members of groups subjected to coercive labor regimes. Historically, caring labor in the homes of more privileged classes was split between wives, mothers, and daughters on the one hand and servants drawn from the ranks of the less-privileged classes on the other.
—Evelyn Nakano Glenn, *Forced to Care*

American society had always defined non-white women as workers and devalued their caregiving roles [to their own children as mothers].
—Premilla Nadasen, Jennifer Mittelstadt, and Marisa Chappell, *Welfare in the United States*

What is not explicitly depicted in the testimonies and reports discussed in the previous section, and yet asserted clearly through their absence, is the stories of care workers. Service deduction and termination do not mean that Medicaid enrollees' care needs magically disappear; they are simply displaced—whether to a gray (under-the-table) or other care labor market or to family and friends—or may experience further debilitation as their care needs are neglected. The shortcomings of and absence of public protection of the right to receive care are profoundly interwoven with the right (not) to provide care.[85] Who is pushed into care responsibilities and labor under the U.S. public healthcare assemblage? How does care as a mechanism of control manifest and materialize as care worker populations are constructed and treated in the care economy? Which people are capacitated to care (figuratively and actually) and how in the racialized, gendered, neocolonial, and disability economies? By addressing these questions, I also articulate how the making of care workers simultaneously creates care receivers and vice versa as such constructions are deeply intertwined. Additionally, this making of care workers through (differential) capacitation shows how the profound divide between two roles and the standpoints (and sit-points) of care workers and recipients is constantly reinstated, as if they are assumed to only be one or the other.[86]

Theorizing the lived experiences of third world women (which includes racially marginalized women in the United States), transnational feminist scholar Chandra Talpade Mohanty described how the care labor force is shaped by the engraved cultural ideas and stereotypes that women, particularly women of color, are naturally more maternal and hence suited to be care providers.[87] This trope undergirds the centuries-old mechanism of the making of care workers as well as devaluation of caring work. In today's U.S. care labor force, a report published by a nonprofit organization, PHI, in 2020 shows that those who occupy paid home care assistant jobs are almost all women (87 percent), and the majority are people of color (62 percent—and 28 percent of them are Black and 23 percent Latinx).[88] Migrant people disproportionately occupy the labor force—31 percent—whereas only 12.9 percent of the entire U.S. population are foreign-born (as of 2010).[89] Almost half of them live under 200 percent of the federal poverty line (while 18 percent of them live under it). More than half of them (53 percent) live with some public assistance, including Medicaid coverage. Even within the occupation of home-based care labor, workers' hourly wages deeply depend on their race and gender—the lowest wages are earned by women of color ($11.13) and the highest by white men ($12.38).[90] Finally, those older than fifty-five are the fastest-growing care provider age group.[91] These numbers show that the caring task is not taken up equitably across populations. Some people's capacity to care is disproportionately amplified as they are (forcibly) capacitated for care labor, which tends to be physically and emotionally demanding with unjustly little and discriminatory compensation.

Feminist sociologist Evelyn Nakano Glenn, whose quote opened this section, adds historical context to these care worker statistics with her scholarship. Approaching the topic of care from an intersectional feminist perspective, she argued that "women are charged with a triple duty to care, on the basis of (1) kinship (wife, daughter, mother), (2) gender (as women), and (3) sometimes race/class (as members of a subordinate group)."[92] I further add how these characteristics of care work are mutually constructed with the devalued nature of care work. In the care economy, the economic marginalization of already marginalized populations who are situated as care workers is further enforced and maintained. In other words, within the care economy, which is not only built on but also further inscribes cisheteropatriarchal, racialized, and class- and migration-based inequality, people are differently capacitated to care.[93]

By centering an intersectional feminist analysis of care, I untangle this differential capacitation within the care labor force by surveying two historical contexts and strands of care worker making. First, I offer a snapshot of how the globalizing neoliberal force expands the U.S. public healthcare assemblage beyond the U.S. border and accelerates the growth of transnational care labor migration—all of which situates certain people as care workers for the United States. I also trace how the history of colonialism and lingering neocolonialism undergird this care worker making. Second, I trace critical race and feminist scholarly works that connect slavery and racist and sexist tendencies within welfare programs for single mothers and families in need to today's care labor formation. The quote by Nadasen, Mittelstadt, and Chappell that opened this section succinctly states that women of color came to be situated strategically as care workers in U.S. history. I untangle these genealogies through analysis of differential capacitation and thus expand and complicate the genealogies by articulating the overlap between the timing of global proliferation of neoliberalism and care labor migration as well as neoliberal turns within the welfare program for single mothers and families in need and Medicaid (aka medical welfare).[94] The history of care worker making is simultaneously a story of determining who occupies care receiver positioning. I demonstrate, therefore, the construction of capacity in the arena of the care labor force that is shaped in racialized, gendered, (neo)colonial, and disability economies.

The Making of Transnational Care Workers

When the United States historically faced care crises with a high turnout of care workers or an imbalance between the number of people who need long-term care and those who take on care responsibilities, it turned to the nations of the Global South as one site from which to source the care labor force. In the United States at large, the number of foreign-born workers (of any occupation) has been increasing (from 13.3 percent of all workers in 2000 to 17.4 percent in 2019).[95] While the U.S. government does not have an official migration recruitment program, a historically available pathway to permanent residency status (e.g., via marriage), among other factors, made the United States a more desirable destination for migrant workers.[96] Particularly with the recent globalization of the neoliberal political economy, such transnational labor extortion accelerates in entanglement with racial and gendered economies. It is overwhelmingly women, in the realm of the care economy, who migrate to take up care responsibilities in the nations of the Global North. In the increasing care labor migration, transnational care industries flourish by recruiting and training those (mostly) women to become care workers, thus by coordinating with governments and care industries in sending off and accepting nations to facilitate and market the migration.[97]

Global neoliberalism fundamentally converted means of living for people in different locales and their local economies (e.g., from agriculture for their own consumption and sale to mass-scale exportation businesses as transnational corporations came to occupy the center of business and financial districts in nations of the Global South both metaphorically and literally).[98] In this conversion and reconfiguration, one area of economy that bloomed was the service labor economy. The neoliberal transition in different locales of the Global South, paired with the rapid growth in care needs within the Global North, fueled the flourishment of service labor (i.e., care work) at the transnational level.[99] In American studies scholar Lisa Lowe's words, "In the search for ever cheaper, more 'flexible,' labor pools, this reorganization [due to neoliberal globalization] . . . produces a greater 'pull' for new Asian and Latino immigrants, especially for Asian and Latina women, to fill the service sector jobs in the United States."[100]

Further, this neoliberal force is built on a history of colonization and neocolonial power imbalance shaped through unjust trade treaties and unfair investment of transnational financial institutions (e.g., International Monetary Fund, World Bank), among other mechanisms. This all means that many formerly colonized nations of the Global South continue to experience ongoing oppressions in the global arena regardless of the independence they fought for and won.[101] In the case of care labor migration going on between the Philippines and the United States, feminist sociologist Anna Guevarra traced how the Christianity instilled in the Philippines during the multicentury-long colonization by Spain (1565 to 1898) laid the groundwork for the mentality expected and demanded of migrant care workers, which includes "suffering, sacrifice, martyrdom."[102] In addition, forty-seven years of U.S. rule in the Philippines from 1898 to 1945 instituted the nursing program based on the U.S. standard and curriculum in the Philippines, which was a precursor to turning the Philippines into a suitable and desirable nation for care labor exports (e.g., nurses and domestic workers) to the United States.[103] Furthermore, global power dynamics and imbalanced postcolonial U.S.-Philippines trading treaties forced unfair trading to the Philippines, which pushed (or forced) the Filipino government to turn to labor migration in order to have economic stability.[104]

At the other end of the transnational migration assemblage, the U.S. government has been facilitating the smooth entry of care workers from Global South nations (including the Philippines) to fulfill the care needs of U.S. citizens by increasing the number of visas to allow workers to enter the United States and loosen the existing policies that were originally placed with an intention to maintain quality care.[105] Feminist economist Nancy Folbre explained that

> the U.S. encourage[s] immigration of nurses, often under terms that reduce their mobility and their bargaining power.[106] In 2002, more than 7,500 nurses were admitted to the U.S. as temporary workers.[107] Conservatives in the U.S. Congress have advocated legislative changes that would expand the number of visas, and eliminate requirements that include English proficiency testing and educational curriculum reviews. Particularly telling are related efforts to rescind the existing requirement that facilities employing foreign-educated nurses only require them to work hours commensurate with those of U.S. nurses.[108] The U.S. health-care industry can use international recruitment as way of avoiding the more costly solution of improving current working conditions.[109]

Folbre not only addresses the reality of care labor importing but also how global inequality and migration-based discrimination are institutionalized and continue in the workplace. While this quote was on a specific form of care work (nursing), it shows that migrant care workers (including home-based care workers and domestic workers) are deeply woven into the fabric of everyday U.S. life, and this reality is built on and shaped by significant historical context as well as complex and multiplying mechanisms of industries and governments. In other words, multiplying and dynamic forces directly and indirectly shape these women's decisions to take part in transnational care labor migration and how they are treated as they perform care labor. Care labor migration is, in other words, much more than a personal endeavor but part of a system developed over the centuries and across the globe.

As much as governments exercise and become a major force for the nation's move toward transnational labor migration, what has also been noticeable with its rapid growth is the private sectors that recruit, train, market, and facilitate care migration.[110] In this transnationally orchestrated arrangement, women from Global South nations are *capacitated* to become the *desirable product* for transnational care industries to market.[111] Such capacitation happens both symbolically, by manipulating how their labor capacities and skillsets are represented and marketed, and at the level of actual bodyminds by training their bodyminds and conditioning them to fulfill the care needs and desires of receiving nations. Both forms of so-called capacitation are profoundly entangled with and rely on the racial and gendered stereotypes that further facilitate the targeted marketing and commodification of those women's caring capacities.[112] In the case of Filipina migrant domestic and care workers, Guevarra has reported, "With employers in the role of consumers, the seemingly top-of-the-line labor commodity that they have purchased (the 'Mercedes Benz' of domestic workers) serves as the family's status symbol, to be paraded by the family and envied by other employers."[113] They are trained and taught to take up multiple professional roles, including as tutors for children, care providers for infants or elderly family members, and chefs familiar with the cuisine common in the employers' culture, and to be overall physically and mentally fit to be envied for their caliber.[114] Even the history of colonization and stereotypes rooted in such history are turned into a marketing strategy to broker Filipinas as ideal workers who are "obedient, submissive, and yet trained within the US nursing education standards to perform US quality care" (given the instilling of U.S. culture and norms through the U.S. colonization of the Philippines).[115]

Within the complex combination of marketed images and training to learn and reconfigure themselves as care workers in order to make a living in the neocolonial and neoliberal political economy, many women of the Global South are primarily turned into commodifiable and marketable "products."[116] They come to be recognized based on or mainly as a labor capacity to be circulated and exchanged for wages (a certain portion of which may be also taxed in their home countries) in the context of the transnationally extending U.S. public healthcare assemblage. Global location and its geopolitical history determine who is considered to be a suitable care worker and set up to take up these responsibilities within the United States and for U.S. citizens among other nations of the Global North. This context simultaneously dictates and shapes the stark division between care worker and care receiver, and who is granted the roles of providing or receiving care.

To unpack the care arranged within the U.S. public healthcare assemblage is to examine the care set up specifically for U.S. citizens. One of the lines that shapes and distinguishes who receives care and who takes up caring labor in the assemblage is, therefore, the national border. National origin and migration status (i.e., whether one is a citizen or not) dictate and determine which role one is granted under the assemblage. The control and inequality exercised through care (i.e., the construction of care workers and care receivers, the devaluing of care work, unchecked quality of care) are therefore merged with the sociopolitical forces of neocolonialism, U.S.

imperialism, and the transnational racial and gendered economies. The amplified capacities of people (and mostly women) to take up care work are commodified and circulated across national borders by the tag team of transnational care industries and the governments of the sending and receiving nations. This care-based inequality is further intensified particularly in the era of global neoliberalism, in which transnational labor migration accelerates as the service economy (e.g., care economy) continues to grow, building on the history of colonialism. By emphasizing migrants as capacitated to take up care labor in the United States, I certainly do not intend to overlook the lives of migrant disabled people who may receive care under different care assemblages (in addition to or without government-funded care) or who may continue working in whatever ways they can within the context of a lack of governmental supports to supplement income and health care, among others. Rather, I draw on the structure of how global power dynamics impacts the care dynamics within the U.S. to delineate whose care needs are prioritized and whose are sublimated as they are primary considered as care workers.

The Making of Welfare-to-Workfare Care Workers

From the 1930s on, each generation of government officials and public
welfare professionals clung to the premise that poor single mothers could end
their own dependency on welfare by maintaining the independence of those
incapacitated through no fault of their own—that is, by performing care
work. They could become rehabilitated in the process of rehabilitating others.
The deserving and undeserving, like the public and private sectors, stood
interconnected rather than apart. [Additionally,] haunting this history was
the legacy of slavery and segregation that racialized the [caring] labor and
defined it as low paid and unskilled.

—Eileen Boris and Jennifer Klein, *Caring for America*[117]

In the 1990s, the major shift in Medicaid with the implementation of managed care began to widely spread across states, while the U.S. major welfare program for single mothers and families in need also went through a major transition with the implementation of the Personal Responsibility and Work Opportunity Reconciliation Act in 1996. These shifts happened while the neoliberal political force continues to become the norm of everyday life in the United States. "The end of welfare as we knew it" came with the termination of Aid to Families with Dependent Children and the beginning of Temporary Assistance for Needy Families (TANF), which signaled the further intensifying of implementation of welfare-to-workfare doctrine.[118] Not only the overlapping timing in the transition of those major U.S. welfare programs (Medicaid and TANF), but the unfolding of how those transitions changed the requirements for those welfare programs demonstrates how the making of care workers and care recipients and the process of their capacitation and debilitation under the U.S. public healthcare assemblage are conducted side by side and mutually affective. The mutuality is clearly stated in the quote by Boris and Klein that opened this section, in which lower-income (and thus working-class and poor) single mothers' dependency is distinguished from that of those who became "incapacitated through no fault of their own," while both are expected (or forced) to rehabilitate. Single mothers' rehabilitation from dependency on welfare hinged on more labor, which often meant care work for *other* families, while these single mothers' need to care for their own children (and themselves) or their children's care dependency on them are entirely dismissed. Meanwhile, other people's (i.e., disabled people's) dependency is believed to be rehabilitated through care supports. What differentiates these dependencies that in/visibly occupy the quote? How did one's dependency on welfare (for single mothers) come to be recognized as their own fault, which is met with punitive labor demands, while another's dependency on welfare (e.g., Medicaid or Medicare) is seen as innocent and deserving of public supports to attend their own well-being (though the rehabilitative assistance provided to them was often experienced as ableist violence and control)? Finally, what does this clear distinction of their dependency do to the current care formation?

This mutual co-creation of care workers and recipients shows that historically, capacitating a certain population to take up care work has simultaneously come with overlook and neglect of their care needs, and recognition of them primarily as (care) laborers often impeded them from claiming disability or debilitated status to receive care on a structural level.[119] In other words, the process of making some people into care workers is also the process of prioritizing whose care needs (or debilities) will be recognized and met in society, under publicly sponsored care services or otherwise. The intent here is not to obscure the different degrees in care needs that people embody, but to pay attention to how racial, gendered, migrant-based, and disability economies or the notions of a *disposable workforce* and the *pitiful and burdensome disabled* who need public protection shaped the recognition of people's durability and labor capacity on the one side and vulnerability and needs on the other. Many workers were and are impaired to the point that they need long-term care and yet are made to continuously work.[120] And many disabled people were and are situated under the care that they call abuse and control over their lives, rather than being embraced as part of the larger society with quality assistance. Such notions get lost in the reductive dichotomy of care provider and care receiver roles maintained within the matrix of in/vulnerable and un/deserving.

Evelyn Nakano Glenn traced the process of racial and gendered making of care workers back to slavery and explains how today's care formations were shaped and built historically.[121] Her works as well as those of other feminist scholars further connect how the processes continue to be carried on through the development of U.S. welfare programs for single mothers and families in need—which leads us to 1996 and presence.[122] All of these historical events can be connected by and demonstrate the racialization and gendering of (care) labor capacity.[123] Their capacitation was also inherently registered as rehabilitation from their dependency on the state to reprovoke the preceding quote by Boris and Klein. In the history of the United States, it is Black women and other women of color who have been exclusively situated as care workers, while their vulnerability, need for care, and hence humanity have been quickly overlooked or considered secondary to their laboring capacity. The term *capacitated* to describe care workers in this case is used quite differently (with some overlap) from the labor capacitation that women of the Global South endure under globalizing neoliberalism and requires further examination. This forcible distinction of laborer and recognition as a disabled person and hence needing supports is, for instance, clearly traced in critical race and feminist historian Sarah Haley's writing. Studying and theorizing the post-slavery criminalization of Black women as a way to exploit their labor capacity in order to build the modern South, Haley noted why she does not use the term *disability* in her book to depict the impairing and debilitating conditions those women experienced in the historic period: "The vast majority of women at the [Milledgeville State Prison Farm] were black and were, accordingly, excluded from the category of disabled. . . . [T]hey were considered to have *a particular capacity* for hard labor and assigned a disproportionate amount of the fieldwork at the fledgling state farm."[124] Here, disability is understood as a government-assigned status and category that is mutually exclusive from being a laborer. She uses terms such as *deviancy*, instead, to signal the pathologization and stigmatization of Black women experiencing impairing conditions to mark how they were denied disability status and the accompanying public supports, and hence regarded as not in need of care.[125]

Going further back in the time period and by tracing and depicting the making of the care worker population in the United States prior to the American Revolution, Glenn reported:

> In the decades leading up to the American Revolution, three-quarters of new migrants were unfree workers: slaves, indentured servants, and convicts. . . . [A] significant proportion of women and children were assigned to household tasks . . . tending to sick and disabled family members [of the privileged].[126]

Shortages of domestic laborers and care labor in more affluent families were at the time addressed coercively by the structure of slavery and other forms of forced labor, where the racialized and gendered making of care workers is deeply inscribed. Even after the end of slavery and legal indentured servitude in the U.S. South, for example, "legislatures used criminal laws [such as vagrancy statutes] to compel labor. . . . And black women were included among those subject to arrest [and then exploited for their labor force]. . . . [Or, even when] married black women [were] supported by husbands, [they were still] assumed to be idle if not working for wages."[127] Those Black women were then apprehended and ushered into servant jobs in order to pay off the fines that resulted from their apprehension, while married white women were trusted to tend their households and families, and their husbands assumed the breadwinner responsibilities. Even in the U.S. North, Black women were largely put to domestic and caring work for the privileged.[128] In the history, these women's (and men's) capacity was marked and activated differently, as staying home of white women is expected and demanded, while that of Black women was criminalized. These white women's capacity to care was, in a way, domesticated for their own families, while Black women's capacity to do so was turned into a public property and for privileged others.

This brief overview of Glenn's in-depth analyses may overly simplify the long and complex history of slavery in the United States and how it continues to haunt the status quo.[129] Nevertheless, it does depict how the current care labor force has a significant history. In other words, care has always been considered unpaid and hence devalued labor in the mainstream United States, particularly when it was conducted by Black women (and other women of color) who were always and already forced to work outside their home. This historical fact also means that U.S. society demanded that Black women prioritize the well-being and care of others, and especially more privileged others, above that of their family members and themselves.

Haley's and Glenn's works, among others, are complex illustrations of how the devaluation of care work, the devaluation of those who are made into care workers, and the making of care workers are all entangled in racialized and gendered economies.[130] To untangle the formation of care and to build care scholarship, therefore, is to recognize how the structure of care has been deeply tied to and built on racial provocation and assumption of capacity to labor care. This sets Black people and other people of color as an exploitable and disposable labor source and always suspect when they claim disability status and express their own needs for care. The historical study of slavery and post-slavery criminalization of Black women simultaneously is, therefore, the tale of care formation. It also speaks to the social position of care for (white) disabled people and other people requiring long-term care. Although this history demonstrates who has been granted institution-alized disability status and viewed as vulnerable and deserving care sup-ports from local governing bodies, it also shows that care for them was considered as being able to be provided by those who are "enslaved" and "convicted." Care work, in other words, was not a priority into which "un-enslaved" and "un-convicted" privileged people's capacities (and particu-larly those of men) were to be poured.

Feminist historians Eileen Boris, Jennifer Klein, Premilla Nadasen, Jen-nifer Mittelstadt, and Marisa Chappell, among others, have traced the geneal-ogy of the making of care workers in the racialized and gendered economies from the time leading up to the American Revolution to the present by look-ing at how welfare programs for single mothers and families in need have been situated to meet increasing care needs in relation to the emergence of Medicaid, Medicare, and other public healthcare programs.[131] Since the earli-est form of public supports for single mothers, Mothers' Pensions in 1911, there has been a tendency to exclude Black single mothers and other single mothers of color from receiving benefits based on assumption on racialized labor capacity: there were jobs available for these populations to take up such as domestic work and field work, which are often reserved for women of color, and hence they are considered as not needing public assistance.[132] While the racist exclusion of mothers of color and racialized and gender-based recogni-tion and de/valuing of their capacities to labor and needs for support continue to shape welfare programs for single mothers and families in need, feminist historians Nadasen, Mittelstadt, and Chappell further explain the shift in such programs. They point out the increasing and intensifying disciplinary and controlling forces within the welfare program, as enrollment by mothers of color increased in the 1950s onward.[133] Such a shift signals the beginning of condemnation of welfare recipients and backlash against the programs (e.g., development and deployment of stereotypes such as *welfare queen* or *underclass*), which further intensifies work requirements for the recipients. Nadasen, Mittelstadt, and Chappell describe the trending attitudes within the politicians and everyday people against welfare recipients as follows:

[S]ocial workers insisted that the [newly and increasingly admitted African American welfare recipients in the 1950s and early 1960s] were afflicted with "social disabilities". . . . [I]n the words of social work researchers they were "immature," "dependent" personalities whose single motherhood and "dependence" on welfare were evi-dence of *pathology*. Beginning in the early 1950s, social workers, liberal reformers and politicians turned to fixing the perceived prob-lems of [Aid to Dependent Children] clients. Their solution was something they dubbed "rehabilitation." . . . The 1956 law [Social

Security Amendments] authorized states . . . to use federal funds for
job training, job placement programs. . . . Pilot rehabilitation projects often directed welfare clients to positions as domestic [work-
ers]. . . . the only jobs open to non-whites.[134]

What is bizarre and crucial to point out here is the strategic use of disability
to pathologize people's needs and dependencies on the state supports. It is,
thus, not anyone's needs and dependencies that are made issue and met with
demands to work in the labor force to "rehabilitate." In the surge of the
racist- and sexist-based condemnation of welfare programs, welfare recipients' stated inabilities or needs are not taken as a sign of vulnerability that
deserves public supports. Their needs are seen as deviancy that requires fixing through punitive and disciplinary laboring requirements and not even
medical and health care which is often seen as the solution to pathology for
other people. Those single mothers' needs and inabilities to perform all the
tasks required for them and their families to live (e.g., child care, earning
wages) are met with the demand to further capacitate themselves somehow
to care more (through care work for other people). Their dependencies are
not *need* per se in the state's perspective but are turned into pathological and
punishable *laziness* which is set to be fixed though labor demands. Further,
those scholars note how welfare programs for single mothers and families in
need were often put to continuous scrutiny and defunding (more punishment), while politicians often rushed to protect welfare programs for (selective) disabled folks (i.e., Medicaid and Medicare).[135] All of them reinstate
how the notions of un/deserving and un/worthy poor were constructed in
the history of U.S. welfare programs to loop us back to the introduction of
this chapter. At the same time, we need to be cautious and contemplate the
notions of *worthy* and *deserving* from critical disability analysis to avoid as-
suming that those who are recognized as disabled and receive public care
supports are necessarily treated as worthy and deserving. Disability communities, on the contrary, have brought up over and over how their dependencies and needs that are read as *pitiful* and *burdensome* are also met with
punitive treatments including eugenics, forced institutionalization, medical
treatments, and abuse under the name of care. Constructions of pathology
or disability and their consequences are shaped in relation to racism, sexism,
and classism, and thus ableism experienced differently based on one's intersecting identities. All of it is embedded in the history of care formation.

This discriminatory tendency throughout the history of welfare programs is said to have been passed on to TANF. The emergence of TANF, which
limited the welfare recipient period to five years maximum in their lifetime (and two years maximum on continuous assistance) and included mandatory work requirements, highlights the ultimate intensification of the

welfare-to-workfare mandate, as its recipients were strongly encouraged—or forced—to enter the workforce.[136] The introduction of TANF and the cap for the welfare recipient period is said to have decreased the number of welfare recipients by 6.5 million, more than 53 percent, in the first four years after it was implemented.[137] Glenn has warned that this statistic should not be read as TANF's success in supporting the financial independence of mothers, though.[138] Those numbers more accurately describe how the state came to cease supports for single mothers and families in need and seized their rights to receive public supports to care for their own families. Among those who were dropped from TANF include the *disconnected* (19 percent of whom are pushed out of welfare), who were pushed out of the welfare supports regardless of their unemployed status, without supports of breadwinner partners or other family members and friends, or their or their children's disabling conditions—all of which indicate that they were not ready to be cut off from the welfare supports.[139] Furthermore, in the first few years after TANF's implementation, 60 percent of its former beneficiaries gained employment—employment that led them into chronic poverty, as their newly tasked jobs paid low to minimum wage.[140] This data indicates that the introduction of cap to the welfare reception period created a large pool of lower-income (or no-income) single mothers who had no choice but to take any job available, including low-wage care jobs.

Historically, care work has been set up as an inevitable and suited designation for the *rehabilitation* of Black women and other women of color, whether from their criminalization or from welfare dependency. Such analyses and theorizations laid out by a number of feminist historians, and their quotes throughout this section, indicate the connections between welfare programs for single mothers and families in need and medical welfare such as Medicaid as a relationship of demand and supply for care. Glenn describes that a nonprofit care agency in New York State, Cooperative Home Care Associates (which administers a number of Medicaid long-term services and supports cases) symbolizes this point as they emphasize their work as connecting those who need long-term care with "women wanting to leave welfare."[141] The latter group does so by engaging in care work for the former.

The mechanisms for the makings of care workers and care recipients are profoundly connected and mutually constructed. Needs of supports for people with various backgrounds and intersecting identities are recognized differently, followed by drastically different consequences, and they intersect at the site of long-term care, some as care recipients and the others as care workers. In this distinct reading and registering of people's needs and dependencies, some who are institutionally recognized as disabled are exclusively considered as vulnerable and thus burdensome when their needs never cease and are considered significant. The needs of lower-income single mothers of color are grossly overlooked and activate, instead, more labor demands. All of them shaped in the complex forces of racism, sexism, classism, and ableism that dictate people's capacity, debility, and needs, as well as worthiness and deservingness of public supports. Changes in Medicaid long-term-care programs, in other words, have impacts not only on the lives of those who enroll in the programs but on those who are hired to provide the care as well. Strategic deployment of welfare policies that require its recipients to engage in labor including that of care for Medicaid recipients continues nearly a century later—today.

Care has been deployed as a mechanism of control through the commodification of people's capacities and debilities in the assemblage of the care industrial complex, federal and state policies on medical and single-parent welfare programs, and much more. Lower-income migrant and nonmigrant women of color are, therefore, not only capacitated to take up care work in the United States, but also rhetorically in that they are assumed not to get sick, disabled, or become frail, and hence not require care for themselves. They have been overwhelmingly excluded from the potential deserving care receiver pool and put into the arduous care laborer pool at a structural level. Furthermore, using the term *capacity* to describe the making of care workers warrants further examination. The capacitation enacted or forced on largely migrant workers and women of color in the United States to be care workers is not simply an enhancement of the power to act, to cite affect theory's notion of capacity. Rather, it refers to a capacity specifically to labor for the U.S. public health and other care assemblages.[142] In other words, one way to deepen the description of the capacitation is to acknowledge its subjugated capacity, in which the labor capacity of those who are situated as care workers is constructed to be extracted to the U.S. public healthcare assemblage, including the transnational and domestic care industrial complex.[143] Additionally, such subjugated (or territorialized) capacity certainly is accompanied by their debility on another level. I will further write about the mutual debilitation of Medicaid enrollee care recipients and their care workers under the neoliberal public healthcare assemblage in the next chapter. Also examined is how the devaluation of care in the historical interaction of racism, cisheteropatriarchy, colonialism, and ableism as well as de/valuation and commodification of different bodyminds and their capacities and debilities manifest and materialize in day-to-day co-engagement on care practices.

Speculative Connections of Care Assemblages in Different Locales

While the focus of this chapter is on the historical and contemporary mechanisms that shaped care formation—and particularly care worker and receiver populations—I would like to emphasize that those people did not passively take up subjugated roles attached to them. The histories of domestic worker and disability rights communities and activism demonstrate the powerful resistance and revolutions that led us to reimagine care as we know it.[144] The opening depiction of "Don't Cap Our Care!" rally is a case in point. And disabled Black women and other women of color were among those who participated in and at times led these activism works. Although the main analysis that took over this chapter was the dichotomized and interwoven making of care workers and recipients in racialized, gendered, migrant, and disability economies, this does not mean that there are no Black women and other women of color whose disabilities are recognized by the state and receive Medicaid care support. They not only exist but are leading more intersectional disability activism.

Further, although my analyses focus primarily on those who are directly situated as care workers and recipients in U.S. public healthcare formations, they are not the only people whose lives are deeply impacted and shaped within them. Family members and care clients that care workers had cared for prior to joining the U.S. public healthcare assemblage, or those that they continue to care for, are some examples of those affected. For women and gender-nonconforming femme people to be overwhelmingly situated as care providers in and outside of their homes, they are likely to have multiple sets of care responsibilities in addition to their paid care labor. These responsibilities may be toward their own children or elderly parents, for example, or care clients they once attended before they left their home countries and towns to join the care labor force in the United States and its metropolitan cities. To be capacitated to take up care labor in the interwoven racial, gendered, migration, and disability economies is, in a way, to receive orders regarding whose care needs must be prioritized.

Sociologist Arlie R. Hochschild has introduced the concept of the *care chain* to illustrate the expansive wave of impact care formations in the nations of the Global North trigger. Illustrating the care chain in the global frontier, Hochschild noted that "global capitalism affects whatever it touches, and it touches virtually everything including . . . global care chains." The care chain is, she continued,

> a series of personal links between people across the globe based on the paid or unpaid work of caring. Usually women make up these chains . . . [that] may be local, national, or global. Global chains . . . usually start in a poor country, and move from rural to urban areas within that same poor country. Or they start in one poor country and extend to another slightly less poor country and then link one place to another within the latter country. . . . One common form of

such a chain is: (1) an older daughter from a poor family who cares for her siblings while (2) her mother works as a nanny caring for the children of a migrating nanny who, in turn, (3) cares for the child of a family in a rich country. . . . Each kind of chain expresses an invisible human ecology of care, one kind of care depending on another and so on.[145]

I would add to Hochschild's suggestion that, at every step, multiplying industrial and governmental gatekeepers oil the chain and make the movement of care labor forces go more smoothly. This analysis is useful to understand how U.S. care workers as well are rarely left with much choice but to leave their sick and disabled family members, elderly parents, or children needing caring supports at home to conduct their work as paid care workers, and are required to negotiate those care demands as well as their own care needs.[146] In the cisheteropatriarchal economy where women and gender-nonconforming femme people are overwhelmingly situated as care laborers, their migrations or entry into the care labor force give rise to additional needs for care to be negotiated, met, or compromised. Critical race and feminist sociologist Valerie Francisco-Menchavez studied the ways in which transnational families reshape their familyhood through fictive kinship and other means in the context of the contemporary Philippines: "Neoliberal structural shifts in induced and sustained migration shape and ultimately change the intimate relations and definitions of care in Filipino families. . . . Migrant and non-migrant family members are tailoring their definitions of the family form based on the conditions of their lives while global processes are restructuring intimate family dynamics."[147] Within the United States, too, feminist scholars Lisa Dodson and Wendy Luttrell have traced how single mother care workers often have no choice but to leave their kids behind to be the breadwinners for their families, while their children are left to attend to one another's care needs.[148] The prioritization of different people's care needs is quickly drawn as that some folks' care needs are attached to financial value—wages for care work.

Drawing on this perspective, I see care chains as a potential area to speculatively connect the lives of disabled people coming from different locales, including those of the Global North or a more affluent class background and the Global South or a less affluent class background. Although Hochschild's concept focuses on care providers, this concept also tells the stories of those who are situated as their care recipients. In fact, it is likely that in order to meet the care needs of U.S. care recipients, the care workers assigned to them may be migrating from the Global South, while the care recipients they used to attend to are now left to reconfigure how to meet their care needs. Also, such migration can happen domestically, as a mother may take up care labor to financially support her family while her disabled parent may need to be attended by someone else or simply wait until she comes home.

These overtly simplified analogies certainly deserve to be more nuanced and featured for their richness. As discussed, for example, Medicaid long-term care is not necessarily promised to all disabled Americans, its quality may not be as good as people expect, and their well-being may not be prioritized in the assemblage. In other words, although conversations about global inequality can be quickly vacuumed into a reductionist comparison between quality of life in the Global North and struggles in the Global South or quality lives for care recipients and uneasy lives for care providers and their families, it is highly problematic given the previously mentioned circumstances that disabled people in the United States go through. It is also troublesome to quickly assume that the lives of disabled and other care recipients and their families in the Global South are primarily filled with struggle. Francisco-Menchavez continues, "I also assert that the social reproductive labor of transnational family members can be a site for hopeful potential in challenging gender roles, pushing back against which currencies of care work count in the family, and even creating new types of solidarity in diasporic sites that center fictive kinship as a form of transnational family operations."[149] With this assertion on generativity, she resists the act of their lives being minimized and imagined solely as hardship or victimhood.

What I want to activate here, instead, is a social imagination to expand our ideas for care justice and to recognize that disabled people of different geopolitical locations, class, and other backgrounds are un/recognized, de/valued, and affected differently in globalizing neoliberalism and through the impacts made by the U.S. public healthcare assemblage. What does it mean in this age to be U.S. citizens whose care needs are deployed in the U.S. public healthcare structure and hence the global care economy? Onto whose back are their care needs structured to fall? Further, what implication does this speculative connection possibly impose on U.S. disability activists fighting for just care? How can the nationwide rally to save Medicaid recognize and integrate the global impact of the U.S. public healthcare assemblage? How can the care justice they imagine expand to include various people whose lives are deeply touched in this care structure? How can U.S. disability rights activism extend its expertise and wisdom in order to engage in care justice work not only to target immediate benefits and rights for U.S. citizens to receive care, but also to entail just distribution of care responsibilities and just care for all globally? What kinds of solidarity can become dreamable? Here, by focusing on disability community care activism, my intention is not to situate the responsibility of global care and labor inequality with them, as they are also exploited in the political economy. My intention is to foreground and be cognizant of the global frontier as well as the deeply ableist, racist, and cisheteropatriarchal U.S. history where the care formation has been developed. Care practice is a site where racialized, cisheteropatriarchal, and neocolonial capitalism intersects and interacts with the disability economy.[150] As people of different regions are examined, exploited, and circulated based on the marketability of their capacity and debility within global neoliberalism, what kind of potential solidarity might also emerge or be needed? How can activism centering care justice expand its web of activism and movement beyond national borders and a single identity category? The Chicago Medicaid rally shows that care injustices hit multiple marginalized communities and that it is only through their solidarity that we can truly ensure just care for all.

2

My Body Pays the Price

Necropolitics of Care

Being disabled IS A JOB! Everyday I put in work! Most people have no
idea how draining the invisible labor of managing a disability in an
inaccessible world really is! . . . All because Medicaid does not cover
[the cost of accommodations I need] and Medicaid REALLY doesn't
want to. This right here is what your tax dollars DON'T pay for. *Instead
my body pays the price.* I'm tired of being required to jump higher,
and run faster, to get less, in a race where they know I can do neither.
I've been meeting able bodied standards in an ableist world for a long
time. I've been surpassing what's expected of me in an America rich
with misogyny and racism my whole life. But *it's wearing on my body,
and my soul.* [emphasis added]
—Angel L. Miles, "Being Disabled IS A JOB!"

"What [care agencies] are doing to [disabled Medicaid enrollees
and care workers is] abuse!"
"They are care pimps!"
[Hysterical laughter.]
"Ahhhhh that's so true! They are pimping us."
"Oh my goodness!!! Care pimping!"

Hysterical laughter took over.[1] Some people were even crying from laughing
so hard. In the sunlit room of a state disability service building, a number
of Medicaid enrollees and a few of their care partners (care workers) had
gathered to discuss their daily experiences under Medicaid and long-term
community-based and home-based care (long-term care provided in the
Medicaid enrollees' own homes). One moment they were sharing advice,
laughing out loud at the pimp joke, and forming friendships and support
systems across the care worker–recipient divide taken for granted in the
care structure. The next moment, the air was heavy. In the center of a long
table, Tyler, a Medicaid enrollee who is a middle-aged Black man in a manual wheelchair, slowly opened his mouth and spoke in an educational tone

about how care workers and Medicaid enrollees are treated by care agencies:

> A lot of times, [care agencies] just hire [anyone], they just need *a body, [to] fill a spot* [emphasis added], because they want to get the money from Medicaid. . . . Agencies don't care, as long as they send someone [to the enrollee's home], and you are covered . . . whether [the care workers] go or not. The agencies are just collecting money, sitting back and doing whatever Medicaid needs them to do.

A wave of bitterness in the room was palpable as Tyler finished his sentence. Both disabled enrollees and care workers shared similar and overlapping accounts of how undervalued and uncared for they were in the current healthcare system. Recognizing it out loud was daunting because it highlighted the contradiction between such reality and prevalent beliefs that public healthcare programs are fundamentally about providing quality medical and health care to lower-income people and setting up meaningful occupations for care workers. Their eyes were turned to the floor. Soon after, though, their faces lifted and they rolled their eyes, and cynically yet with a sense of familiarity called this treatment what it is: their daily reality. The energy in the room was buoyant and heavy. The supports and care for one another that were inevitable in the space coexisted with bitter critiques and articulations of care-based oppressions they encounter. It was an array of visceral reactions—anger, frustration, jadedness, a sense of familiarity, as well as resilience and resistance through humor—that filled the room and bound us together. This unreducible atmosphere mirrored the daily care practices in which these Medicaid enrollees and their care partners co-engage daily. The next two chapters trace the complex and nuanced realities of how the current care structure shapes the day-to-day lives and well-being of care workers and Medicaid enrollees.

With stories and affect, including wisdom and pain narrated by those who embody care experiences, I theorize today's care structure, assembled within the neoliberal public healthcare realm, as necropolitical. Care workers and receivers (i.e., Medicaid enrollees) are brought to *mutual* and *constant debilitation* under the disguise of state-funded care as nurturing and life-making—for either workers or enrollees. When care is highly commodified and turned into a mechanism of social control and oppression in this neoliberal climate, how do such commodification, control, and oppression manifest in these people's bodyminds, and how do they materialize in their daily care practices? The narratives of care workers and Medicaid enrollees add depth on care as taking place at the micro level, as they are primarily recognized and valued based on their financialized capacities and debilities (or needs for care assistance), while their stories reveal the human(e) connections, capillaries of joy, solidarity, and humor through and across monetized dynamics of neoliberal care.

In this chapter I address how both care workers and Medicaid enrollees are structurally left uncared for, debilitated, and further marginalized, while the assemblage of U.S. public healthcare programs—including the care industrial complex—flourishes. By doing so I continue to articulate the overlapping and intertwined structure of care injustices that those who are situated as care workers and receivers experience. I do so with a hope that such articulation can provide further analysis of how social oppressions falsely put multiple marginalized communities into antagonistic relationships and thus nurture the ground for their solidarity and collective-care justice visions. Using relational analysis of care workers' and Medicaid enrollees' care narratives and experiences through critical disability, race, and feminist perspectives, I challenge the dominant dichotomizing belief in care studies that it is either care workers *or* care recipients who bear the unjust and at times violent treatment on behalf of the others, who in turn thrive under the name of care.[2] I also illuminate how structural oppressions, separately analyzed, indeed interconnectedly shape the everyday lives of these populations. Care workers are impacted by the care injustices that Medicaid enrollees are embedded in, and enrollees' daily lives are shaped by the injustices their workers are subjected to. Putting forward the argument regarding the mutual and constant debilitation of care workers and Medicaid enrollees also promotes the claim that many care workers are becoming disabled or are already so, which illuminates how different disabled people are situated differently in the public healthcare realm—some as recipients of publicly funded care and some as laborers of that care. Simultaneously, this chapter's opening quote by Black feminist disability studies scholar Angel L. Miles reiterates that the public supports for disabled people rarely meet enrollees' needs and expectations comprehensively. Many who are situated as enrollees of public healthcare programs as well are subjected to not necessarily capacitative but at a time debilitative care. Zooming in on the daily lives of Medicaid enrollees and their care workers shows a different picture than the prevailing notion about public healthcare as a safety net that also offers meaningful occupation.

I investigate this reality of care practices by juxtaposing, weaving, and un/folding together the experiences of those who are situated as care workers and recipients, which may seem contrasting and even antagonistic at first glance and yet are entangled and constructed in relation to each other. Care is nested in the web of racial and gendered capitalism as well as the global neocolonial neoliberalism and disability economy.[3] Within this multilayered oppression, care workers and care receivers experience exploitation in both overlapping and distinct ways. Care-based injustices enacted in such political economies trickle down, embedded and embodied in the daily care practices that are co-conducted and co-negotiated by them. Those who are situated as Medicaid enrollees and care workers spend most of their waking time together too. This means that they co-experience almost every moment together and their daily lives are interwoven. Their well-being and the unjust treatment they face can also relationally and interactively affect and shape their care partners' well-being. Or the care injustices they individually experience can materialize and be enacted in each other's hands as they are made enactors of the structural oppressions (here I am considering both cases, of mistreatment delivered in the hands of care workers and enrollees). Engaging in this relational analysis further reveals that liberations and justices for both groups are interconnected and mutually dependent too, which sheds light on the potential and much-needed solidarity and affinity between care worker and care recipient populations and communities.[4] In a way, relational analysis is in radical opposition to the binarification and dichotomization of public-sector care workers and enrollees of public services without erasing the unique and different capacities and needs for care they embody as well as overlapping and mutual yet distinct historical development of care injustices that are inflicted on them. What are the new understandings of the mechanism of care that this approach illuminates, and what are the kinds of activism it activates?

Necropolitical is how I describe care arranged in the current assemblage of U.S. public healthcare programs. Constant weathering is the embedded component of caring and being cared for within the assemblage. Constant debilitation has been an unavoidable component of living for many. The term *necropolitical* is used here to denote the sociopolitical power that controls people (and especially marginalized populations) by deploying and regulating their proximity to death. I am building this argument in contrast to the notion of *biopolitical care* that is widely assumed in much of the care scholarship.[5] Instead of foregrounding the dichotomy that disabled Medicaid enrollees are *made live* at the expense of a weathering care worker population and vice versa, to call care necropolitical is to argue that *both* care workers and enrollees experience constant debilitation in the shadow of a flourishing healthcare assemblage.[6] In other words, what is primarily invested in and valued is the economic structure (the assemblage of U.S. public healthcare itself), and actual humans—situated as care workers and enrollees—are turned into mere *parts* to sustain the structure. Given the increasing numbers of those who need public care supports and those who take up care labor in the U.S., enrollees and care workers are, in addition, turned into as if *disposable* populations.[7] This disposability relegates these populations into the formula not to *make live* but to *let and make debilitate* (and acutely die, particularly during the COVID pandemic).[8] I explain the current care structure as necropolitical particularly by bringing together theories touching on the theme of death and debilitation as a form of control and the consequence of social injustices.[9]

The word *death* (as in *necro*politics) has such a strong connotation. Disability, race, decolonial, feminist, and queer studies and communities have deep insights regarding the notion of death as they continue to debunk stereotypes where disabled people are frequently situated at *worse than death* status and fight against life-taking state violence targeting them (e.g., police brutality, lack of healthcare supports).[10] Against this backdrop, necrotheory was developed and deployed in critical race, queer, decolonial, and disability studies to depict, analyze, and fight acute violence and the debilitating nature of social injustices.[11] My primary use of necro-theory-related terms—slow death, debility, and deterioration—is to explain the *setup* or the current state of the public care assemblage and to theorize its devastating consequences. I do *not* use necro-theory, therefore, to depict and reduce the lives of those who are situated as Medicaid enrollees and care workers as mere passive victims. Instead, I write of creative resistance and the revolutionary collectivity they nurture in the chapters to come, whereas in this chapter my focus is to illuminate the *structure* of how care is assembled in the current social formation and how it impacts and shapes the well-being and vitality of those who are situated as care receivers and workers in an intertwined manner.

Biopolitical Care and Its Limitations

At the turn of the twenty-first century, as globalization and the neoliberal political economy intensified, philosophers Michael Hardt and Antonio Negri, among others, theorized the transition of industry from material to immaterial labor. Under immaterial labor industry, products are "knowledge, information, communication, a relationship, or an emotional response," which gives rise to the *affective labor* industry, which "produces or manipulates affects such as a feeling of ease, well-being, satisfaction, excitement, or passion."[12] The industrialization of care is core to the affective labor upsurge, where affective experiences of care are packaged and sold. Further, Hardt and Negri conceptualized affective labor as biopolitical labor to emphasize the life-making and at times controlling aspects of care practice and how the commodification of care also entails the shaping of life itself for those who are situated as care receivers. Care (or biopolitical care), in other words, is described as inheriting "the power to 'make' live and 'let die' . . . the power to guarantee life. [It] is . . . a matter of taking control of life and the biological processes [by regularizing them]."[13] Here, care is theorized as a modality to control lives through the intentional subjugation and devaluation of some lives.

Additionally, the notion of biopolitical care is implicated in care studies in regard to the question of who are made live and who are not, which inadvertently reasserts the dichotomy and the divide between populations who are situated as care workers and care receivers. An extreme example is narrated here by feminist sociologist Pamela Abbott: "the cost of normalizing life for mentally handicapped [sic] children is to de-normalize it for their mothers."[14] Feminist studies on care at large diligently assert that the gendered nature of care labor means that (female and gender-nonconforming femme) care providers are often taught to put their own lives and well-being aside to prioritize that of others and specifically those who are positioned as their care recipients.[15] Additionally, the commodification of care at large inherits the capitalist consumer model and its associated power dynamics between care workers and their care recipients or clients. Care receivers (i.e., client or consumer) in general are expected to use their consumer power to purchase care labor, which simultaneously determines how the workers' lives are shaped and impacted by their occupation.[16] The multiplying social forces that bring *certain* women and gender-nonconforming femme people to take up care labor (e.g., neocolonialism and global neoliberalism, racist cisheteropatriarchy) as well further reinforce the unequal power dynamics normalized in these care practices. Many care studies invoke images of care workers from lower-class backgrounds tirelessly serving children or elderly people who come from more affluent families that can afford to purchase care labor.[17] In other words, in feminist care studies, it is granted that care workers are the ones whose capacities and hence lives are consumed and weathered under the biopolitical care that allows care receivers to thrive.

By contrast, analysis of biopolitical care is infused in many disability studies on care to understand how the lives of those who are situated as care recipients are inherently subjugated and shaped by care workers, where care is used to objectify disabled people positioned as care recipients.[18] Care, in this context, entails the care workers' in/direct power to manage and control the quality of care and ultimately the quality of life for those who are situated as care recipients.[19] The Independent Living Movement and activism regarding a direct-payment policy, for example, have been developed precisely to resist such care-based powerlessness that many disabled people are subjected to, and to re-imagine the care worker–recipient relationship as that of a worker and client (instead of patient).[20] Here, disabled care recipients are considered as the ones who weather and "let die," while care workers thrive in their care jobs. To negotiate and shift this version of bio-political force of care is, therefore, a fight the disability community has been tackling.

The argument I build in this chapter (and throughout the book) is nurtured in and built on these dedicated analyses of care injustices and how feminist disability studies continually bridge them. When we expand our focus to analyze how the larger structure of care shapes these individual experiences relationally—that is, the structure in which care workers are consumed also depletes those situated as care recipients—what kind of new care studies gets activated? I put forth the notion of necropolitical care, as I believe it portrays the current care structure more accurately, particularly when it is carried on in the U.S. public healthcare assemblage, which is entrenched in neoliberal political forces and an interlocking system of oppressions. Care funded by U.S. public healthcare, in particular, offers a unique case. It is an outlier, because it is not necessarily the care recipients and their families who dictate the business and management aspects of care work (e.g., wage, sick leave and vacation days, overtime), even under the direct-payment policy.[21] The state and care industries ultimately dictate and direct care as the main authorities in the commodification of care. They determine how much and what kind of care Medicaid enrollees need and deserve as well as compensation and benefits for the care workers. In other words, Medicaid enrollee care recipients do not possess the authoritative power to which many who privately purchase care labor have access.

Becoming Care Workers and Medicaid Enrollees

Becoming a Care Worker

"When I was younger, before I came to this country, I take care of my aunt. . . . Do everything for her. When I come here, I say, 'Maybe I could do [the care work]. Try and do it!'" Tia is a middle-aged Black woman who migrated to the United States and has worked as a care worker for most of her adulthood. In our conversation, she described her choice to enter care work as being based on her experiences of having been a care provider for her family members before, as well as the fact that she had to find a way to survive and thrive in a new place. I felt her sense of pride and hope in the exclamation point that punctuated her speech. Such choice, hope, and pride embodied by her and other care workers gets absolved into the larger socio-political forces. Echoing the quote by Tia, another care worker, Alisha, explained, "I had a grandmother who was invalid [sic], and she couldn't do anything. . . . I was living with her, so I had to kind to chip in and help." Alisha is a middle-aged, second-generation Black migrant woman and mother. Her and Tia's sentiments demonstrate that the entrance to care work is paved by gendered, racialized, and globalizing occupational expectation and division.[22] Stereotypes associated with care work—a deprofessionalized occupation that can be conducted by anyone and especially those with the maternal love that is often associated with women of color—mixed with the care industries' minimal eligibility criteria make care work more inviting particularly for women of color or migrant women, as well as for those with less institutional education.[23] Recalling her initial entry into care work, Alisha continued,

> [Care labor] is still a big demand. . . . When I took the class [on care work offered by a care agency], I didn't have any skills. I never attended a college, so [care work] was the easiest way for me to find a job [because it has no eligibility restrictions].

Many care workers I talked to brought up how their previous experiences of providing unpaid care labor to family members prompted them to enter this job. Further, Alisha added,

> You have to do what you have to do sometimes. . . . I was a single parent. I had children to provide for. I have people depend on me, so I didn't have a choice [but to take any job available to me].

Alisha's testimony not only traces the relative lack of occupational choices that she and others experienced, it also signals the sentiment of urgency or desperation that some people I talked to experienced as they were looking for jobs and eventually entered care work. When the path to care labor has already been constructed in relation to intersecting gender, race, and migrant stereotypes and expectations as well as the divided labor structure, and when those women experience a sense of urgent responsibility to provide for their families and make a living in a new country, the agencies' minimal eligibility requirements offer the final push for them to take on care labor. In the shadow of choice, pride, and hope are also the urgency, frustration, and vulnerability that are socially formulated under the occupational division.

These sociopolitical forces—intersecting xenophobic, classed, and gendered racial stratification—determine the jobs to which these women have easier access and simultaneously ensure that precarious, physically taxing, and lower-paying occupations are reserved for certain women under these forces and occupational segregation.[24] These affective and material factors work in the agencies' favor to fulfill their need for employees who will take on low-wage care work, which can lead to higher revenues for the agencies,

as they receive per-capita funding from the state under the newly implemented Medicaid managed-care programs.[25] Finally, given the undervalued
and low-paying nature of care work, the reality that the paths are paved for
specific women to enter care work can be also interpreted as a way to use
care occupations to reensure the economic marginalization of this specific
already marginalized population.[26]

Becoming a Medicaid Enrollee and Care Receiver

> Medicaid application, I open it up, and they close it. . . . I open it up,
> they close it. . . . I can't stand the cycle [of opening the case and hav-
> ing it be shut down]. . . . Over the years, sometimes you have to
> memorize stuff [like the spellings of words I need to know to apply
> for the public services]. And sometimes I forget how to spell my
> own address, and I've [lived at that address] twenty-something
> years. (Anton)

> Social Security turned me away a bunch of times. The question was
> always "What kind of disability you have?" [although I have a visi-
> ble disability and use a wheelchair]. . . . [Those examiners were]
> sayin', "What is [your disability]? Oh, can [the disability] go away to-
> morrow?" . . . Or "You don't sound disabled. You don't really
> look disabled. . . . You don't look disabled *enough* [emphasis
> added]." (Keisha)[27]

In contrast to the smooth (and sometimes forcible) entry for care workers,
becoming a Medicaid enrollee was described as tiring, defeating, and humiliating by the experts (i.e., focus group participants) I talked to, who are
mostly lower-income, Black and Brown disabled adults.[28] In the preceding
quote from Anton, a Latino middle-aged man with a learning disability, he
asserted with frustration that in order to start a Medicaid application, one
needs to know the process of how to apply. From there, one needs to know
how and be able to fill out one's basic information, which can be challenging
for many disabled people for various reasons, without supports of family
members, friends, or social workers to assist them with the process. Department of Health websites in general are complex and hard to navigate, to say
the least. Thus, the selective recruitment and retainment of Medicaid enrollees operated by some care industries means that not everyone is encouraged
and supported to apply for Medicaid programs.[29]

The process of applying for Medicaid continues to be complex. In the
expert discussion (i.e., focus group), many participants explained how rigorous the interview and examination that led them to Medicaid enrollment

were. Thus, they described the rigorousness as becoming indistinguishable from humiliation and dehumanization. Keisha asserted this point clearly in the second quote and how she was suspected of lying and malingering to take advantage of the state. Keisha is a disabled Black middle-aged mother to disabled and nondisabled children. Before she passionately finished her sentence, Rick joined in with enthusiasm on the shared experiences of being regarded as lying about his needs; their voices overlapped and resonated with one another: "I'm standing there in front [of the state employees examining me for my qualification], it's obvious that I have [a] disability [since it is visible and I use a scooter] . . . I mean, it's obvious that I have a disability!" Rick is a middle-aged Black man with a progressive physical disability. From time to time, raised voices and heated discussions took over the expert discussions, as people spoke or yelled over one another to share how their experiences were even more horrendous, scandalous, and unbelievable than the testimonies just shared by others—it was as if I could see steam coming off of their heads, as they added emphatic exclamations of "A-HUM," "YUP," "OH YEAH," and "AMEN!" to each other's testimony and followed with their own: "I've been told *that*, and I was 'wow.' I don't look disabled to you *now* [emphasis in original]. . . . My disability is a progressive disability. It's gonna get worse. It's not, in [a] million years, gonna get better!" These experts shared stories about their interviews with state agents who examined and determined their eligibility for and enrollment in Medicaid programs among other public services. Their stories tell how they were judged, un/recognized, and de/valued against the agents' ideals of a disabled person: what an average and deserving disabled person is supposed to look and sound like.[30] According to their experiences, one needs to be disabled just the right amount, and deserving and worthy of public supports—in fact, Keisha, Rick, and others were interrogated with suspicion for not looking and sounding disabled *enough*.

Applying for and being granted medical welfare and other forms of public supports is never straightforward, and exclusion of certain disabled people from the public supports is not new. And yet the neoliberal political economy intensifies it by implementing more profit- and industry-centered solutions to meet the care needs of those who have no choice but to rely on publicly funded care supports.[31] This intensification, intertwined with the ever-threatened public healthcare budget and the ever-increasing population that requires long-term care, implies that not every disabled person gets support and protection from public services—let alone quality and comprehensive care.[32] The agony of becoming enrolled in Medicaid programs was apparent in the expert discussions with disabled Medicaid enrollees and their care partners (i.e., care workers), where they shared never-ending testimonies on tiring, defeating, and humiliating encounters they had when applying for, or appealing for continuation or increase of, their long-term care.

Indeed, what does an ideal and deserving disabled person look and sound like from the perspective of the state, and how is this ideal reinforced and maintained in the process of Medicaid and other public welfare enrollment examinations? Based on the testimonies of these individuals and cases of malpractice engaged by judges for public services, I speculate that such an ideal is molded at the intersection of racism, ableism, xenophobia, and other social formations.[33] This assertion can be corroborated by the historical development and flourishing of rehabilitation sciences (e.g., rehabilitation psychology), which centered on returning (white, male, physically disabled) veterans after world wars as well as the overrepresentation of white disabled people as leaders and the faces of U.S. disability communities historically, and by these experiences of being the targets of profound suspicion having been narrated mainly by disabled people of color.[34] Another contributing stereotype is the vicious portrayal of people of color as inherently frauds—for example, as *welfare queens*—who may fake their needs for benefits, and therefore do not deserve the public supports.[35] The ideal of the acceptable and deserving disabled person has been shaped historically and continues to haunt Medicaid and other public services enrollment examinations and beyond.[36]

The disabled experts I talked to were painfully aware of the socially constructed and enforced ideals on disabled Medicaid enrollees; they repeatedly asserted how they felt and were reminded that they did not fit the social image that Medicaid examiners expected. Such an ideal evoked various affects among those I talked to, including hopelessness and humiliation, as they discussed their entry into Medicaid programs. It is arguable that these affects, in a way, contribute toward the continuation and maintenance of the public healthcare assemblage, as they mark and further establish the power dynamics between so-called examiners and disabled applicants: examiners are considered to be experts on disability, and they legitimate applicants' disabilities, degrees of debility, and care needed that are profoundly shaped in the notion of their deservingness and worthiness for publicly funded care. Disabled people, conversely, are expected (or forced) to go through such investigations more or less passively in order to fit into the ideal of a docile and deserving disabled person, with the hope that it will bring them to the end goal of Medicaid enrollment.

At the end of the day, it is a painful truth that lower-income or no-income disabled people need to be legitimated and qualified for their incapacity and idiosyncratic needs in order to receive services and stay in the system—which is the only way for many of them to receive some form of long-term care. Further, receiving services and staying in the system mean surrendering to surveillance and control by the government.[37] For example, to receive Supplemental Security Income from the government—which can lead its recipients to receive Medicaid long-term care—applicants' and enrollees' personal possessions are scrutinized by the state to justify that they need and deserve these social services.[38] As Rick described, "[The] Social Security [Administration, which manages supplemental income] wants to be your sole income. It's so that they tell you, you can only put less than two thousand [dollars] in a bank." Keisha continues, "Yeah, if it's there too long, they take it. Yes, if it goes over two thousand one [dollars], they take it." Paula added her own personal example:

> ssi [(Supplemental Security Income)] saw that I have too much money in my account for the whole year 2012. So they see [my bank account] for the whole year of 2012, and they automatically cut me [off from ssi] . . . and they make you *reapply* [emphasis in original] to get the services back. But they said that I can't re-apply until I prove what I spent the money for. . . . How the hell do you live on two thousand dollars?!

Identifying as a middle-aged Black woman with a physical disability, Paula has received long-term care for her entire adulthood. Here, she reiterated and explained that to be eligible for ssi, one's total financial possessions needs to be under $2,000, which means that Medicaid enrollees are forced to live in poverty in order to maintain services.[39] This poverty forced on Medicaid enrollees is recognized by their care partners, too. A care worker, Tia, said, "Sometimes they [(enrollees)] have no food. They don't get enough food stamps. It is never enough money."

These narratives illustrate accounts of how those Medicaid enrollees perceive and make sense of the situation they are put to. Entering the public healthcare (or any social service) sector means to them surrendering their financial and social conditions to the state, and thus depending on them for their sole income and healthcare services. As much as disabled populations and their care needs (i.e., debilities) are essential in the assemblage, governments' constant efforts to suppress and reduce public healthcare expenses as well as the increase in the number of people needing long-term care mean that entry into the assemblage is heavily policed. Finally, it all indicates that once someone is in the system, they often experience continued dependence on the state and subjugation to its surveillance and authority, instead of receiving adequate supports for their financial independence and full self-determination.

In the midst of this reality, nonetheless, the expert discussions were rife with open critiques of the public healthcare assemblage. The evidence was clear, for example, in the quote on care pimps that opened this chapter, that these disabled people do not passively accept the structural injustices they face. They articulated how they are financialized and used as pawns for industries to receive state funding. They critiqued the structure by making fun of it with cynical humor.

Forgotten Bodies: Mutual Debilitation in the Name of Care

> [Agencies] are not gonna hire all quality people. [Agencies] are there just *for bodies to fill positions* [emphasis added], so they can get money from Medicaid. They [say] they offer service training, but [it's so low quality and] they don't have people like us [disabled Medicaid enrollees] to come in and help with training. . . . It's just staff there [training those future care workers], and I'm like, how you gonna teach somebody to take care of us, when we know what we need. We should be there also, tell them what we need, how to care for *our* [emphasis in original] needs; not so-called experts, because they went to a college and got a degree. Our degree come from being in this [disabled] position every day. I offered the agency to come in there, free of charge, and help doin' service [training]. They said okay, then they changed their mind [and turned down my offer]. (Tyler)

One of the most heated topics during the expert discussions among Medicaid enrollees was on the poor, and at times dangerous, quality of care they received—which was complexly woven in with discussions on the quality of *care workers* they encountered. These enrollees offered endless examples of things their care workers did wrong or did not know how to do: from cooking and cleaning to assisting them to safely get in and out of their wheelchairs. Some care workers even joined the conversation during the discussions to critique their unqualified colleagues. It seems harsh at a glance to overgeneralize care workers, yet this kind of issue was also discussed in a more matter-of-fact tone to point out that care work is not for everyone. This critique on quality of care is a structural analysis the experts offered. While public health policies and laws mandate that managed long-term-care organizations (i.e., agencies) develop quality assessment and performance improvement programs, the testimony of these experts who are living in the system day-to-day shows how quality of care and enforcement of such measures are not always perfectly implemented.[40] The quote from Tyler emerged when he and others were framing their comments to address the injustice and malfunction at the structural level, for instance. They attributed issues of the low-quality care they faced to the agencies' careless hiring, low-quality training, and negligence toward both care workers and Medicaid enrollees. While care workers are required to take an initial forty hours of classroom training offered by agencies in this specific state, their comments show that this training is not necessarily enough and does not match with the real-world and unique care demands of individuals.[41] Additionally, when long-term care is given at an individual residence, there is a limit to monitoring of it, which is left to those who are situated as care workers and care receivers to negotiate. In other words, there is an inevitable gap between what is happening in everyday care practice at the micro level and what is set up at policy levels, as actual bodyminds and their needs constantly defy what is penned on paper. What is primarily focused on here is the perspectives and understandings of those who engage in care practice day-to-day that may not be captured at the systemic level and that may differ from what is written in policies.

When care is commodified and the long-term-care structure becomes heavily privatized, the quality of care that enrollees receive seems to become more and more pushed into shadows. It seems particularly so in the realm of the public healthcare assemblage, where those who are situated as care receivers do not have the same kind of consumer power as those in private care do. This situation can mean, for instance, that care agencies can fail to gatekeep those who are not qualified to be care workers from entering care work, according to these experts I talked to. Care workers I talked to as well repeatedly brought up that care work is *not for everyone*, but rather one needs to be caring and loving to continue working in this occupation, especially when it is a low-wage and physically taxing job. Medicaid enrollees painfully observed how agencies hire *anyone* who walks in the door, regardless of these applicants' motivations for and attitude toward care work.[42] The expert discussions were, therefore, heavily occupied by conversations on how the public healthcare sector is filled with unqualified providers who cannot or do not know how to provide quality care for their clients. Maria, a disabled elderly migrant Latina woman and Medicaid enrollee, cynically portrayed her numerous encounters with the care workers her agency has sent as "a comedy, it's a tragic comedy." She did so with a defeated laugh, while adding that many workers she has encountered "are there just for [the] paycheck." Tonya, an elderly disabled Black woman who receives her long-term care under Medicaid, inserted her experience as well:

> [A care worker sent to my home from an agency once told me that] "I haven't worked for many years, and I'm working now [as a care worker] only because I have to get my benefits [unemployment

checks] back. [In order to get the benefits back,] I have to do this [care work], this many hours." So [the person] just went the week, . . . and that's it, [she was] gone.

Others fervently agreed that this neglectful hiring can facilitate devastating results such as stealing and abuse. Many enrollees echoed one another, saying that within Medicaid-provided long-term care, stealing is unfortunately not an uncommon practice. Paula said, "[My past care workers] stole from me. They took things that they wasn't supposed to take. . . . And it was a strain on our relationship. . . . It was just hard to figure out: why this happened. . . . It's a very vulnerable situation." She finished her sentences with a mixture of disappointment and frustration. In this vein, Medicaid enrollees in the expert discussion repeatedly mentioned how the intimate nature of care practice can mean that they can feel a care worker's emotions such as frustration, as that frustration is immersed in the intricacy of care. Whether they called it mistreatment or abuse, these Medicaid enrollees and care workers began to share what they have experienced or witnessed. A young Medicaid enrollee, a white woman with disabilities, Amy, articulated that "when [care workers] got angry or aggravated or [were] having a bad day, they took it out on me [through care tasks]. . . . I didn't feel safe." A care worker who is a middle-aged Black woman and is a child of migrant parents, Isabella, explained what she has witnessed and heard: "Some [care workers] are frustrated. . . . They had their own problem[s] at home, and they come to the job, and some jobs are difficult. . . . They just take it out [on their clients]. . . . Some of the workers are very angry . . . don't care about the patient [sic]." Particularly under long-term care, Medicaid enrollees and their care workers spend most of their waking hours together. Just as enrollees explained how they experienced their care partners' moods directly, care workers too witnessed and at times experienced the projection of a variety of moods that their care partners (i.e., Medicaid enrollees) were going through. Or lack of quality care training does not only negatively impact those who are situated as care receivers. Care workers as well are subjected to a high risk of injury and being infected with airborne and blood-borne diseases because of insufficient training.[43] While there are overwhelming accounts of interpersonal conflicts, all people who joined the expert discussions attributed these incidents to the negligence of agencies and thus shared their desire for better structural supports and safety: "[Agencies] just don't seem to care, and the stories of abuse and theft are getting worse, it's not getting better. It's getting dangerous. . . . All of us [Medicaid care receivers] are abused one [way] or the other." Here, Maria reminded us that the interpersonal conflicts are never solely personal but are highly impacted by and shaped within the agencies and the larger U.S. public healthcare assemblage and are therefore political. She provided important context to Medicaid enrollees and care workers' experiences.

Finally, the care agencies' negligence regarding hiring qualified providers, providing rigorous training, and taking care of the care workers they hired caused Medicaid enrollees to go through a number of care workers before meeting ones who would stick around and who were capable of providing the care that they needed and desired or that was good enough. Maria, for example, recounted, "In four or five years, I went through at least sixty [care workers]." This high turnover is common, according to Medicaid enrollees I talked to, as agencies continued to send unqualified and uncaring providers, and as care workers were exploited and worn out and thus became incapable of providing quality care to all the care recipients they were assigned to. It then becomes Medicaid enrollees' job, instead of the care agencies', to identify care providers who can provide quality care, or else bear the constant turnover of care workers.

Between descriptions and examples of horrendous care, Medicaid enrollees and some of their care workers also critically analyzed how the care structure has been becoming profit-centered, as well as how and where they were situated and what roles they were given in it. Tyler's narrative, which opened this section, contained a deep cynicism on how the capacitation of disabled Medicaid enrollees through care seemed not necessarily the priority of the agency or the larger assemblage. Tyler interpreted such disregard for quality and negligence in general as a sign of how care workers and enrollees are treated as *mere numbers* or *tokens* to be exchanged and circulated with the per-capita funding provided from the state and federal governments to care industries.[44] In other words, these experts I talked to articulated that disabled enrollees were left to bear the burden for the lack of rigorous hiring and training of workers conducted by the agencies. This view of how enrollees' well-being is actively forgotten or put aside under the assemblage is further amplified in contrast to the way Tyler viewed himself and fellow disabled people as *experts*. He asserted that those forgotten disabled Medicaid enrollees are actually experts and wisdom holders of care practices, and that they are most suited to train care workers, because their credentials come from daily lived experiences and not from educational institutions.

Tyler continued this critical interpretation of enrollees' circumstances under the public healthcare assemblage:

[With the low wage care workers receive, they] are not gonna end up caring about the job that much. . . . If you have good workers, they are wearing off so far. . . . They are not gonna be able to keep the pace up too long. They get worn out just trying to make ends meet.

As he finished speaking, it became clear that although these disabled people and their care worker partners described many workers as *unqualified* or *uncaring*, they were also addressing the reality that the workers were not necessarily unqualified per se but instead were profoundly exploited and left without any mental or physical energy to carry out the kind of care they desired to provide. By connecting the injustice happening to them and to the care workers, the discussion among enrollees began to illuminate how the shortcomings of the care industrial complex and the interlocking system of oppressions trickle down to *both* care workers and care recipients in separate, overlapping, and somewhat interwoven ways.

The care workers I talked to individually confirmed this point in conversations that often entailed a sense of hopelessness, despair, and frustration as well as their critical analyses of the circumstances that care workers endure. They characterized their care work as involving low wages and extensive labor hours, and hardship of the work is unnecessarily intensified by the care agencies' negligence regarding their working conditions and well-being. All of the care workers I talked to disclosed with frustration and cynicism that they worked twelve hours a day and six days a week *at least*: "It's not enough money. If you work for nine dollars or eight dollars an hour . . . you've gotta do twelve hours to bring the money home." Granting that care labor is a low-wage occupation, Tia told me with a sentiment of desperation that working long hours was the only way to support her family. And these extended work hours are not adjusted during holidays, as Alisha explained—"I used to work holidays. . . . I'll be with [care partners and their family] . . . away from my kids and family"—or extreme weather situations: "We come in the snowstorm, all kinds of stuff. If there's a storm, you get stuck; nobody is coming to relieve you. They [agencies] don't wanna compensate for that. . . . It's a lot. . . . I think that's kind of . . . slavery. I don't wanna use the term, but that's kinda like [slavery]." Here, Alisha is also touching on the lack of comprehensive protection offered under the Fair Labor Standards Act, which includes overtime payment and was offered to all workers except home-based care workers and agricultural workers at the time of the interview.[45] Sofia, a middle-aged, migrant woman from South America, did not anticipate the long hours of work ending in the near future: "I [will] finish [doing this care work after] twelve years . . . because [Social Security] told me sixty-five . . . that's [when] Social Security told me [I can retire and receive a pension]." Another care worker, Isabella, summarized the sense of frustration and defeat common in my interviews with care workers: "We just get the little scram. . . . We do a lot, but we don't get paid. Doing home care is very hard and less money."

This reality of low-wage care work was recognized and brought up by those who were situated as care recipients, too. Many Medicaid enrollees discussed the low pay that their care partners received for the care they themselves receive. Tyler shared, with frustration, what he found out when he did some research on how Medicaid funding is distributed:

> [The] agency gets around twenty-five or twenty-seven dollars an hour [from the state] for [an enrollee] that [they are] supposed to be caring for. They pay the workers seven-fifty [$7.50] an hour or eight dollars an hour. . . . They get about seventeen, eighteen dollars [while] a person that [is] doing the work or that they hire to do the work gets the lowest wage. . . . So it was like [care workers] work twelve hours a shift, seven-fifty an hour. It's probably a little bit over a hundred dollars they are making for the day. And [the] agency gets another two hundred dollars. So they get twice as much as the workers get for not doing anything.[46]

Medicaid long-term-care program enrollees can download their individual funding allocation breakdown from their state Department of Health website, Tyler mentioned, as he broke down that the majority of its funding goes to the care industry—often 200 percent of what care workers receive—before it reaches the workers. Hence, care workers are seldom left with a choice but to extend their working hours. Researchers Annette Bernhardt, Siobhan McGrath, and James DeFilippis, studying unregulated labor forces, echoed this quote by explaining that the low wage of care workers can be traced to how "home health care in New York is contracted out to agencies, sometimes in multiple tiers, which in the end can take as much as 50% of the public funding for overhead and administrative expenses" and hence lower wages for workers.[47] While the researchers also emphasized the challenges of finding out how Medicaid funding is exactly spent within agencies, all who joined expert discussions shared that care workers are paid close to or below minimum wage, especially given the lack of comprehensive overtime pay at the time of the interview.[48] The injustice of low wages and the sense of defeat shared by care workers become even more obvious when one considers what care work entails and how it does not necessarily end and cannot be compartmentalized into set labor hours. This is particularly true when we take emotional care more seriously; it can leak into time when care workers are not with their care partners but continue thinking about them.[49]

Tia described her responsibilities as a care worker: "I've gotta do *everything* [emphasis in original] for [my care partner]. . . . You need to do everything [including cognitive work such as remembering things for them], 'cause sometimes, they [are fine] remembering, [sometimes] they are not." Care workers are trained to provide a wide range of care (e.g., physical care, household chores).[50] In particular, though, their emotional care for their clients often extends their sense of responsibility to fulfill the shortcomings of care agencies on their own. This can mean that their partners' emergencies become their personal responsibility. Sophia explained to me, "In this job you have to love the person [who is your care partner]. You have to love this job. [If you] don't feel the kind of love to help people, [then it] is better [that you] don't come to this job." She then continued with a story of unpaid overtime work with great pride:

> When [it's] eight o'clock finish, [time for me to leave,] and the client moves the bowel. . . . What do you do in the moment? . . . I take off my coat, it's time to work [again]. When I finish, maybe thirty minutes after or forty-five [minutes later], I feel happy. [Do I get paid for the overtime labor?] No.[51]

On the one hand, her narrative was full of contentment about the way she prioritized her care partner and her job principles, and the meaningfulness of that work to her beyond an exchange of labor and wages. Indeed, she described her work with pride throughout the interview and situated herself as a professional of care work. In her interview, care work is prestigious and care workers are experts in human well-being. On the other hand, though, our discussion also indicated that agencies continue to function regardless of the lack of overtime pay (at the time of the interviews) by relying on and exploiting their workers' sense of responsibility and capacity to empathize with their care partners.[52] The situation forces upon workers an unsatisfactory and exploitative choice—either they or their care partners bear the consequences for the lack of supports from the agencies (e.g., workers work overtime without compensation or Medicaid enrollees spend the night in soiled underwear). Both choices place care workers and Medicaid enrollees in a scenario of mutual exploitation and debilitation, and simultaneously relieve agencies of facing the dilemma and claiming responsibility. In other words, the U.S. public healthcare assemblage and flourishment of care industries are carried on while the structural negligence regarding providing quality care for enrollees and just compensation to workers are turned into care workers' and enrollees' personal responsibility by taking advantage of their genuine, affirming care for one another.[53]

Both Medicaid enrollees and care workers continually brought up the physical and psychological consequences of the low-quality care they received or their low-quality work conditions. Although care practice naturally involves intimacy and embodies vulnerability for both care workers and enrollees, in overlapping yet different ways, all the care workers and Medicaid enrollees I talked to explained that the experiences of vulnerability were amplified by the structural negligence that is often pointed out in terms of how they are treated by the agencies. Alisha brought up, "How can you care for someone else if you're not okay? Agencies need to have a little more . . . caring and compassion toward the [care workers]." This statement summarizes the frustrations and desires all the other workers I talked to shared. In addition to workers' dissatisfaction with their employers, this quote also implies that this lack of support can lead to their continual debilitation, while just wages, comprehensive compensation, and more genuine care and supports at structural level could potentially recapacitate and sustain these workers and thus allow them even to flourish. As much as these workers were once (forced to become) energized and capacitated to enter the care labor force with training and so on, the ongoing demand to provide care without structural supports can slowly deteriorate and debilitate workers. Additionally, the emotional ties and sense of responsibility some care workers develop with their care partners (i.e., recipients) means that they capacitate themselves each day just enough to get back to caring for their partners. Yet the question remains whether in this context workers are left with sufficient capacities and energy to provide the capacitating and quality care their care partners desire. Their capacities to work and to care lose distinction with the constant draining of their energy—debilitation—working for U.S. public healthcare programs.

Both enrollees and care workers repeatedly asserted that the consequences of low-quality care and lack of sufficient support from agencies can be doubly life threatening. Alisha talked about her concern that the agency ignored calls from her care partner and failed to return both of their calls in a timely manner. Here, she spoke faster and faster, spitting out her accumulated frustrations toward the agency:

> [Medicaid enrollees] call, and [staff at the agency] don't return [the] client's call at all. It doesn't matter if [care workers] call [on behalf of their care partner], still they don't pick up the call. And that *is* [emphasis in original] dangerous. [Medicaid enrollees] may be calling for [an] emergency.

The topic of life-threatening experiences in Medicaid long-term care was also repeatedly brought up by Medicaid enrollees, and they all attributed these incidents to the negligence of agencies. Maria addressed the ultimate consequences for the inattentiveness of care agencies at multiple levels:

> [Some care workers] really don't know what to do [in case of emergency]. If something happens to you in the house, they don't know who to call, they don't know how to go about it. 911 becomes a big issue. Really, it's very dangerous. There are so many people that have

died, those you never find out. . . . I remember falling on the floor once, out of a [wheel]chair. And I told [my care worker] to please put me on the bed. And the person began to talk to me in [her native language which I do not understand]. And I'm going, "Oh, god." All I know is that the person . . . sat on the floor with me. I was frightened. "Please take me to the bed. Please just drag me to the bed. Try to put me on anything, on a sheet and drag me. Anything!" She sat on the floor with me. . . . She didn't know what to do.

Alisha and Maria both narrate the danger and actual deterioration (and risk of acute death) that disabled enrollees go through under the care structure and shed light on how those enrollees' vulnerabilities are constructed in the assemblage. Additionally, these narratives also illuminate how the vulnerability and deterioration of enrollees are complexly entangled with or not without impacts on care workers. Their vulnerabilities are woven into one another's and interactively impact their distinct and yet somewhat overlapping debilitating experiences. Alisha's point about unanswered calls reveals her frustration and also fear regarding a seeming lack of safety net set up by agencies for Medicaid enrollees and also care workers, as both of their calls were ignored regardless of the content. In the second quote, Maria echoed this lack and the similar despair experienced by her and in some extent by her care partner—both of whom were left on the floor, one without a means to get off the floor, and the other without a means to intervene in the emergency situation. Thus, these quotes crystallize the multitudes of affects unfolding between enrollees and care workers as well as reflecting the affects shared during the expert discussions and individual interviews: frustration, hopelessness, insecurity, vulnerability, a cynical sense of familiarity, and resilience and resistance. These affects further reflect these Medicaid enrollees' fundamental lack of choice regarding another, better-quality healthcare program. Medicaid is the safety net provided by the state and often the last resort for many lower-income disabled people to receive necessary medical and other forms of care that they are otherwise unable to afford. With that said, I also want to emphasize that the relational analysis unfolding here is not to equalize the vulnerable circumstances that enrollees and care workers are placed in or to erase the crucial differences in them, including the differences in how one can physically get up and exit the situation (for care workers) while others cannot (for enrollees). What is untangled here is how the structural injustices that Medicaid enrollees and care workers are subjected to overlap and are somewhat intertwined, while their consequences are experienced differently in distinctive magnitudes.

Care workers, as well, repeatedly brought up the physical and psychological stresses they experienced: frustration about the lack of time spent with their own families, the emotional devastation of not receiving care for themselves, and physical deterioration. Many told me with frustration and fatigue in their faces that the extended hours as well as the exhausting nature of care labor left them without energy or time to mother their children. Their sense of anger and defeat was prevalent across interviews: "When I [gave birth to] my daughter, I took [an] extra workday just to make extra money. But even that wasn't much extra [money]." Isabella finished her sentence with a sigh. Here, she depicted the contradictory prioritization she was forced to make: caring for her newborn financially meant taking an extra workday and spending less time with her baby. Tia shared a similar sense of defeat regarding not having a choice but to take exploitative care work for income: "It was a lot of compromise to do with my family. . . . The [work] hours are long, but what you gonna do? It's work." Alisha further addressed the fundamental contradiction and dilemma of prioritization in which many care workers found themselves: "The people that provide a lot of care, they don't get the care themselves. It's kinda like you neglect yourself . . . [and] you do [so] without even realizing." I remember in particular the painful moment when her eyes filled with tears, when she initially could not come up with a response to my question, "Who takes care of you?" Isabella further asserted, "You don't have no life. You don't have time for yourself. [Even on your day off] you have things to do, you need to run around [to get errands done], and by the time you're done [with] all of that, you're tired." This accumulating stress of the exploitative labor—in addition to the (gendered and racialized) responsibility to prioritize another's care—have consequences for the providers' own bodyminds. Tia explained the physical deterioration she went through: "Sometimes you don't eat. I lost a lot of weight," which was echoed by other care workers in a study by Bernhardt, McGrath, and DeFilippis, who all brought up the fact that the irregularity of care needs often meant that they could not take meal breaks.[54]

The exploitation and debilitation of care workers are keenly observed by their Medicaid enrollee care partners too, who framed this debilitation in its larger context and attributed it to the lack of healthcare supports for those workers. Tyler explained how agencies "are not taking care of workers. . . . Regular healthcare [agencies] don't offer that [comprehensive benefits]. . . . Because you see a lot of home attendants with no teeth. You be like, 'Damn, you need care more than I do.'" Another enrollee, Maria, commented on what "a terrible dynamic it is to have a job where you are providing healthcare where you are not getting your own health insurance. . . . Agencies are abusing these people that are coming in." Echoing such observations, a nonprofit care worker training and research organization, PHI, states that only 38 percent of home care workers receive their health insurance from their employers or unions.[55] Furthermore, what these quotes among others are signaling is how Medicaid enrollees care for their care worker partners by paying close attention to and attending to their well-being.

In other words, caring by paying attention circulates between care partners. Amy, a Medicaid enrollee, highlighted this point by explaining the times when the line between care worker and care recipient got blurred:

> A lot of the [care workers] that I had also had their own physical issues. They couldn't do something that I needed because they don't get [quality] healthcare. . . . Once [my care worker] would come sit down and every time she got up, you could tell she was in pain from standing. And it gets to the point where I [a disabled person receiving long-term care] was, "It's okay, you stay, I'll manage."

This quote depicts the multilayered reality of long-term care conducted under the neoliberal U.S. public healthcare assemblage. For one, it tells the story of the debilitating physical stress that care workers go through and how some people with disabling pain (have to) take jobs taking care of others, which are physically demanding and thus further debilitating.

This discussion invokes the questions I addressed in the previous chapter: What is the mechanism that situates some disabled people—including those who experience chronic and acute pain—to receive public healthcare supports, when other disabled people continue to be constructed and (over) worked as care laborers? How do the interlocking forces of racism, cisheteropatriarchy, xenophobia, and neocolonial globalization impact the mechanism by identifying deserving and undeserving disabled citizens? Additionally, as Amy described, sometimes she provides care for her care partner and does not necessarily receive the care she requires in that moment. In other words, both those who are situated as care recipients and care providers are inadequately cared for at structural, interpersonal, and individual levels under the current public healthcare assemblage. In the neoliberal political economy, where the meaning and experiences of care are rapidly shifting and further shaped by intensified social oppressions, those who are situated as care workers and recipients experience mutual deterioration through separate and overlapping mechanisms of exploitation in the name of care.

Necropolitical Care

To better understand this insidious care setup under the neoliberalization of the U.S. public healthcare assemblage, I turn to the theory of necropolitics. Political philosopher Achille Mbembe described necropolitics as "the power and the capacity to dictate *who may live* and *who must die*. Hence, to kill or to allow to live constitutes the limits of sovereignty, its fundamental attitudes."[56] He put forward this theory because "the notion of biopower is insufficient to account for contemporary forms of subjugation of life to the power of death."[57] Other scholarships that similarly emphasize death as the focal point to decipher the current sociopolitical power repeat how "the phenomenon of mass physical attenuation under global/national regimes of capital structure and subordination and governmentality . . . is simultaneously an extreme and in a zone of ordinariness, where life building and the attrition of human life are indistinguishable."[58] Debilitation and thus disposability are increasingly becoming the norm and are further enforced against marginalized communities, particularly those who are deemed unworthy or useless to the political economy.[59] These debilitating realities are intricately stitched into efforts to make a living (e.g., engaging in care work to feed one's family or subjecting oneself to the state's evaluation to receive long-term-care services and supports). Life-making is debilitating, and debilitation is a requirement to *live* for many in this neoliberal world. The constant debilitation pushes people closer to (further) disability and injury, or ultimately death.

I claim that it is a false dichotomy to assume that care recipients are thriving on the backs of their care workers and vice versa in the circumstances of the neoliberal public healthcare assemblage. How control is exercised in the name of care is not necessarily through the force of making them live or regulation through life alone. As people are pulled into the assemblage and exploited based on their labor capacities or needs for care, their actual well-being is not necessarily prioritized. As discussed, enrollees of Medicaid described not receiving quality, life-making care, and care workers are not given sustainable supports or accumulating skillsets and structural capital to advance themselves, let alone sustainable work conditions. These challenges are only exacerbated by the abundance of people who require public healthcare supports to meet their care needs as well as those who are available to take up care labor in the Global North and the United States—thus accelerating the rendition of those populations as disposable.[60] Furthermore, since it is those who are already marginalized in the mainstream society who are turned into care workers and recipients within the U.S. public healthcare assemblage, interlocking systems of oppression also accelerate their further marginalization. Both populations are, therefore, largely neglected structurally in the larger U.S. public healthcare assemblage and left to debilitate within this framework. The dichotomizing assumption that care workers are nondisabled and thus hypercapable and care receivers are the disabled ones does not always hold, when one closely looks at the circumstances and realities of today's care assemblage.

The public healthcare assemblage is prioritized to the detriment of care workers and enrollees. Both populations' humanity is turned into tokens to be exchanged and circulated alongside the flow of funding from federal to state governments, and then to care industries, based on the financialization of their capacities and debilities. The extensive hours that care workers put in and the intensity and demanding nature of care labor—while their emotional ties with their partners continue to bring them back to the work— deteriorate them without adequate compensation or means of sustaining their caring capacities. In reality, the idea of life-making through this caring occupation is losing its relevance, as care workers accumulate more debilities than versatile labor capacities that would allow them more occupational mobility and options or to provide quality care they aspire. This labor reality, then, shapes the quality of the care that Medicaid enrollees receive. The care workers being pushed so much can mean that they rarely have adequate energy or mental strength left to care well for their Medicaid enrollee care partners. Medicaid enrollees, as well, are further debilitated, as they rarely receive life-making, quality care. The constant debilitation of workers, for example, can trickle down to impact the quality of care that enrollees receive, on top of the general neglect toward this population by the care industries—further debilitating enrollees. This debilitation of enrollees can manifest in sickness at times, which can then lead to more demanding tasks for care workers, which further pushes them to stretch themselves thinner. The risk of going down this negative, debilitative spiral together is constructed in the assemblage and haunts both populations in their daily care routines. In addition, as I explained in the previous chapter, under the neoliberalization of Medicaid and transition to managed care, many Medicaid enrollees are assigned fewer hours of daily care than they need, if they are granted any publicly funded care at all. The constant debilitation these workers and Medicaid enrollees experience shows that the meaning and function of care shifts in this given circumstance. Care is functioning and intensified as a mechanism of oppression and exploitation that alter people's bodyminds. The line between care provider and recipient is increasingly blurry too as providers are getting sicker and disabled through exploitative labor and disabled care recipients are further debilitated. Many former care workers are, indeed, becoming the new enrollees in public healthcare programs.[61]

What Is There beyond Necropolitical Care?

It is certainly not news that a practice of care gets turned into a practice of mistreatment or even abuse and violence for those who are situated as care providers and recipients. Critical race and feminist historian Premilla

Nadasen, for example, has offered a historical analysis to draw a lineage between the domestic work of enslaved women and today's care labor force (alongside their uprisings).[62] Critical race and feminist theorist Kalindi Vora, as well, untangled the colonial background of care-labor migration that fulfills the current demands of U.S. long-term care.[63] Others have reported horrendous murders of disabled people by their care providers, which is often called as *mercy killing*. Such cases of murder often end up being rationalized via empathy for those who killed the disabled individuals and without fully holding them accountable for their action.[64] Nevertheless, today's neoliberal political economy adds additional twists to the practice of care as it accelerates the flourishment of the care industrial complex and the private management of public healthcare programs, which have led to the further mutual debilitation of care workers and Medicaid enrollees that I have centered here.

Further, by continuously emphasizing the mutual and relational debilitation that care workers and Medicaid enrollees go through, my intention is not to flatten their distinct circumstances or equate them. They experience vulnerability differently, for instance. Care or lack thereof can have direct implications for an enrollee's life. For them, taking a break from their care partners or long-term-care routines is not an option, whereas taking a break from care work for a day or being late to it does not necessarily hit care workers with similar acuteness and intensity of devastation. Nevertheless, what I have tried to put forward in this chapter is the structural overlap and mutual implications that these populations are subjected to—the mechanisms of oppression that care workers and Medicaid enrollees experience hand-in-hand and of which they share some parts. In other words, these overlapping and hand-in-hand aspects of the care injustice mechanism are key components to fully understanding the care-based oppressions that care workers and enrollees experience and to imagine and fight for their liberation and care justice.

Structural injustices pose devastating consequences for these populations. They are, nevertheless, not mere victims. Underneath this structure, people are asserting their resilience, resistance, and other complex and nuanced responses that came up throughout the expert discussions and interviews. In the previous sections, for example, I brought up the words of Medicaid enrollee Amy, who witnessed the pain her care partner was going through and acted upon it by helping the care partner. I used the quote as an example of the mutual debilitation that care workers and enrollees experience and thus the ways in which both of them are (becoming) disabled. Indeed, the web of white supremacy, cisheteropatriarchy, ableism, neocolonialism, and global neoliberalism deeply shapes the construction and recognition of one's capacity and debility, in which some disabled people become Medicaid enrollees while others may be situated as care workers. Nonetheless, building on this layer of reality, I also recall Amy's words here to highlight yet another layer—the interpersonal and to some extent interdependent support used to negotiate and engage in care routines. The experts (Medicaid enrollees and care workers) with whom I spoke sometimes transgressed the divide between care worker and care recipient roles prescribed by the care industries by caring for one another outside of the care tasks assigned by the industries. This description does not justify or cancel out the injustices that care partners mutually go through. Nevertheless, it also shows that there is more to the daily lives of care workers, enrollees, and the two as a collective than their individual and simultaneous debilitation in the public healthcare assemblage within which they are embedded and circulated.

As the book proceeds, I investigate the other forces of care that the relational analysis will uncover and illuminate. By recognizing that the circumstances and well-being of care workers and disabled enrollees are contingent on one another and deeply intertwined, can solidarity be forged between these populations, rather than situating care workers or enrollees as sacrificing themselves for the other or antagonistically contrasting their experiences and perspectives? Can this shift in framework ignite more relational activism toward care justice and build stronger solidarity between feminist and disability communities? Such solidarity must acknowledge that some of us are disabled women and engage in care work while receiving care. What is care justice? Who is embraced under such justice? I use the rest of this book to explore and unfold care justice from multiple perspectives. At this point, what is clear is that care cannot be a mode of debilitation and further marginalization of already marginalized communities.

3

Affective Collectivity

Beyond Slow Death and toward Haptic Relationality

The interdependent relationships between disabled people and the people who provide care for us are often messy and fraught with power imbalances rooted in racism, sexism, homophobia, transphobia, ableism, and capitalism. These imbalances frequently cause abuse and neglect for the person receiving care, low wages and exploited labor for the person providing care, and harassment flying in multiple directions. *And yet interdependence exists whether it's laced with easy banter and mutuality or with struggle, hierarchy, and exploitation.* [emphasis added]

—Eli Clare, *Brilliant Imperfection*

An attendant [care worker], who is not only an attendant, but a person who you coincide with in so many ways. . . . They see you when you are good and when you are bad. . . . There's a lot of things you share with them that you don't really show . . . to anybody else. It's one of [those] things where they can *sense* when you don't feel good. They can *sense* certain things no other person can sense. Because they are with you so much, in so many circumstances . . . [and it] is the closest relationship you have in the world, really. . . . The love and care you feel for them. They probably would never know, but it's really "thanks" that you don't know how to tell them. [emphasis added]

—Maria, Medicaid enrollee

Care is an ambivalent site, holding various forces flying in multiple directions, whether they be exploitative and debilitative, loving and affirmative, or a mixture of anything between and beyond these forces.[1] The bodyminds of those situated as care workers and care receivers together witness, experience, and embody the multilayered truths embedded within the care they circulate among themselves. The preceding quotes by those who have firsthand knowledge of (long-term) care shine through and complicate the narratives on the debilitative care structure they are embedded in.

In my conversations and interactions with those who work as care workers and those who receive their long-term care under Medicaid, both of
them repeatedly suggested the complex and nuanced realities of being part
of the U.S. public healthcare assemblage. On the one hand, their narratives
reflect the ways in which neoliberal U.S. public healthcare programs have
exploitative and debilitative impacts on both groups. On the other hand,
they simultaneously insist that there is more to their daily lives and care
practices than the exploitative reality. They demand that their lives and care
practices be understood as more than passive victimization by the neoliberal care formations, and they also assert themselves as the agents of its
destruction. This chapter highlights this complex reality by applying and
further contributing to the core of disability studies: to recognize and illuminate the complexity, nuances, occasional resistance, and richness of the
lives that disabled, injured, sick, and tired or debilitated people continue to
weave and live in the middle of the violently exploitative and debilitative
status quo. I bring in this perspective to attend to those lives that are often
simply theorized as (by)products of the violent political economy and social
stratification and left there without being recognized as more than that. My
particular focus is, then, how these rich lives continue by and through the
collective of debilitated individuals and how such collectivity is forged
through *affective* (i.e., sensual) relationality among them.

Is it possible—and if so, how—that nurturing relationships emerge between those who are situated as care workers and Medicaid enrollees (i.e.,
care receivers), when they are simultaneously embedded in the deteriorating
care assemblage—where their life-building through care work or the long-
term care they receive are intertwined with their debilitation? What does
such a relationship do to them or to the larger public healthcare assemblage?
What are the political interventions that such relationship and collectivity
insert? Or, in critical disability and feminist race theorist Nirmala Erevelles's words, "How do we [and can we] forge a collective struggle [between
those who are situated as care workers and care recipients] without destroying [these] people we really care for?"[2] I address these questions by developing an idea of *affective collectivity*. I do so by exploring care workers' and
recipients' collective interruption of the U.S. public healthcare assemblage.
Such collective interruption is engaged through the micro care they co-
conduct and co-circulate over and over among themselves and through the
relationships they build and nurture together, instead of imagining the resistance as an individual act or emerging exclusively from either care worker
or disabled care recipient communities.[3]

The significance of affective collectivity is further evidenced in the context of care industries banning care workers and their care partners (care

recipients) from developing any meaningful connection such as friendship or comradeship. This ban is enforced for the sake of liability, according to the care workers and Medicaid enrollees I talked to. Therefore, breaking the ban is met with serious penalties including sudden termination of the care partnership. Rick, a Medicaid enrollee, explained:

> If the agency finds out [that care recipients and care workers are building friendship against the agency's rules], [agencies] take [those care workers] out [(he claps his hands)]. All of a sudden somebody [new] is at your door, and they won't tell you why. They just say, "Oh, the old lady [(previous care worker)], she is gone."

As illustrated in this quote, the ban highlights how Medicaid enrollees and their care partners are actively and structurally divided, separated, and managed.[4] And this divide is additionally enforced by the racial, gendered, global migrant, and disability economies that firmly set up who will be tasked with care labor and who will be objectified under the role of care recipient. The individualist divide between care workers and Medicaid enrollees is therefore further engraved in and through the U.S. public health-care assemblage. To forge affective collectivity during and through care practice is, therefore, inherently resistive. Also, I develop the idea of affective collectivity against the backdrop of neoliberal and necropolitical theories that understand the status quo and its controlling aspects in a totalizing manner, as if everything (including people's resistance, for example) is eventually sucked into and taken advantage of by neoliberal political economies, often by incorporating necropolitical strategies. Affective collectivity, then, complicates such a totalizing view of society and people living in the status quo with attention to how such interpersonal connections enact micro and molecular resistance and resilience that can form the undercommons—a destructive collective destroying oppressive institutional and hegemonic structure from within—an idea developed by critical theorists Stefano Harney and Fred Moten.[5]

By affective collectivity, I am referring to a bodymind or ontological connection forged as people adapt to one another haptically (i.e., sensually). In the context of care structures, I illustrate how repeated encounters and interactions facilitate the growth of such collectivity. An example is how some pairs of Medicaid enrollees and their care workers come to preconsciously move their bodies in sync to accomplish care tasks.[6] I argue that by co-conducting care tasks day after day, they accumulate haptic memories and knowledge of one another's bodyminds including bodily touches, movements, rhythms, breath, heat, odor, gaze, and sound as well as each other's distinct capacities, needs, paces, and even desires. All of these elements circulate as parts of care between, beyond, and within the bodyminds of care workers and enrollees. This circulation highlights the *sensual* connection of bodyminds in the shadow of how human connections are understood and normalized as happening in more cerebral or cognition-based manners. Particularly in academia and elsewhere, the ways people relate to one another have been theorized as primarily happening through conversations, reading and reacting to body languages, and assessment of the similarity and differences between them.[7] This cerebral and cognition-centric way of relating is hegemonic and thus expected as a way for people to relate and connect. What I want to push forward with the idea of affective collectivity is, therefore, that there is more than one way for people to connect and develop relationships; however, noncerebral ways of connecting (e.g., through touch) are often quickly dismissed or read as signs of unsophistication or even primitive.[8] The term *affective* in *affective collectivity* comes from affect theory and the affective theorization of body, to be discussed in the following sections. It is a way to emphasize the sensual, haptical, or ontological nature of the connection I illuminate, and not to signal affection or affirmation necessarily.[9]

Encounters of bodyminds can bring friction and debilitative outcomes, as conflicts between care workers and Medicaid enrollees are also a reality. In this chapter, though, I focus more on how such affective collectivity can be co-capacitative as well. Following the narratives of care workers and recipients I talked to, I trace how those who are situated as care workers and Medicaid enrollees turn their passive positionality in the care assemblage into an active one by forging affective collectivity. To do so is also to complicate their positionalities by demonstrating that they are more than mere pieces to be circulated in the assemblage and are also interruptive and destructive forces. Given the context where they are not allowed to forge any kind of friendship according to care industries, the building of such relationality interrupts and resists the flow and guidelines of public healthcare programs.

Finally, I end this chapter by connecting affective relationality with a praxis, undercommons—how people who are oppressed under systemic oppressions interrupt and disrupt the system from within to abolish it.[10] Bringing these ideas together points out the possibilities of affective collectivity to become a foundation for collective revolt and alternative ways to care for one another, instead of simply accepting and aspiring toward neoliberal demands: to be individualist and independent, or to passively be disciplined within the necropolitical care structure that constantly debilitates them. Also, it suggests and explores what kinds of social change and more just-world can become possible, when affective collectivity is recognized and embedded as the foundation for social change activism building. With the notion of undercommons, I conclude by resisting the totalizing (i.e., zero-sum) notion that the resistive power of affective collectivity is entirely vacuumable and appropriatable by the larger neoliberal force. Instead, I argue that such power, activated and embodied by affective collectivity, is transgressive and enacted in multiple assemblages simultaneously and not exclusively consumable by the U.S. public healthcare assemblage. As the chapter proceeds, it is crucial to note here that in highlighting how affective collectivity is nurtured within the public healthcare assemblage, my intention is not to romanticize the U.S. public healthcare assemblage—which is undergirded by layers of social injustice—or to let governments off the hook for not supporting the care needs of their denizens, distributing care responsibilities more widely, and justly compensating care workers. Nor is my intention to refuel the dichotomy of *bad* versus *good* forms of care or good and bad care partnerships. Labor exploitation and care-based mistreatment are realities in Medicaid long-term care. Not all care workers and enrollees reach the point of conducting care immersed in an affective collective manner. In reality, care partnerships are disrupted or terminated at the discretion of care industries all the time. Despite these realities and structural limitations, though, some *do* develop and nurture forms of collectivity that sustain one another and their relationality through interdependent care in the context of the neoliberal public healthcare assemblage. The care workers and enrollees I talked to, in fact, discussed sporadic, restorative moments that they co-experienced within the unjust structure of care in which they are embedded. Care, in reality, is ambivalent, contradictory, and a site of multiple affections, intentions, and effects. Highlighting such restorative collective moments—as sporadic as they may be—is crucial to expand on the complexity of power that emerges through collectivity. These moments occur against the backdrop of the necropolitical, neoliberal social formations that deploy the totally opposite strategy: deflation of collective power by enforcing individual competition as well as capacity- and debility-based exploitation—and hence, insurgent.

Beyond Slow Death and Cerebral Connectivity

I put forward the idea of affective collectivity as the breakthrough or line of flight from the status quo that has been increasingly theorized as neoliberal and necropolitical. Critical theorists from ethnic, disability, and queer studies have described the subjugation of marginalized populations to different paces of debilitation and in relation to the changing prognoses of their lives, particularly in the context of state-sanctioned racialized and cisheteropatriarchal violence (and other interacting social issues).[11] Societal obstacles keep emerging and making it difficult for marginalized communities to continue their meaningful lives uninterrupted. To write about social injustices, therefore, often means to write at length about notions of violence and also death and proximity to it.[12] Public healthcare is one of the areas where the phenomenon of slow death manifests and is enforced, as those who are situated as care workers and care recipients both are exploited and experience mutual deterioration.[13] Theories of debility and slow death have been developed to describe the life-affecting social formation and how hard it is to distinguish slow death from the process of life-*building*.[14] These theories foreground the frustrating and totalizing feeling of having no way out from this violent neoliberal control but to go the route of the debilitation.[15] Depicting neoliberalism as "the current stage of racial capital" and describing the deployment of sexuality within it, critical race and feminist theorist Grace Kyungwon Hong connects and describes the necropolitical aspects of neoliberalism:

> I define neoliberalism foremost as an epistemological structure of disavowal, a means to claiming that racial and gendered violences are things of the past. It does so by affirming certain modes of racialized, gendered, and sexualized life, particularly though invitation into reproductive respectability [i.e., complicity with the neoliberal standard], so as to disavow its exacerbated production of premature death.[16]

Simultaneously, though, with queer of color critique scholar Roderick Ferguson, she also writes, "Out of these contradictory conditions of devaluation and death arise ways to imagine different aspirations for our political projects, aspirations not limited to recognition, visibility, or legibility."[17] With this statement, Ferguson and Hong complicate and add nuances to the everyday lives of those who make a living in the middle of the unjust, neoliberal, and necropolitical climate. They illuminate the reality that there is more to the lives of those who are deemed marginalized and debilitated. What can emerge and be nurtured in such sites are vision, aspiration, resilience, resistance, and revolution. Motivated by this insight, I put forward my conversations and interactions with care workers and enrollees to argue that resistive and nurturing collectivity can spring up in the middle of the exploitative care structure; affective collectivity between care partners is an example of this emergence. In the violent status quo, where care workers' own care needs and impairments are pushed aside, disabled people are not considered as contributing to others' well-being, and the two are firmly prohibited from forming any kind of connection, care workers and enrollees un/intentionally develop a collectivity. The process of the collectivity-building and -nurturing entails potential insurgence, as small as it may be.[18]

Additionally, I would like to pay particular attention to the significance of the sensual or affective (hence ontological) nature of affective collectivity emerging in some care practices. In academia and elsewhere, how people connect and relate (e.g., romantic relationships or political solidarities) are often understood primarily as a function of cognition or intellect, dividing the interwoven nature of body and mind by privileging mind over body.[19] As I mentioned briefly earlier, the privileging of and primary understanding of human connections as being forged through more cerebral and cognitive assessment and approach—and, thus, capacity to forge connections in this manner—is normalized and demanded. People are, in other words, expected to carry on conversations based on logic and rationality by decoding body language and other cues that another person emits, or by assessing each other's similarities and differences.[20]

With this privileging and separating of mind over body, other ways of relating are rarely imagined, explored, or valued.[21] This normalization of human connections thus dovetails with the disregard for other ways that people connect and discriminates against those who are deemed incapable of communicating in normative ways. Many developmentally and intellectually disabled activists have articulated how incapacity for and resistance to engaging in normative communication (e.g., verbal) leads to further pathologization and stigmatization of this population. Disability activist Mel Baggs, for example, describes through typed speech how communicating in any way (e.g., typed communication) but normalized English format often automatically contributes to the dehumanizing treatment and attitudes to which Baggs was subjected.[22] In other words, connecting through spoken and normalized communication is often seen as the hallmark of being human.[23]

In the following, instead, I lay out many examples of how care workers and Medicaid enrollees relate in a haptic manner. I do so to emphasize that there is more than one way for people to connect. And it is happening always and already at the site of everyday care practices and elsewhere. What does this affective collectivity do to the larger public healthcare assemblage and beyond?

Affective Collectivity

The First Encounter

As we sat in the corner of a fast-food restaurant, Tia, a middle-aged Black migrant care worker, told me keenly yet with despair,

> Supervisor [at the agency] gives you the case, but they don't tell you
> where you're going. . . . Sometimes it's hard for me. Tears coming to
> your eyes, because you don't know where you're going. . . . Some-
> times you get robbery. You're scared to go. [Supervisor] don't tell you
> nothing about patient [*sic*]. So when you reach their house, patient
> gives you the attitude [for not knowing basic information about
> them]. You have to calm them down [by] saying that "You know
> what? I didn't know."

She continued to narrate how sometimes tears come to her eyes, as she was
exhausted and intimidated about entering Medicaid enrollees' homes without being clearly informed or having a sense of being fully supported from
agency and being left on her own to encounter her clients and their families
and enter their homes.

This conversation with Tia provided me insight into care workers' experiences as they enter a care arrangement with a new client. Tia's sentiment
immediately brought me back to the similar faces of exhaustion and frustration I encountered a month ago. This time, they were coming from other
side of the first encounter: disabled Medicaid enrollees. Maria—an elderly
Latina migrant woman with disabilities who received her long-term care
from Medicaid—spoke: "The agency is sending [different care providers]
sometimes three or four [times] a week who [you] don't know. . . . You are
admitting this person to your home. . . . They know everything about you,
but you don't know anything about them which is [an] upsetting setup."
Paula—a Black middle-aged woman with disability who received her long-
term care from Medicaid—echoed the sentiment: "With [the] agency, you
never know who's gonna come in your house. You have to go with the
flow. Because if you don't, you're not gonna have the help for the day." In
both spaces, care workers and Medicaid enrollees shared overlapping
sentiments—fear of unpredictable encounters due to the lack of information
and despair at having no other choice but to go with the setup—although
they shared these sentiments separately.

Leading up to the very first encounter, vulnerability heightens in both
the Medicaid enrollee and the care worker on the other side of the door—a
worker outside and an enrollee inside. This vulnerability in anticipation of
the first encounter is more than what one generally expects in any first encounter. It is further induced by external factors such as the care industries
that arrange and manage the structure of care, and social oppressions and
associated power dynamics that intimately manifest in care practices. Those
external factors materialize in the lack of information and communication
from the agencies, the rules enforced by the agencies that include never

forging any sort of connection with one another, and stereotypes based on past experiences of care worker personalities or the attitudes of Medicaid enrollees.[24] In care partners' bodyminds and their encounters, these external factors manifest and shape their anxiety-filled first encounters.[25]

Many people whom I talked to attributed their anxiety and vulnerability to the care industries. Care industries—in the shape of agencies—assign care tasks and coordinate care worker–enrollee partnerships as well as occasionally monitoring the care practices conducted between them. Care agencies are the primary factor, according to those I talked to, that directly shapes the foundation of care practices with their administrative authority. Both care workers and Medicaid enrollees discussed, for instance, the fact that the agency withholding information is one of the roots of their heightened vulnerability. They also noted that subtle power dynamics between those situated as enrollees and care workers are structured and seeded by care agencies, whether through the trainings they assign to care workers or the rules and guidelines they enforce for both populations. In other words, a care routine conducted between a disabled enrollee and their care provider is never without interference by care agencies.

Remembering the initial training that care workers were required to take, Alisha—a middle-aged Black woman who is a care worker—described her experience:

> [At a training set up by the agency, instructors] just talk to you, walk you through with do's and don'ts. [They tell you,] "even if the client yells at you or they are little annoyed which they can be, all you have to do is just talk to them. . . . You have to still *give them a little independence* [emphasis added]." So, [the agency] talked to us about that.

In the training, according to Alisha, fundamental power differences are established and inscribed. The preceding quote demonstrates how the training constructs Medicaid enrollees' ability (or lack thereof) to navigate life independently in the given society as well as what kind of attitude care workers should bring to their care practices. Affective expectation and imagination are set up and occupy care practices even before the care workers and Medicaid enrollees encounter each other—which are part of what is assembled at the first encounter. Further, although care workers are taught to tolerate mistreatment by Medicaid enrollees (i.e., their care partners), they are simultaneously informed that they have ultimate power over their care partners and that the well-being of these partners is in their hands, as they are situated as the agents of controlling how much independence is given to their disabled counterparts. Paternalistic dynamics are anticipated by and instilled in the care workers at the training. They are, in other words, capacitated to be the stereotypical disciplinary yet loving and caring figure in the care practices to come.

In the expert discussions with Medicaid enrollees, as well, many of their narratives reflected how interactions with care workers were structured and governed by care industries. Maria offered an example of such experiences: "If you tell [a care worker], 'Could you do me a favor? Please could you just clean that spot over there?' And [the care worker] calls the agency and says, 'She wants me to clean,' and you talk to the coordinator [who tells you whether she can clean the spot or not]. I'm always wrong and [care workers and agencies] are always right." She ended her comment by raising her hands in the air in a gesture of defeat.[26] Here, she shared her dilemma of how the agency is set to dictate and manage the care dynamics accumulating between her and the care worker (i.e., her care partner). Other enrollees also voiced vividly how the agency is situated as the ultimate authority to establish the infrastructure of the care practice and to judge who is right and who is wrong. These quotes show that care practices are never simply an engagement by and between care workers and enrollees. The shadow of care agencies is present in care practices constantly.

In this control and regulation of care practices, social stereotypes also materialize in first encounters and in the early state of care practices. Care workers I talked to often remarked on how disabled people are "human too, just like them": "I have respect for [my client], *even though she may have a disability, she's still a person* [emphasis added]. So, I do respect her, I do care for her." How the reaffirmation and recognition of disabled people as human is turned into a reason why they deserve care workers' respect and care is alarming. It can be read to mean that disabled people are generally considered to be *less than* human or *non*human, and thus recipients of justifiable ableist violence or otherwise undeserving of equal treatment. The fact that almost all care workers I talked to expressed this sentiment shows that care practices do not begin on equal ground; rather, they begin as if the disabled care recipients are less and the care workers are the liberators to recover the humanity in their care partners. These narratives and sentiments of the care workers are not the only place that such oppressive stereotypes manifest. Disabled people also enter their care practices by bringing the capitalist notion of service provision with them: how care practice should be, what they are entitled to, and how their care workers should behave and hence what sort of attitude is allowed and demanded. Particularly as they are not mandated to take training on how to work with their care partners—as care workers are—how they work with and treat their care partners is left up to them. Isabella, a middle-aged, Black, second-generation migrant care worker, addressed this situation to me as we sat down in the corner of her agency's empty room during their holiday party. On the one hand, she described at length the lasting relationships she has with some of her past care partners even after their formal care arrangements have ended. On the other hand, though, she also explained,

> Some of [the Medicaid enrollees I worked with] don't think [about] our lives, just be with them, only. Just to work, work, work, work, and take care [of] them. . . . You tell them [that you] have a kid, but they don't even care. Just want me to be there for them only. Just to do for them, them, them.

Here, according to Isabella, her care partner (i.e., a Medicaid enrollee) aggressively asserts their authority as a care client and disregards Isabella's whole humanhood. In other words, the disabled enrollee is enacting the stereotype of an exploitative boss as normalized in the capitalist sphere, where such self-centered attitude is not only permitted but also seen as a sign of effective authority and employer. Some care workers are, in other words, situated as if they have two bosses: care agencies and Medicaid enrollees.

In the case of both care workers and Medicaid enrollees, the larger social injustices and the intersecting control and exploitation effected by the U.S. public healthcare assemblage trickle down and manifest through care setups and circulate between care partners and through their bodyminds, since they are the ones who are situated to encounter each other and spend their daily lives together. Within this context, the vulnerability and related frustration experienced at the first encounter, which is induced by external factors, are often directed toward each other. The mistreatments that care workers and enrollees experience are often delivered through one another's hands. Care workers and enrollees are generally left to negotiate the care-based injustices crystallized in the encounter, which often forces them into an antagonistic position at the beginning of their care practice.[27] Both enrollees' and providers' bodyminds are already affected by a number of predisposed expectations and assumptions. Key components for the development of the relationship are, then, whether and how care partners come together to undo the power dynamics seeded by agencies and other external factors.

Recursive Encounters

> Being able to anticipate just enough, not too much. And that's tricky, that growing, organic thing that develops over time. . . . [My care partner] could *anticipate* [emphasis added] just enough to be

[helpful] to a point. She didn't need to be directed or asked; but not too much so that she took away my independence. (Bill)

Care practice begins as external factors haunt and shape the care arrangement. By care practice, I mean the daily encounters of care partners, their co-engagement to fulfill the care plans assigned by the agency, and all other caring or ways to maintain and improve each other's well-being that circulate between them.[28] The care workers I talked to work for Medicaid long-term care and conduct the assigned care activities for twelve hours a day, five to six days a week, in order to make a living. And enrollees receive a range of hours of care: from a few hours a day to around-the-clock care. Care routines are repeated daily, and enrollees and care workers reencounter each other every morning. From there, they co-engage the same set of care routines that they did the morning before (e.g., getting out of a bed and into a wheelchair, with some variation day to day). This repetition of care routines continues on until their care partnership ceases. Regardless of how long-lasting their care partnership may be, they negotiate, adapt to, and at times learn each other's unique needs, capacities, desires, and rhythms through recursive care routines.

Just doing what [my care partner (Medicaid enrollee)] asked of me, no matter how many times she asked. And just doing it. She said that it takes a lot, a lot of patience. This is what I dealt with every single day. . . . Sometimes I did it the right way [in making the bed], but she'd say, "But I don't feel it right, so you've gotta do it all over again." [Laughing out loud sarcastically]. Woof! I really, really learned.

Here, a care worker, Alisha, illustrated with a laugh and sarcasm how constant trial and error were exchanged among herself, her care partner, and the bedsheet. At a glance, Alisha's illustration might be interpreted as a care worker being overworked with unrealistic and unreasonable demands. Yet disability can also involve chronic pain or heightened sensitivity, which means a subtle bump or a rough surface can be experienced as pain. Also, the bed is a crucial space in which many disabled people spend the majority of their lives. Hence, care practices are required and requested in a visceral way—for example, whether the bed feels right to the enrollee. Learning and adapting to a care partner's needs, capacities, and desires certainly takes repeated practice and patience. Thus, it is not only the care worker's job to learn and adapt to their care partner's needs and desires.

[Agencies do not want you to have a relationship with your care worker partners], but it's hard. When you're working with a person six hours, eight hours, nine hours, four days a week, five days a week, seven days a week, you start to know who these people are. What their habits are, you know what their *needs are*—you can almost *anticipate* [emphasis added] what their needs are. (Rick)

My conversation with a group of Medicaid enrollees was filled with mentions of a variety of subtle and not-so-subtle care *they* offer their care worker partners in order to co-conduct care tasks effectively. Rick, a middle-aged Black man with a progressive physical disability, voiced the care and adaptation to his care partner that he came to embody in the preceding quote. Care circulates as enrollees too adjust and adapt to their care partners, including the pace of how fast or slow they work together, as Rick pointed out how he anticipates what his care partner needs. In other words, care is never a one-way gesture given from a care worker and received by a Medicaid enrollee. It is co-conducted. They come to learn and adapt to each other together as they move from a bed to a wheelchair, for example. As much as a care worker *lifts* the enrollee's body from a bed, the enrollee as well may rest their head in a certain way on their care partner's shoulder, or their muscle may tighten in anticipation of the lift. They meet in the middle to accomplish care tasks together over and over, day after day.[29] A white disabled Medicaid enrollee, Bill, whose story opened this subsection, also emphasized the circulation of the anticipation as well as the embodiment of care tasks experienced by both him and his care partner. Although it is not easy to articulate how care is sensed and care practice is conducted at an embodied level, the following quote by affect theorist Couze Venn addresses this aspect of care practice: "The concrete, experiential forms of non-conscious and proprioceptive communication . . . take place through touch, smell, the gaze, movement, sound, taste occurring directly between bodies, and sensed as a tacit knowledge of oneself and the world that doubles as an embodied way of being-with others."[30] Tacit knowledge is accumulated through care practices: from how each body moves to how the movement feels, to the point that care activities are conducted in sync. Based on the unique ways each care worker is shaped and moves, Medicaid enrollees change up their body movements, posture, and tempo to meet their care partner in the middle, to smooth the conducting of care. Such tacit or haptic knowledge sometimes is co-developed as unique sensory communication by care partners:

[Akemi: He gives you the wink to communicate with you?] Yeah. . . . He can't move [his body to conduct normalized verbal communication], but he can move the eyes: makes his eyes so big [(she demonstrates how he opens up his eyes)]. Last Sunday, his beard grew already. I asked him, "You don't mind if I shave again?" He said, "Nooooh." So, I did. . . . I take my time, I have fun . . . [doing] that. He puts like that [(demonstrating his eye movements to communicate with a big smile to indicate that he was content)], eyes so big.

Sophia, a middle-aged migrant woman from South America, uses all her body parts, facial expressions, and Spanglish to demonstrate her unconventional, haptic connection and the communication she co-developed with her care partner.[31] Her description of her care relationships with her care partners itself was largely communicated affectively with her smile, varying tones of voice, body language, and everything in between during my interview with her.

Care practice, on paper, seems to be a rigid, clear-cut list of services that care workers are assigned to perform for their clients and check the box as they complete each task. In reality, though, it is more like a mixture of spontaneous and simultaneously well-rehearsed dance happening at sensory and corporeal levels. Each task requires the choreographed collaboration of both bodies on multiple levels to adapt to the needs and capacities of both enrollee and care worker in terms of bodily movements, pace, desires, capacities, and needs. Such adaptation is thus facilitated and nurtured as they repeat their encounters and care practices day after day, and as they circulate and accumulate haptic knowledge of one another—their shared heat, sound, odor, gaze, texture, and more. Daily care practices require them to communicate by feeling one another, beyond what is communicable with words or rationally understandable.

Shared Vulnerability

Care practices begin with the awkward and vulnerable first encounter. In the repeated encounters to follow, though, each encounter inserts different affects to the relationality between care partners and accumulates within it to alter the relationality itself and future encounters. During the sensual process of learning and adapting and co-experiencing daily life, the relationship between workers and Medicaid enrollees sometimes slowly shifts, and so do the affects circulating between and beyond them. They both, for example, start witnessing, acknowledging, and co-experiencing the vulnerability their care partners experience:

[My current care worker] was about to quit [right before she began working with me]. . . . She was not gonna take anybody's mends. If I had said anything wrong, it was gonna go down. . . . I was nice, I just asked her to do my laundry on the first day [which is considered an easier task]. (Rick)

You know what, there are a lot of good [care workers] that do the work, and they don't get acknowledged [by care agencies]. (Anton)[32]

Here, Medicaid enrollee Rick and applicant Anton sympathetically illustrated a variety of snapshots of how negatively care workers had been treated within the U.S. public healthcare assemblage. Rick described, with a smile and a friendly laugh, one of many encounters he had had with assigned care workers in the first quote. Rick was well aware of high care worker turnover and viscerally cognizant of care workers' exhaustion and frustration, based on which he decided to look after his new care partner by adjusting the care tasks for the day. Many similar sentiments were brought up during the conversations with Medicaid enrollees. Their comments began to show their frustrations *for* their care partners, as many called themselves advocates and firsthand witnesses to the experiences of their care partners. The second quote, from Anton—a middle-aged Latino man with learning disabilities—indicates that care workers' capacities to engage in care work do not necessarily mean that they are invincible and immune from emotional and other stresses. Anton thus recognized and acknowledged the structural injustices that many care workers endure during their exploitative labor.

Not only do enrollees and care workers acknowledge each other's vulnerable moments, but the extensive amount of time they spend together means that they encounter and experience each other's vulnerable moments together and through one another. With a glimpse of exhaustion, a care worker, Tia, described the time both she and her care partner were fed up with an argument going on in the household where they were co-engaging in care routines and co-conducted an escape to take care of one another: "It was better for [my Medicaid enrollee care partner] and better for me [to leave her house]. Because if [the enrollee's] family members start arguing, that's too much, too frustrating. . . . So we say, 'Let's go. Can we just go watch a movie?' We go, and we laugh. It'd be better for both." Witnessing, acknowledging, and sharing vulnerable moments, in some cases, gave rise to a sense of empathy for each other as well as intimacy and moved care partners to tend to one another, which further nurtured their relationalities. Empathy and care for their care partners going through vulnerable and unjust moments was present in all my conversations with care workers and Medicaid enrollees I talked to.

Alisha, a care worker, explained the situations her care partners go through in the following narrative. Her tone of voice and recognition of the vulnerable setup that many disabled people who are situated as care recipients endure reminded me of and resonated with the tones of disabled Medicaid enrollees' narratives, who also discussed this vulnerability from their own perspectives. Alisha said: "What [disabled Medicaid enrollees] are going through is not easy. It takes a lot for people to ask somebody to wash them up. That's not something to get easily adjusted to do. That's a total stranger, somebody you don't know have to come in to do everything for you, [though] you don't know [the person] yet. Your body is a temple, it's private. . . . It's a lot for [the enrollees] as well." Throughout her narrative, her voice embodied her irritation, resentment, and disappointment about the lack of structural supports she felt as she witnessed and co-experienced the vulnerable moments between herself and her care partner. Alisha described this not as a way to compare to and highlight her able-bodied privilege; rather, she spoke out of frustration and empathy for her care partner, articulating the injustice in the structure that further intensifies already and naturally vulnerable practices of care.

While care workers and Medicaid enrollees embody distinct capacities and needs, or ways to communicate and move their bodies, and despite how they are acutely distinct in the public healthcare structure as care provider and recipient, they also adapt and nurture ways to relate, communicate, and sympathize sensually and collectively. Care starts circulating between them, rather than exclusively being sent from a provider to their recipient as the agency and society enforce and expect. A Black female care worker, Terri, illustrates the care she receives from her care partner, who is a Medicaid enrollee: "I do receive care from [my care partner with developmental disabilities]. She appreciates things. . . . She gives me hugs; she tries to do a little thing. Or sometimes she shares things. . . . She shares some foods sometimes." Paula—a Black, middle-aged woman with physical disability receiving her long-term care supports from Medicaid—discussed in a lively way how she and her care partner also developed enough trust to build their own routine of care practices suited better to them rather than exclusively following the routine set by the agencies: "We built a pretty good relationship. Like [my care worker partner] fixes me food or anything. She'll probably take [some food] for herself. That's how we do things. I don't mind, as long as you don't take it for granted. [Sometimes my care partner asks], 'Paula, today I have to leave early, because of another case.' And I'm like, 'Okay, can you make sure you finished [the task]? Can you come back later, or can you finish that next day?'" During the co-experience of vulnerable moments and in the circulation of empathy, nurturing care comes to be materialized. And although care agencies impose the guideline not to form any kind of connection between care workers and Medicaid enrollees, and thus turn care tasks into a checklist that is clear-cut, dry, and quantifiable, it seems inevitable for some of them to build intimate and unique bonds over time. As the opening quotes of this chapter illustrate, care workers and disabled Medicaid enrollees become the "closest person, the closest relationship . . . [where] they see you when you are good and when you are bad. . . . It's an unbelievable relationship."

Affective Bodymind

Bodymind and particularly body have been understood in various ways. An affective understanding of body is one of them and frames the body as open-ended, dynamically modifying and being modified.[33] According to such understanding, the body is composed of different elements and temporalities that constantly reconfigure their arrangements and relationships based on external and internal forces. It is ever in formation and extends beyond its skin as its border.[34] Even before the popularity of affect theory, such an understanding of body and thus bodymind was nurtured in critical race, disability studies, and elsewhere.[35] Audre Lorde's writing on the erotic, for example, explores the affective body:

> The erotic [embodies] the power which comes from sharing deeply any pursuit with another person. The sharing of joy . . . forms a *bridge* between the sharers which can be the basis for understanding much of what is not shared between them. . . . [T]he erotic connection . . . open[s] . . . fearless underlining of my capacity for joy. In the way *my body stretches* to music and *opens* into response hearkening to its deepest rhythms, so every level upon which I *sense also opens* to the erotically satisfying experience, whether it is dancing, building a bookcase, writing a poem, examining an idea.[36]

Whereas Lorde describes the erotic as the affective modality through which people forge connections beyond their bodymind boundaries, my focus is on how care activates the connection. The experience of the erotic, she writes, fundamentally changes the configuration of the body, and it expands the body's potential and capacity by opening up her "fearless underlining of capacity for joy." In the extension of a bodymind to its surroundings, it forges relationality and transgresses the limit of the individual bodymind.[37]

This affective understanding of bodymind as open-ended provides alternative ways to understand the encounter of bodyminds and the conceptualization of relationality among them. By expanding our understanding of bodyminds to include how their parts pre/consciously connect, relate, and adapt to other bodyminds, their movements, and the larger surroundings, how the encounter of bodyminds is understood also demands expansion.[38] An encounter is experienced beyond what is cognitively registered or empirically understandable. The encounter is collective becoming, inheriting both the capacitative and debilitative potentials for encountering bodyminds and their relationality—to follow affective understanding of bodymind. It integrates constant making of themselves (i.e., the bodyminds) and their parts in each other's presence. Past bodily or bodymind memories as well as surrounding sociopolitical forces come to shape the collective becoming. In critical Mad studies scholar Rachel da Silveira Gorman's words, "[Affect is simultaneously] the product of repetition and sedimentation of ideology, rather than of 'preindividual bodily capacities.'"[39] One way to theorize the collectivity developed and nurtured between some care workers and Medicaid enrollees, therefore, is to illuminate how such collectivity grows as they connect haptically, primarily through practices of care that they co-conduct day after day in the context of the U.S. public healthcare assemblage as well as the surrounding web of social injustices and intricate political economic forces.[40]

In the repeated and collective practices of care, care partners haptically sense and adapt to one another's bodily shape, movement, rhythms, habits, heat, odor, sound, texture, sight, capacities, needs, desires, and eye movements.[41] They feel each other and experience their surroundings through one another: a process that entangles both bodyminds beyond the boundaries of their own skin. Additionally, the repetitions of the encounter and the practices of care routines are how the affective connection of bodyminds further grows and collectivity evolves.[42] Through this haptic learning, bodies accumulate ontological knowledge of one another. My definition of *learning* goes beyond the cerebral, which is assumed to be the foundation of learning. On the contrary, learning happens through various senses and ontologically.[43] As evident in the opening quote of this chapter from disabled Medicaid enrollee Maria, care recipients and providers adjust slowly to each other's working styles to move their bodies in sync to accomplish care tasks: they come to anticipate the moves preconsciously. The collectivity is embodied, as there is an "interpersonal sense of connectedness written into our bodies."[44] Such accumulation of ontological knowledge is also sedimented over preexisting knowledge from past care practices and affective collectivities that workers and enrollees forged with their previous care partners.

One by-product of affective collectivity is the enhancement of care partners' capacities to accomplish their care practices smoothly. The narratives of the care workers and Medicaid enrollees I have explored throughout this chapter describe with nuances how such affective collectivity can also immerse each of them in empathy and other affirming feelings for one another. However, I also want to caution that encounters and care practices have the potential to negatively affect both workers and enrollees as well as their care practices. In reality, care practices and encounters are affected and shaped by various factors, including the well-being of a care worker or enrollee on a given day, which may manifest in their attitudes toward one another, or general distrust of care workers or enrollees constructed via the care industries and shaped through the exploitative commodification of care. Such factors can diminish their capacity to care for one another or to collectively accomplish care routines. Political philosopher Gilles Deleuze says, "When a body encounters another body, [they] combine to form *a more powerful whole* . . . [and] our power of acting is increased or enhanced. [At the same time, though,] when we encounter an external body that does not agree with our own, it is as if the power of that body opposed our power. . . . it may be said that our power of acting is diminished."[45] In addition to the possibility of encountering bodyminds to experience debilitative dismay, expectations and demands for positive and emotionally affirming care that are particularly put to care workers can further deepen their exploitation in care industries.[46] Care practices filled with affective collectivity itself can be further instrumentalized by the neoliberal political economy as well, which I further examine shortly.

While acknowledging negative connotations associated with affecting bodyminds via care, nonetheless, the care workers and Medicaid enrollees with whom I interacted described how the continual co-conducting of care tasks can strengthen their relationships in the long run. As enrollees and care workers repeated care practices, spent extensive hours together, and better learned about and adapted to one another, the feelings that circulated between them sometimes came to change too: from individual and defensive vulnerability, to collective and shared vulnerability, to empathy and intimacy. In this relationship, disabled enrollees who are situated as care recipients begin to look after their care partners (e.g., by sharing food) as much as care workers come to witness and co-experience the vulnerable moments their care partners go through, which was not taught at care worker trainings. In affective collectivity, care becomes dialogical, and such collectivity is a communal becoming that contains the potential to increase their collective bodyminds' capacity or power to act: "The embodied and shared micro-political moments as movements . . . are the vital relational circuits through which negotiations, capacities for responsible and effective agency and change can most tangibly be grasped, explored, expressed and understood."[47]

Further Contemplation: Co-capacitation and Undercommons

What does affective collectivity forged in daily care practices do beyond its impacts on the interpersonal relationships I laid out earlier? Under the racialized, ableist, and cisheteropatriarchal political economy, people's labor capacity and its attached value are constructed and exploited as the care labor force, while their own emerging impairments and care needs are actively overlooked.[48] Additionally, this political economy shapes and makes use of people's debility to feed into the care industrial complex.[49] In the U.S. neoliberal public healthcare assemblage, bodyminds are capacitated and debilitated to be commodified as labor capacities and care needs; in other words, care providers and recipients are reduced to mere capacity and debility to be capitalized within the assemblage.

In that context, what does it mean that affective collectivity can be and has been co-capacitative for the care providers and recipients I talked to? A number of critical thinkers depict neoliberalism in an absolutist manner, by explaining that both capacitation and debilitation of bodyminds is totally and entirely manipulated and exploited under the political economy.[50] In reality, and on one level, the capacity that is born out of affective collectivity is sucked into the neoliberal U.S. public healthcare assemblage. Such relationality or the bond is part of what keeps care workers returning to care work and has them filling the ever-existing gap between what care industries narrowly assign as care tasks and what disabled enrollees actually need (often more than what the industries assign). For example, although care workers do not receive overtime pay, many workers I talked to explained that they stayed and worked extended hours for their care partners, as unforeseen incidents and needs appear at the last minute (e.g., a bowel movement by their care partner who then needs to be cleaned). Many Medicaid enrollees as well often settle for the shortcomings of care—due to the gap between the care offered to them by care industries and what they actually require—out of their concern for their care workers' well-being. Affective collectivity, therefore, can be understood as further sustaining and enhancing the assemblage.

Additionally, given the ban of any form of bonding, such collectivity building entails risk. Acknowledgment of how affective collectivity simultaneously entails an extension of care and compassion by both care partners for one another as well as how it can partially fulfill the need of the public healthcare assemblage to be run smoothly is crucial to avoid an uncritical and romanticized perspective. Affective collectivity should never be used to justify the oppressive nature of the neoliberal public healthcare assemblage.[51] While I foreground the investigation of care-based injustices at the macro level in previous chapters, I further engage in the co-capacitative nature of affective collectivity in the rest of this chapter.

Co-capacitative Force of Affective Collectivity

Power—and capacity—has been studied as manifesting in multiplying and various ways. Political philosopher Baruch Spinoza, for example, conceptualized power as two different modules: *potentia* and *potestas*.[52] I bring up Spinoza's conceptualization of power briefly here because it often underlies and shapes today's affect theories that lay ground for this book. Potentia is the indwelling power of acting, inherent to one's existence: "being able to exist is power."[53] In contrast, potestas is externally induced and born out of friction with other bodies, and it entails domination of one over the other or one's interference with the other's potentia or power to act: "Lack of power consists only in . . . that a man allows himself [*sic*] to do what the common constitution of external things demands, not what his own nature, considered in itself, demands."[54] This differentiation and highlighting of multiple kinds of power and capacity is critical to further understand the possible co-capacitative nature of affective collectivity. Certainly, the capacity born out of affective collectivity can be, partially or otherwise, subsumed into the macro political power of exploitation (i.e., potestas), as I briefly traced earlier. Nonetheless, affective collectivity can also be a way to enhance care recipients' and providers' power to act and exist (i.e., potentia). Lorde's words that I quoted earlier echoed this underlying power of connection. It is through people's connections to dancing, building a bookcase, or examining an idea that their underlying innate power emerges.[55] In other words, I am thinking of power born out of the affective collectivity in a more multiplying or layered—rather than absolute—manner.[56] What is happening in care practices and through affective collectivity is more than what the neoliberal U.S. public healthcare structure can incorporate and exploit.

In the U.S. public healthcare assemblage, on one level, care recipients and providers are territorialized or subjugated as they are individualized and turned into a mere degree of capacity and debility to be managed.[57] Affective collectivity is, on another level, a way for those who are made care workers and enrollees to deterritorialize, or regain, their collective agency and potentia. Thus, such collectivity can be transformative, having the potential to interrupt the assemblage. Going back to the linear notion of debility and slow death reviewed earlier in this chapter, there is so much more to the everyday lives of those who are situated as care workers and enrollees at the molecular level than the necro-theories that account for the molar level assume.

Affective Collectivity and Undercommons

In their collaborative book *The Undercommons: Fugitive Planning and Black Study*, authors Stephano Harney and Fred Moten developed the idea of *undercommons* to illuminate forms of destructive forces igniting underneath oppressive social systems "underground, the downlow low down . . . where the work gets done, where the work gets subverted, where the revolution is still black, still strong."[58] Commenting on the book, another critical theorist, Jack Halberstam, interprets and further expands on the undercommons, saying that it

> cannot be satisfied with the recognition and acknowledgement generated by the very system that denies a) that anything was ever broken and b) that we deserved to be the broken part: so we refuse to ask for recognition and instead we want to take apart, dismantle, tear down the structure that, right now, limits our ability to find each other, to see beyond it and to access the places that we know lie outside its walls.[59]

With this concept, Harney and Moten sharply critiqued how institutions are built on a bedrock of racial and other interacting social injustices, and they engage in dismantling of it instead of receiving recognition, legitimation, and ultimately protection from that very institution.[60] Without the eradication of the system, we cannot imagine and lay out different, more-just ways to live together. These scholars shed light on how people who are embedded in the system can simultaneously engage in the destructive work within it collectively through interactions and hang out (what they call *study*).

Considering how forging affective collectivity itself rejects the guidelines enforced by care industries, the care workers and Medicaid enrollees who bonded through affective collectivity entail the potential to disrupt the flow of the assemblage from within bit by bit. They thwart the assemblage from territorializing or subjugating themselves into agencyless bodies of care workers and care recipients: mere capacity and debility to be capitalized in the assemblage. As they destroy the flows, they deterritorialize themselves by circulating care between themselves and beyond against the ban. Throughout this chapter, haptic connection was described as a means through which to forge affective collectivity—a form of human connection that is often pushed aside in terms of how the connection is understood and normalized. Disabled communities, alongside care worker communities, often find such hapticality in their everyday realities. Collectivity and relationality are often the primary way that disabled people navigate their lives in ableist society by co-conducting their daily activities with and through others.[61] Affective collectivity born out of haptic connection in a way depicts the inherent dependencies each person embodies to different degrees—beyond their disability status. Affective collectivity is the basis for the undercommons of lower-income disabled people and working-class, (non) migrant women of color, who are too often situated as care recipients and care workers. They tap into non-normative or nonstandard ways of getting to know each other and connect. However non-normative these ways may be, they also insurgently foster connections that threaten care industries, which then ban these connections because of liability concerns.

Many scholars who write critically about neoliberalism put forward such collectivity as an antidote to the neoliberal political economy that enforces individualism.[62] Affective collectivity fundamentally breaks the individualism entrenched and enforced in the neoliberal political formation. As the undercommons involving disabled people inherently entails an affective, relational caring nature, because it is often the only and main way for many disabled people to participate in collective resistance, affective collectivity should be woven into the undercommons and other acts of resistance.[63] Affective collectivity is, after all, a way to create accessible and inclusive insurgence to all by centering people's dependencies and by practicing and embodying collectivity, not regardless of but because of differences in one's capacities or needs.

4

Living Interdependency

Desiring Entanglement in Messy Dependency

[Shifting from the ideological sphere to everyday lives accompanies] a
lot of hard work toward figuring out how exactly to practice
resistance in material terms of struggle and perseverance. This is
work that feels mundane and not so exhilarating, because it's about
daily life, little things, everyday all-the-time decisions and actions,
and it can feel impossible sometimes, and so much easier to rely on
old paradigms and strategies—but this is the work we have to do.
—Johanna Hedva, "sick woman theory: an interview"

In my experience, when access intimacy [which is interdependence in
action] is present, the most powerful part is having someone to
navigate access and ableism with. It is knowing that someone else is
with me in this mess. . . . Access intimacy is knowing that I will not
be alone in the stealth, insidious poison that is ableism. . . . The power
of access intimacy . . . [is its asserting] that there is value in disabled
people's lived experiences.
—Mia Mingus, "Access Intimacy, Interdependence and
Disability Justice"

E very week from 2011 to 2015, I visited my friend Riley, a disabled artist. I commuted to her metropolitan apartment on Wednesday nights
to exchange conversation and updates while we engaged in collective
care.[1] She was one of a few people who consistently provided major emotional care for me, and she also offered cognitive care, as she was the English
copy editor for my graduate schoolwork. From my end, I offered physical
care for her night routines. I visited her around her bedtime; she always
welcomed me with a soft hug, asking me if I wanted tea, water, or wine. We
shared lots of laughs and updates as I kneeled to take off her shoes and
socks. We co-facilitated care tasks, as she got ready to shower and go to bed.
While she assisted me by shifting her body or positioning her legs in certain
ways, I lifted her body so we could co-conduct multiple transfers together.
As she lay on her bed at the end of the evening care routine, I sat in her
wheelchair as it charged next to her bed, and we continued to share every

detail of our week: a mixture of many feelings, laughs, and sometimes tears. I recharged myself emotionally with Riley's help, as I hope she recharged herself too. Riley often offered me a hand massage, as my disabled hand would be tired and in pain from the academic labor of typing. Or we talked about care labor and the never-ending questions of fair labor bartering, or if there even is such a thing. We circulated emotional care among so many other forms of care between us.

We were part of the larger care collective that Riley initially organized with a group of her friends and strangers that she recruited who provided physical care for her nightly and for whom she provided a wide range of care as well. Members of the collective were assigned a day of the week to visit Riley, and each of us developed our own unique relationships with her as well as with one another. It was a collective experiment to actualize and practice interdependence in our everyday lives intentionally, extending from Riley.

The preceding excerpt is from autoethnographical notes on an interdependent care collective I was part of. Care collectives—community-based mutual-care structures—organized by disabled people and their allies emerged throughout North America in the 2000s and on (while such forms of care have always been present throughout history, which I will discuss shortly).[2] Such collectives were initiated by disabled people who were fed up with the injustice entrenched in the hegemonic ways that long-term care was structured, particularly under the neoliberal care industrial complex. Some disabled people started care collectives in order to fill the lack of care they were experiencing within public healthcare assemblages or because they did not have access to family-provided care (as families are often situated as the major care provider and manager for disabled people). Some forged collectives as they visited conferences or other events and wanted to experience and move together throughout the events.[3] In whatever ways they came to experience care collectives, these disabled people were eager to collectively endeavor to create different and more-just ways to meet their care needs and honor their caring capacities. In many ways, the emerging disability justice movement and its advocacy for the idea of interdependency inspired many to actualize this social justice ideology by forging care collectives.[4] The preceding excerpt, therefore, is a snapshot of one such layered story. It tells a story of friendship as much as exemplifying the social changes that were happening in our bedrooms by reimagining long-term care and intentionally practicing interdependency. It illuminates how social change and visioning can happen through care, and thus care is the foundation for social change work. What it obscures, though, is the challenges, conflicts, and trial and error that are equally present in the overlap of friendship, care, and social change work, which the openings quotes of this chapter touch on. How can we translate and interweave social justice ideology like interdependence into every breath of our lives? What is it like to live the ideology in the middle of the status quo, which instead values and enforces *in*dependence?

Interdependency is one of the ten principles that disability justice activists put forward to reimagine not only how we engage in activism but also how we live our everyday lives and how the larger world can be organized in more-just ways.[5] Disability justice activism emerged in the early 2000s as the term *disability justice* was coined and used by activists who were trans, queer, gender-nonconforming, disabled people of color, and thus many of them were migrants themselves or offspring of migrated people (including Patty Berne, Mia Mingus, Leroy F. Moore Jr., Sebastian Margaret, and Eli Clare, along with Stacey Park Milbern, Leah Lakshmi Piepzna-Samarasinha, Lydia X. Z. Brown, and many others).[6] They have been reframing disability activism by putting forward disability, Mad, neurodiverse, sick, and Deaf knowledge and wisdom nurtured within racialized, trans, queer, feminist, migrant, fat, poor and working-class, Indigenous, and other marginalized communities, as leading activists of disability justice also occupy these communities and their activist work (as much as they also build cross-community solidarities with disabled people who are doing disability justice work in these communities).[7] A leading activist, Patty Berne, with disability justice art organization, Sins Invalid, have described interdependency as follows:

> Before the massive colonial project of Western European expansion, we understood the nature of interdependence within our communities. We see the liberation of all living systems and the land as integral to the liberation of our own communities, as we all share one planet. *We work to meet each other's needs as we build toward liberation*, without always reaching for state solutions which inevitably extend state control further into our lives.[8]

Politically, interdependency is a way to value community-based collective and mutual care in critique and resistance against the ways state-sponsored care is deployed as a mechanism of surveillance and control. Additionally, the practice of interdependence is indicated in Berne and Sins Invalid's quote as a way of decolonialization and toward the collective liberation of people and lands. I also believe that interdependency is resistance work that pushes against the independence-driven and individualist demands enforced within the United States and through U.S. imperialism, particularly since such drive and demand are further intensified in current neoliberal political force. On a more inter/personal level, another leading activist in disability justice, Mia Mingus, has explained that "interdependence moves us away from the myth of independence, and towards relationships where we are all valued and have things to offer."[9] Reflecting this assertion, interdependent care is often imagined as and sprouts from the core belief that everyone is dependent on one another and requires care as much as everyone contributes to the care and well-being of others. In other words, care is circulated rather than only given unidirectionally from designated care provider to care receiver, and thus, independence is a myth.[10]

Ideas of interdependency as well as community and collective care are not necessarily new, but different versions of it have been used as a method of surviving and thriving for many marginalized communities historically.[11] When marginalized communities have been deprived of necessary institutional care supports (e.g., medical treatments at hospitals) as a form of state violence, community-based collective care has been a crucial strategy for them to keep each other alive and nurtured.[12] This strategy manifested in the health justice wing of the Black Panther Party, which provided care to its community members when the government denied institutional care to Black communities.[13] Interdependent community care also shows up among chosen families and other kin formations that trans and queer communities have developed to support one another when they have been pushed out of or escaped the family-based care structure or government-sponsored ones.[14] The Street Transvestite Action Revolutionaries (STAR) is one example; Marsha P. Johnson and Sylvia Rivera provided home and nurturing care for trans and queer youths of color needing the supports.[15] More recently, Houston Health Action (which is a pseudonym) is a collective of disabled, undocumented, and uninsured migrant people coming together to care for one another, when xenophobic policies do not allow them to access affordable institutional care (e.g., medical care at hospitals).[16] In short, the interdependency and care collectives I put forward in this chapter—which have emerged from disability justice activism—are built on and through these histories as much as being part of the histories. Disability justice has in particular been developed by those who are parts of multiple marginalized communities and brings together wisdom from various racial, trans and queer, migrant, feminist, and Indigenous communities to rethink disability activism at the intersection.[17]

I started my research into interdependent care collectives originally because there is little scholarly writing on the topic of *how* culture or social relation can be developed and nurtured so that interdependence becomes the norm; in other words, how interdependence is un/intentionally embedded in the everyday lives of disabled and other folks. This is so, although scholars have certainly recognized the significance of interdependency as a

key resistance against neoliberal political force and intertwined social oppressions as well as a crucial tool for collective survival and to enable other-
world-making.[18] Also, this research forms one way that I contemplate and
work to contribute to disability justice work from my stand- and sit-point.
Although the praxis of interdependence has been sustained over decades in
multiple formats, here I explore exactly how interdependence manifests in
the everyday lives of disabled people and what it takes to intentionally form
a collective around the idea. What does it feel like to practice interdependence and form a care collective that embodies a totally different formation
of care from the way care is organized currently at the institutional level?

Actualizing and practicing the ideal and vision in our everyday lives
certainly brings layers of complexity. As the opening quote by artist and
scholar Johanna Hedva eloquently summarizes, it is hard to enact the vision
of other-world-making in the middle of and against the grain of the status
quo.[19] When I was in conversation with those who participated in care collectives to practice interdependence, the conversations were filled with the
never-ending challenges they faced as much as the joys. Although they had
initially pictured interdependence largely to be a harmonious and nurturing
engagement that affectively reflected what living in a just world would feel
like, they also mentioned how messy it was in reality. My fascination was
piqued, therefore, when they shared their desire to reclaim and illuminate
their *dependency*—their entanglement in each other's messy and unruly
dependency—in addition to interdependency.

Messy dependency is a term I use to explore this desire, particularly
against the backdrop of how interdependency has come to be imagined as a
clean-cut reciprocal relationship when the idea was translated into everyday
practice and actualized in the care collectives I looked into. Here, I build on
the conceptualization of *mess* offered by critical anthropologist Martin F.
Manalansan vi, who illustrated messiness as the reality and portal for
queer migrant futurity against the backdrop of how neat categorization and
measurement of populations have been used as a colonial and capitalist
mechanism for controlling and disciplining queer migrants.[20] Based on my
autoethnography and interviews with those who have participated in interdependent care collectives, I develop the idea of messy dependency as political interventions to the neoliberal status quo and a way to widen disability
activism and particularly care activism enacted by disability communities.[21]
I ask, what does it mean for members of care collectives to desire and reclaim their and other disabled people's dependencies, when independence
is inherently valued and enforced in the United States (and elsewhere)
historically?

The idea of independence has formed the foundation of the United
States and its American-ness over centuries—and has been, hence, deployed

as the social norm and aspiration.[22] The inability to embody or perform independence, therefore, has been met with various forms of social stigma and deprivation of dignity and agency of those who are labeled as dependent, contingent on who bears the marker of dependency (e.g., babies, elderly people, disabled and sick people, and so on).[23] Particularly in the case of disabled adults, the inability to perform independence (through activities of daily living) according to ableist social standards has been used as a justification for dehumanizing treatments against them including institutionalization, eugenics, and all the other violent management exercised under the name of care.[24] Understandably, then, one way to interpret the history of the disability rights movement, including the Independent Living Movement, is to name it as a history of fighting for independence or distancing themselves from the stereotypical notion of disabled people as *burdensome* dependents.[25] What does it mean, then, for those disabled people I talked with to yearn to reclaim their dependency and embrace its messiness? What kinds of possibilities arise when we shift our focus to reimagine our lives and societies in a dependency-centric way? What would the notion of messy dependency contribute to the idea of interdependency that disability justice activists nurture? Or, is the idea of messy dependency and the desire for it mere romanticization of ableism (when dependency is used to oppress disabled people)?

Dehumanization in Valuing of Independence and Devaluing of Dependency

Independence has historically been the foundational virtue and value in the United States.[26] It is the expectation and aspiration that shapes our everyday lives. It is more than expectation but also functions as demand. It has been deployed as the measurement to categorize and hierarchize people along the human and dehumanization spectrum that undergirds social oppressions enacted in the United States.[27] I am bringing forward this notion of a human and dehumanization spectrum, which I learned from the works of disability activist Mel Baggs. Baggs has articulated how not using verbal or other normalized communication (i.e., speaking formal English) and having a developmental disability diagnosis automatically turn the person into someone not quite human, hence dehuman.[28] In other words, being cognitively independent by expressing one's logical and rational thoughts verbally is held as an important measure and marker of being human.[29] Within disability studies as well, Nirmala Erevelles inserts materialist criticism of how liberalist notions of citizens—rational, autonomous, and competent—are used to inherently discriminate against people with "intellectual/severe" disabilities, which results in the material deprivation and dehumanizing treatments the population faces.[30] Feminist philosopher Eva Kittay illuminates how she brings a dependency critique to the scholarship of care: "[The notion of] democratic liberal nations [is understood] as an association of free and *independent* equals.... [T]he conception of the citizen [is therefore forged on the notion of independence and] to whom [human] rights [are] attach[ed]."[31] Critical race scholar Sylvia Wynter (among others) also traces back and adds how independence was a key criterion to construct and enforce "civilization" against the notion of "uncivilized" at the time of the Renaissance and colonization. The notion of independence is, then, used to define human (i.e., "Man") and place people of different backgrounds on the human-dehuman spectrum, which has been used to justify various forms of atrocity.[32]

Independence is also deployed as a keystone of capitalist and neoliberal political social formation and its mechanism to discipline and control the population.[33] Individual competition, for example, is set up as a way that success is sought and determined within the neoliberal political economy. Individuals are turned into each other's competitors and encouraged (or forced) to explore ways to enhance one's wealth and access to resources for individual survival and gains against others.[34] Additionally, since public supports (e.g., various welfare programs) have been shrinking under the political economy, the ideology of individualism has intensified such that one's access to various resources necessary to maintain oneself as independent and productive (e.g., healthcare, quality education, secure housing, and employment) has been turned into an individual responsibility. People are forced to perform independence, and their care and other needs are actively looked over. The long-term-care needs of disabled and other people are expected to be met by family members and friends, the newly flourishing care industrial complex, or worse, left unmet.[35] It is as if the degree of constructed, amplified, and embodied *certain* dependency we each hold determines our location on the spectrum of human to dehuman. Here, I emphasize *certain* dependency, because not all dependencies (e.g., affluent people's reliance on domestic workers) are devalued equally, since some dependencies are naturalized as they are believed to enhance the depending person's productivity and ability to compete, while the others (e.g., disabled people's dependencies) are pathologized and criminalized.[36]

Independence-based de/humanization is one way that ableism manifests and materializes and to which disability communities assert critical analyses.[37] The expectation and enforcement of independence is profoundly interwoven with the mechanism of ableism and vice versa. *Ableism* is exercised not against any ability or inability but specifically against the inability to fit social norms and orders, including the ability to behave within its standards and to satisfy social virtues including independence. These social norms and orders are shaped in the web of racism, cisheteropatriarchy, settler colonialism, and other interlocking systems of oppression.[38] Failure to demonstrate (certain) independence has, then, laid grounds for disability categorization and discrimination. Disabled people's exclusion from society has been justified based on their inability to attain independence; thus, medical and rehabilitative industries were established to help or force disabled people to attain independence (which also comes with profit and medical authorities for the industries).[39] Against this backdrop, care has an intricate relationship to the notion of independence. Care has been situated as a structure to enhance the independence of disabled, elderly, and/or young people who need daily assistance. Care and care labor have also historically been used to assign caring responsibilities to welfare recipients with an expectation for them to gain financial independence and therefore terminate their dependencies on state welfare programs. Care at the structural level is, in this sense, a mechanism to manage and suppress the dependency of marginalized populations with the goal of turning them into independent and productive citizens.

Given the intricate (and seemingly cursed) tie between the notions of independence, ableism, and de/humanization, disability communities and scholars have developed in-depth analyses on the notion of in/dependency. As disabled people have been automatically classified as dependent, and in particular *burdensome* dependent, disability community activism has been historically centered around debunking the stereotypes and gaining independence.[40] In other words, gaining independence has been seen as a key to attain equal ground with nondisabled people, since the fight to gain independence is equated with gaining rights for self-determination and assertion of their agency and humanity.[41] One path that disability rights activists have taken to achieve this goal is, therefore, to rethink and shift how care is understood and practiced.

The U.S. Independent Living Movement, for example, has advocated for the term *assistance* to replace the word *care* since the late 1960s.[42] They critiqued the paternalistic connotation embedded in the term *care* and how it is used to stigmatize them. And hence, they preferred the term *assistance*, since it naturalizes their needs (removes the suggestion of burden) and is used generally to address the help nondisabled people receive.[43] To advocate for the term *assistance* was their way to make an intervention in the power dynamics exercised in and through care by emphasizing and maintaining the agency of the assisted person and to detach disabled people from the stereotype of dependent and hence passive receivers of care. The term also amplified their authority to manage their personal assistants as independent beings.[44] This movement for independence was crucial to transform the dehumanizing living conditions many disabled people experienced in and outside of residential institutions. As disability activism has evolved, though, many disabled people came to meditate on this aspiration to be independent. Disability justice advocates, among other disabled people, began to question this investment in independence and acknowledge that absolute independence is a myth.[45] Regardless of disability status, who is completely independent? In particular, disability justice advocates (i.e., trans and queer disabled people coming from racialized, and migrant communities) were perplexed by this aspiration to live U.S. virtue, which was built on its settler colonialism and interlocking system of oppressions and its incongruity from what other communities they are part of valued and embraced (i.e., collective reliance on one another).[46] These activists, therefore, began to put forward the notion of interdependence, which was followed by the enactment of the idea through care collectives.

Given this context, what is it like to embrace and collectively try to live interdependency in one's everyday life, while also being embedded in—and expected to perform independence in order to survive and thrive in—the larger hegemonic society? It is, in a way, to go against what the neoliberal political economy enforces and rewards; thus, it is what we are taught to aspire to and desire. And finally, what does it mean for the disabled people I spoke with to desire messy dependency and to reclaim their dependencies, while they are already and always and historically assumed to be overtly and burdensomely dependent?

Care Collectives in Action

> Interdependence to me is mutual support and exchange of care. . . .
> Life giving. . . . Sort of quality of life supports. (Erica)

The reasons why those I talked to turned to care collectives are as numerous as the ways they understood interdependency and care collectives. Broadly speaking, care collectives are community-based mutual-care structures where committed community members and their allies engage in the circulation of long-term and other forms of care. They are volunteer-based and conducted outside of or in addition to state- or family-structured care. Some people turn to care collectives because the long-term care they receive under Medicaid barely covers their care needs. Others do not have close ties with their families to anticipate care supports from them. Of the people I spoke to for this research, these factors certainly were among the reasons that influenced their choice to participate in care collectives. Latina disability activist Jocelyn explained,

The reason that we had to sort of cobble together this collective is because we never had the resources that we needed [whether in terms of Medicaid long-term care or otherwise]. . . . There [are] lots of situations in which [care workers] just don't show up. . . . It is just bound to happen. And even though these agencies are contracted and are supposed to cover this care, a lot of times it just doesn't happen. And the onus ends up on whatever family or support circle the person has.

Woven between these practical reasons was their political curiosity and commitment to practicing the idea of interdependency promoted by the disability justice movement and to co-navigate the world together—which Erica's quote at the beginning of this section touches on.[47] Hearing and learning about how other disabled people engaged in care collectives encouraged many of those I talked with to actualize this practice on the ground. Drawing on the ideas of interdependency, they reconstructed the care they experience from the basis that independence is a myth (hence people are inherently dependent) and everyone needs care as much as everyone can contribute to others' well-being through care (hence the circulation of care). They were all yearning to explore more-just ways to engage in long-term care and followed in the footsteps and wheel traces of disability justice activists to turn sites of care into sites for social change.

Some collectives covered in this chapter were constituted solely of friends and allies; some included professional paid care workers. Some collectives had more formal structures with set schedules, while many care tasks were also done in an ad hoc or spontaneous manner. In the formal ones, people started collectives by describing their care needs as well as the kinds of care they could provide and by scheduling care rotations (like the one that opened this chapter). In more informal ones, caring interdependency was interwoven as part of disabled friends hanging out with one another (e.g., sharing dinner), because meeting each other's care needs together was the only way to be with one another.

As I entered interviews with people who were part of different care collectives, they explained over and over how engaging in interdependent, collective care brought them joy—the joy of experiencing surprising discoveries and steep learning curves. While the main focus in this chapter is to trace and theorize messy challenges and the realities of trials and errors they faced in their respective care collectives, I want to start this section with some snapshots of what I read as joys. Care collectives were certainly more than just challenges but a complex mixture and interweaving of joys, challenges, resistances, and visioning.

The way in which I feel better about [being part of the care collective] is that I know that I'm contributing to the collective. It's taught me a lot about how to be in the world. Sometimes I feel like . . . [exclusively] a person that requires care, because I'm disabled [and receive long-term care]. But then I stop and I say to myself, "Well, I am also providing care to people in this group, to friends, [to] this care collective, who are not identifying or perceived as disabled." (Jocelyn)

The significance of intentionally engaging in interdependence was brought up by all the care collective members with whom I spoke. They described joys they experienced as making new friends who genuinely cared about them; disabled people recognizing that they contribute to the well-being of others, contrary to the ableist stereotypes recognizing disabled people exclusively as care receivers; and everyone learning to recognize and accept that they do need care and it is okay to ask for supports. Although Jocelyn, just quoted, is a feminist disability activist and well aware of contributions she makes to the world, when it came to care, it took her some time to learn and assert that she does provide and contribute to care for others. Being part of a care collective helped her to halt and break through the social assumptions put on her and to recognize and reconstruct the multiplicity of herself and her roles in the collective. She continued:

I had to [learn to] open up, I had to let people in . . . so [I had to] bust down those walls and bring people in and trust them to various extents. . . . It shifts that conditioning that I [was accustomed to that] only family is gonna take care of you because society's not gonna take care of you. . . . And a lot of the time it still is scary for any of us to ask for help. None of us is good at asking for help, I don't think.

Her migrant family of origin, she told me, instilled in her the value of self-sufficiency, mainly due to the lack of public supports available to migrant families and the state's blunt xenophobic tendencies. Given this background, she asserted, learning about care collectives and meeting strangers who genuinely cared about her and wanted to engage in caring relationships with her was a surprising shift in her life.

Intentionally learning and shifting the way they operated their daily lives occupied a big part of the joy that members found in care collectives. Echoing Jocelyn, another care collective member, Dani (who identified as white, queer, gender nonconforming, and with disabling conditions) stated, "[Participating in a care collective] got me to ask for help better . . . [to] learn to ask for help. That's a really hard lesson, you know?" As much as it seemed like a simple gesture, many were surprised how hard and vulnerable it was to consciously admit that they needed help, to open up and share the fact, and to rely on others to respond to their needs. Their accounts showed how care collectives were turned into a space for members to experiment with different ways to circulate care; to break through the social expectations that framed them as *either* care giver or care receiver or expected them to perform independence; and to instead embrace their embodied needs for care. In other words, care collectives and their efforts to engage in interdependency were more than an alternative care formation but also a catharsis to reexamine and reimagine how collective members related to their bodyminds' needs and how care is set up in society.

Challenges in Care Collectives

The subject of challenges came up in the conversations I had with members of care collectives as much as they were a reality in collectives I was part of. It shows that embodying and materializing a vision that goes against the currents of the status quo are destined to face some challenges. This will become clearer with further theorization; such *challenges* are simultaneously the resistance and process of other-world-making through care. For now, these challenges are framed and described in terms of how the *limit of care* is drawn—which is to examine who and which care need is prioritized or put on hold and which need is met with care and which is not. Many people are often stretched thin with competing responsibilities, and it is certainly true to those collective members I talked with.[48] For example, some of them work multiple jobs, while others multitask by handling care collective scheduling while calling care industries and other governmental entities as they wait at a doctor's office—all in addition to their commitment to participate in care collectives. Thus, competing responsibilities are intensified by social stratification and further stretch those who are socially marginalized, in particular.[49] In Sam's words,

> [To be part of the collective means that] you're making a commitment to try to be at the same time, the same place, and also to respect how that evening [with a care routine] fits into a person's entire life. . . . Providing care for the other person [involves] not only when we're physically together in the same room, but also to think about how that two to three or four hours [of doing collective care work] affect[s] the person's week.

Sam, a white disabled queer woman, traces here the mundane yet crucial factors of being together at the same place and time for care collectives, and how such coordination can have ripple effects. In reality with competing responsibilities, not all care needs and desires were necessarily met immediately in full (both quantity- and quality-wise) within a collective alone, particularly when the needs for care surpassed the capacities to care—hence the limit of care emerges. I write about this limit as the material and affective terms of challenges, to invoke wording in Hedva's opening.

Material Terms of Challenges in Care Collectives

> I think sometimes the "inter" part of interdependence is really emphasized. (Sam)

> I feel usually when people use that word [interdependence], it's kind of like reciprocity, "Oh, I'll do something for you, and you do something for me." . . . I don't know if this necessarily has to be that way. (Sara)

The material terms of challenge address the tangible difficulties of meeting the care needs that emerge in a care collective. The notion of care—what is recognized as a care need or dependence and what is acknowledged as caring labor— as well as the concept of interdependency have each been constructed historically and impacted by the commodification of care. Such impacts stubbornly haunt us and dictate whose caring labor in the collectives are recognized and appreciated and whose are overlooked, whose care needs or dependence on others are amplified and prioritized, and whose needs are trivialized and invisibilized. In addition, the idea of interdependency is far too often interpreted and translated into expectations for *equal reciprocity of care*, which has become the goal of care collectives that those I spoke to participated in and reflected in the preceding quotes. For instance, Sam recalled how the collective she was part of started: "When I was having the one-on-one conversations with people to set up the care collective, [I asked,] 'what is care that I can provide you?' It was asked [in a] barter or skill share way, but not in a way that could be more expansive." Here, Sam's primary attention was on how to *exchange* care. Her retrospective concern was that she has started the care collective from the foundation of interdependency as a synonym for bartering of care tasks. This led those in the care collective to question how to engage in this bartering or reciprocity in an *equal* manner. Sam continued, "The challenge of [a care collective is] feeling like I didn't [engage in] an *exchange enough* [emphasis added], [like, not thanking collective members] for the care . . . that was given to me. But also feeling like I'm not thanked in other ways. . . . [Care I provided was] not acknowledged or appreciated. . . . [The assumption was] that one person builds up like a surplus and another person builds up a deficit." This sentiment from Sam was echoed by other disabled people I talked to who require long-term care and have more complex care needs, like Jocelyn, who mentioned, "I worry that I'm not doing enough for people that have done things for me. And sometimes it's human nature [to also] think, 'Well, I did all the stuff for this person. I don't feel like I'm getting much in return.' But then, that's where it becomes important to stop and say, 'Okay, I need to talk this out before it starts to fester and turn into a resentment.'"

Similarly, nondisabled people and disabled people without long-term care needs I talked with echoed the narrative in the following manner: "Part of my internalized ableism [is that I] think [about] whose feeling and emotion are allowed to be discussed more openly [in the collective]. And whose feeling needs to be more private because of that kind of privilege I have over [other collective members who have more complex care needs]." When I mentioned this sentiment during an interview with Dani, who is also disabled but does not need long-term care, they immediately responded, "Yeah. That's how I feel too!" What underlies Sam's, Jocelyn's, my, and Dani's sentiments is how normalized ideas of care labor and care needs have dictated the ways that interdependence have been practiced in care collectives. All quotes refer to different ways that people's caring behaviors are recognized and valued or overlooked. Further, they demonstrate how a ranking of emotional needs has carried into collectives and impacted members' decisions regarding whether to share their needs with others.

Sam and Jocelyn, as discussed, received mostly physical (and long-term) care and provided emotional and cognitive care. Jocelyn, for instance, provided care to others by "disseminating information. If people need to know how to get something done, particular within medical or social service stuff locally, they tend to ask me." Regardless of how she and Sam contributed to this circulation of care, they both articulated that certain caring labor was recognized and appreciated over others based on the types of care provided or who provided them. While physical care is easily registered as care labor by many in the care collectives, for instance, nonphysical care such as emotional and cognitive care was not as readily noticed or lacked the framework to be valued as caring labor. Also, care collective members I spoke to were constantly working to resist automatically recognizing disabled people (particularly those with long-term-care needs) as recipients of care and not providers, while care provided by nondisabled people and disabled people without long-term-care needs was quickly registered as care. In my conversations with Riley (who identified as a white, queer, disabled woman), I recalled all sorts of nonphysical care she had provided—which I started this chapter with. While both of us identified as disabled, I do not require long-term care, which Riley did. I stated during my conversation with Riley:

When I was doing the care collective with you, because we had the barter system where you were doing the [copy] editing [of my graduate school assignments, we often talked about the editing as if it were the only care you provided me.] But also, you're so aware of the needs that I'm not even aware of myself. You offered to massage my [disabled] hand, and I [didn't] even realize that I needed it, and it was [actually] much needed. My body needed it. So, I kept [wondering even after I left the collective] how much emotional and cognitive labor [it was] for you to keep paying attention [to] what the person needed and [offer] the care.

Riley as well as other disabled people with long-term-care needs described how they constantly paid close attention to how their collective members were doing and how they could be supported. They also engaged in cognitive care by organizing and scheduling the collectives by reaching out and checking in with members. Normalization and standardization of care deployed and further enforced in its commodification (as care is regulated under public healthcare programs and through care industries) means people tend to internalize it and bring it to the collectives. One consequence is that although many disabled people with long-term-care needs I talked to constantly gave emotional and cognitive care to the point that they experienced burnout from time to time, it was rarely recognized, while their idiosyncratic movements, needs, and paces were amplified and quickly registered as signs of needing assistance.

The combination of rarely recognized care that they kept providing and their disproportionately amplified care needs then put pressure on many of the disabled people with long-term-care needs I talked with to give back more, to compensate for the physical care given to them in order to fulfill the reciprocal expectations embedded in many collectives. In this context, where their needs are spotlighted and their caring labor is overlooked, mutual or reciprocal exchange of care seems next to impossible, especially when the exchange is imagined or expected to be done in a more or less equal manner. Thus, it seems to be drifting further away from how interdependence was originally imagined in disability justice activism and elsewhere. Jocelyn, who receives her long-term care from a combination of Medicaid and a care collective, articulated how such expectations reminded her of the demands for productivity enforced in the larger capitalist political economy:

I feel better about that I'm contributing to the collective [as a disabled person]. At the same time, even if I wasn't, that's still okay. And that's another thing. Even within [the] disability community, you have to give back. You have to do, do, do. It's okay, people are still worthy of love and care, even if they can't reciprocate it.

What is raised here is how the obligation to give back to be a good collective participant could increasingly resemble the expectation for productivity, which is enforced by capitalism and deeply interwoven with ableism. Jocelyn brought up her concerns about how the tendency to equate people's productivity or capacity to give back with their value can bleed into disability communities and interdependent care collectives as well.

Further, different collective members I talked to echoed the concern about whose needs or feelings could take up space in collectives and whose tend to be put on the back burner. The latter is a sentiment shared by those without disability or those who are disabled but do not require long-term care. The white, queer, nondisabled ally Sara, who along with her partner was part of a care collective, elaborated on this point:

> There was this false dichotomy between people who were providing care and people who were receiving care. [Providing care] was still really, really challenging for [my nondisabled partner who was providing care to others] emotionally and physically. It felt like [this hardship] almost didn't matter because [she] wasn't technically disabled at that point. . . . [She was] just supposed to be really strong and awesome, [and] be this *super able-bodied person* [emphasis added] who could do all that stuff.

In this quote, she succinctly illustrated how the capacities and abilities of seemingly nondisabled people are quickly recognized and prioritized as the capacity to labor care. This recognition, along with the privilege associated with their physical capacity, is accompanied by Sara's and her partner's deprioritization of their own needs for emotional supports. The difficulty and feelings Sara's partner was going through were kept private and not necessarily recognized and pursued in the collective.

Priority of care is established both in the larger care structure and at the level of care collectives. Care needs are often quantified within the state-sponsored care structure, for instance, in order to determine the care priority. How, then, can care collectives further expand and complicate the notion of care priority, as they endeavor to acknowledge and value all collective members' needs and contributions to care—without losing sight of how we all experience care needs and urgency differently? How can the notion of interdependency intervene to seriously acknowledge everyone's caring contributions and needs for supports without dictating that people embody either one or the other?

Challenges shared by those I spoke to seem to be rooted in ways that care is constructed as quantifiable and without regard to the subjective aspect of the care experience. Dani earnestly pointed out, "I sometimes don't like when interdependence is posited [as if] it presumes that things are commensurable. It gets trapped in the same kind of exchange-based idea as . . . money does." As care is increasingly and further commodified in the rapid development of the transnational and domestic care industry complex, physical care comes to be the default and definition of care. Care became conceptualized as quantifiable and hence barterable. Medicaid long-term-care service is, for instance, measured in hours as well as in the format of simplified, checkbox care tasks (e.g., assisting with showering) solely based on the quantifiable activities of daily living. In other words, care has been tasked to care workers as labor stripped of emotional, cognitive, spiritual, and other substance. Or one's care needs and dependencies are perceived as compartmentalizable and somehow stop at the end of the care labor shift. Additionally, care is set up as if it is given from one person to another in a one-way direction, ignoring the reality in which care is given, received, and circulated in complex and rich ways. I included Sam's description earlier of how people are categorized in economic terms of either surplus or deficit based on their productivity for care labor or abundant need for care. Challenges that those collective members shared with me as well as how they interpreted interdependency in their collectives all illuminate the fundamental limit of how care is set up in the hegemonic society. In this case, a significant challenge has emerged: they imagined interdependency primarily as a reciprocal exchange of care, at least when their care collectives were initiated; however, care needs and the act of caring itself are rarely contained enough to be measured for *equal exchange*, per se.

Similarly, to further tease out the impossibility of reciprocity in care as narrated by members of care collectives, I would like to emphasize that people's needs for care or dependency are socially constructed and exacerbated. Needs for care are not only embodied but amplified in inaccessible environments as well as in the normative pace and manner in which people are forced to function and carry themselves in society. Any deviation from the narrowly set standards can then be labeled as incapacity and inability to engage in activities of daily living independently, and hence disability and *burdensome* dependency. When disabled people's care needs and dependency on other collective members are understood as socially constructed, such as needing supports from others to enter an inaccessible building, for example, what does it mean for the disabled person to be expected to engage in reciprocity with the person who assisted? Capacity to care is constructed as well, as not everyone is equally socialized to notice and attend to others' needs for care, particularly in this cisheteropatriarchal society where care work is highly gendered, racialized, and classed. Erica, a white, queer, disabled collective member, recalled many moments when one specific member of her collective tended to go above and beyond to care for Erica:

> She always takes on more work than she was [asked for] ... that's just who she is. If you ... tell her that your care needs are X, Y, and Z, ... she will cover the entire alphabet ... which is 1) draining for her, 2) it also sometimes would create inner personal problems because I would get frustrated at not being allowed to do things for myself... and 3) I think it meant that other [collective members] didn't learn how to do stuff because she would just do it. .... And then she would get to a point where she was crashing [from overworking].

This quote highlights how people are building care collectives and practicing interdependency on the ground where their care needs and capacities to care have been already sociopolitically shaped.

Care as we know it and how we engage in it are highly dictated by the historical making of what is considered care, whose care needs are denaturalized or considered a social burden, and who is made responsible to meet care needs. This historical making of care is profoundly infused with and intensified within the neoliberal commodification of care and intersecting social injustices. To dream and enact interdependency and other-world-making in this context, therefore, seems to require the groundwork to radically reimagine care. It is a part of collective building to unlearn every building block that constitutes our everyday lives and to reimagine every step. Our challenge is, therefore, to reimagine and embody care in the environment that continues to enforce ableist-capitalist norms and customs of care. How can we interpret the *inter-* part of interdependence in a way more aligned with disability justice politics and without demanding equal reciprocity, when some people are made more dependent and some are trained more to care for others, or when one-way dependency or the notion of unidirectional care is the environment in which care collectives operate? Disability justice activism has conceptualized interdependence in a way that emphasizes *all* people as dependent beings and possible contributors to one another's well-being. This approach challenges the ableist perception of disabled people's dependencies as a burden alongside the naturalization of nondisabled people's dependencies. Building on this strategic emphasis, there is yearning to further tease out how we are *differently* equipped and situated in relation to dependency and care contribution, and how this recognition can enrich our understanding and practice of interdependency even more. In discussing the practice of interdependence in care collectives, those I talked to began to dive into the details of how this ideology manifests in their everyday lives.

Affective Terms of Challenges in Care Collectives

> [I don't want care collectives to] be [where people consider that] disabled people who can build really good interdependent relationships are the ones who are worth living or something. I don't want that. (Sam)

With the increasing popularity of disability justice activism, the notion of interdependence has come to be recognized and celebrated more widely. Interdependency is, in other words, a way to enact and embody social justice and other-world-making in our daily lives, particularly in the context where individualism and independence are enforced and further intensified under the neoliberal political economy. This root of care collectives, then, has unintentionally shaped an expectation for a certain atmosphere within the care collectives that those I talked to were part of. Particularly given that social justice work is posited as transformative of the violent status quo and a pathway to a more-just and more hopeful society, such work is often expected to embody the opposite kind of affect than that which we feel in the status quo (e.g., desperation, anger, depression, despair). A sentiment expressed by Sara depicts the affective norm infused in care collectives: "[Interdependent relationships and care collectives are] imagine[d to be filled with] a kind of harmony or something like that . . . kind of relation between two consenting people [which] can be like really beautiful." This sentiment was echoed by others I spoke to and signals that the expectation for a hopeful, harmonious, or nurturing atmosphere (i.e., affective norm) is prevalent in many care collectives, as people came together to practice interdependence. This expectation could then backfire, when it was turned into a demand and norm of the collective.

At the opening of this subsection, Sam described her concern about how a member's successful fulfillment of the affective norm and expectation of the collective is implicitly presumed to translate to the member's value. She continued: "I'm an introvert. . . . And I would sometimes feel like I couldn't be my introvert self [in the collective with the presence of its member next to me and wonder] how can I get [my care] needs met without being stressed out [about] having someone next to [me] all the time. . . . [I was feeling the pressure that I had to] make [the care collective] a good positive experience for [everyone]."

Additionally, since care is subjective (whether in terms of caring or being cared for), the ability to fulfill the collective norm and affective expectations was not unrelated or without impact on the quality and quantity of care granted—indirectly shaping, for example, whose care needs were prioritized or not. In other words, a politics of likability can bleed into and distract interdependent and caring relationships. I have observed and also heard about how likability, or the ability and capacity to engage in interdependency in respectful and harmonious ways, unfortunately shaped the circulation of care within collectives. One can accumulate likability by reading and understanding the atmosphere of the collective correctly and sensitively, and by participating in and contributing to a collective's affective norm. Likability, certainly and inevitably, shapes and is core to any relationships besides care collectives. We tend to enter and commit to form friendships and other forms of relationships with people we like. What I highlight here is, then, the complications that the notion of likability can bring to care relationships forged in care collectives and rooted in collective members' aspiration for interdependency. In other words, these relationships are not mere friendship but also involve care that deeply dictates people's well-being and even life at times. Not receiving care or *good* care can mean not being able to fulfill daily plans and having to forgo any opportunities and responsibilities that come with them. Here, I am thinking of it as *politics* of likability to emphasize that likability is deeply entangled with the desirability that is formed with interactive forces of racism, cisheteropatriarchy, xenophobia, fat phobia, ableism, ageism, and much more that dictate who is to be desired and who not to be. Politics of likability is not detached from many normalized skillsets (i.e., reading and responding to one's body language accordingly), as the ability to perform the skillsets is quickly interpreted as un/favorable traits of the person, and such normalized skillsets for interpersonal interactions can easily become ableist demands.[50] This is to say that one's likability is deeply mediated and determined by the sociopolitical context. This ability and capacity to perform and conform the codes to be likable are then often turned into the hallmark to dictate who is suited for membership in a care collective and worthy of community care and even love, and who is not. Care is and can be easily influenced or dictated by the affective attachment or detachment that people experience regarding one another and their collectives.

Below, Ruby, who has depth of insight on living with psychiatric disabilities and trauma, asserted another layer of reality on how likability could shape care circulation within a collective:

> Think about trauma survivors here. [They] may have drug problems [or] might [be] super sexually promiscuous. . . . They might be a kid who makes up a lot of stories, [or] bully other kids[, and] are trying to heal. But when they come into a community where [community

members] say, "we always have to be respectful, and we never use these terms, and we never do these things. If you act in this way, you're not part of the community" . . . that kid might immediately be rejected from [the community]. [It is not that] what they're doing is unhealthy [but] it's their body and mind's attempt to adapt to something that was done to them. . . . People most in need of healing are often the ones who are the most *messy* [emphasis added]. Especially in a disability [community] . . . and care collective units, you have people who have been multiply oppressed . . . and many of us have very deep trauma histories and we bring that shit . . . and how we act things out and how we enter into relationship with each other can be a lot of mind fuckery.

Ruby is a white gender-nonconforming person with disabilities and illuminated the reality that we live in a messy and unjust society where people are treated oppressively and sometimes traumatized. She went on to explain that she had seen many people, particularly from multiple marginalized communities and including herself, who had gone through oppressive and traumatic experiences and engaged in behaviors that could be read as "acting out." Some mental disabilities, she noted, could also induce mood swings, impulsive attitudes, and behaviors that are read as aggressive.[51] Further, disabled people in general might "act out" as a form of resistance and push back against ableist infantilizing treatments they receive.[52] Regardless of the reason behind it, this "acting out" can result in a person being ostracized from communities or care collectives, as they are considered to be breaking the community's or collective's harmonious unity and respectability code. Ostracization from care collectives or communities can, thus, entail these ousted members losing the care they once received. The stakes of conforming to a harmonious affective norm are, therefore, too high. Additionally, this reality narrated by Ruby addresses how ableism bleeds into social justice organizing and the work of other-world-making. Ableism in this case is happening through the mode of an affective norm and is about valuing or discriminating people based on their capacities and abilities to conform and contribute to the affective expectations of the collective. Ruby further explained,

I think we frequently include or exclude people based on ideas of whether they're living up to our ideals or not . . . sort of culturally accepted or validated ideals within that niche. But the real work [of a care collective] is to figure out how to be interdependent with people who aren't living up to [the ideal] and how to continue to participate in that [collective] when we ourselves are the ones who can't meet that expectation. . . . The challenge of interdependence is [therefore] to (A) be there for those people, . . . (B) to allow those people to grow and give them opportunities to be there for others, . . . and also, how to keep everybody safe in a world where all of us are caring.

Disability has been defined historically as a marker to divide deviancy from the norm. In other words, the forming and enforcement of norms happens hand-in-hand with the pathologization, criminalization, and marking of certain bodyminds as deviant and hence disabled. In the preceding quote, Ruby pointed out the danger and reality of how care collectives have the potential to internalize affective norms and dictate members' inclusion in the collective based on their abilities to meet the norm—which also shapes whether they receive necessary care or not. What does it mean that the care supports one requires might hinge on one's likability or ability and capacity to meet the collective norms and expectations? How can people practice interdependency when not everyone is on the same page politically or when they engage in attitudes or behaviors that can be registered as acting out? Is a care collective reserved only for those who are familiar with disability justice philosophy and also capable of enacting this philosophy? Additionally, Ruby ends their quote by bringing up the notion of safety. The idea of likability can easily commingle with a sense of care-related safety, intimacy, vulnerability, and trust. Nonetheless, I want to carefully tease them out and ask how can we build a caring collective for all without vacuuming these senses and feelings into likability. The goal is to ask and explore how we can be there for one another and hold each other to collective accountability supports, while circulating necessary care without using withdrawal of care as a punishment to treat those who do not fit in the affective norm as disposable; how we can forgo the sense of absolute harmony to share and be in vulnerability together; how we can move beyond overtly and exclusively reading each other's disrespectful behavior as a risk to collective safety, undeserving of care, and antonymy of trust?

Tracing how interdependency is intentionally practiced and how care collectives are organized and experienced brought up challenges and more questions than answers. Narrating these challenges also reveals the shortcoming of how care is conceptualized and structured in the larger society and articulates issues of likability and negative consequences for not living up to it—and how it can emerge even in spaces dedicated to social change and justice. The stakes are high, as access to care is profoundly interwoven with those challenges. Needs for care are way more unruly and unpredictable than these existing structure or affective norms can account for and not fully reciprocatable. Endeavoring to find more-just ways to live and connect with one another is not always harmonious and nurturing but can be risky, scary, or unpleasant or entail disrespectful moments. It is messy! It is messy to enact ideologies of social change in our everyday lives and collectively. The challenges I laid out in this chapter simultaneously show that people's desires and demands for people's care needs to be not only met but centered within social transformation work.

Desires in Care Collectives

> I like dependence, [b]ecause I like to think of need as desire. . . . If we could think of [need and dependence as] desire[,] not as lack . . . something you don't have, that you want to have. (Dani)

> I am actually more interested in dependency than I am in interdependency, because . . . even though we can say everyone is depen dent, just as we can say everyone is interdependent, I think there are ways that we can talk about *specific dependencies* [emphasis added] that get a little bit closer to the kind of power [that] disability [and] disabled life [have]. (Sam)

In the middle of the joys and challenges, there was desire. Care collective members with whom I spoke were becoming more interested in reclaiming their and other disabled people's *dependencies* in addition to or rather than interdependency—which was clearly communicated in the quotes by Dani and Sam. They are painfully aware that their and other disability community members' dependency is as much constructed in an ableist society as it is idiosyncratically embodied; thus, it is used to justify various forms of ableist violence against disabled people. And yet they suggested revisiting, reimagining, and thus reclaiming the dependency they embody as powerful and unique insights that disabled people and communities can offer to the world. Although they were up front that dependency was messy and considered burdensome, they still insisted that messy dependencies on one another seemed to be the more accurate description of how they stayed together, survived, and thrived collectively in this ableist society. Contrasting with how interdependency was translated and practiced in the collective, Dani talked about dependence: "I would rather be entangled [with one another] even when it's messy and hard and scary, because that's what [disabled people are] dealing with all the time [to navigate ableist society]. . . . That's what it was to be friends [with other disabled people]." Sam further elaborated on why she was intrigued by dependency:

Interdependence [is considered and set up in care collectives as] something you could pull back [and take a break] from, whereas we know that dependency doesn't work that way. [The never-ending nature of dependency is] a beautiful, complicated thing. Sometimes the formal construction of interdependence looks like two or more people coming together for a certain time and then leaving [it at a time of] their own choosing. *The reality of need and dependency is much more entangled, and it is not so individuated* [emphasis added].

Dani and Sara echoed this view in their conversation:

SARA: [Interdependency often assumes that] two people who are independent in some way, even though they're dependent on each
other, agree to be dependent. Whereas I feel the kinds of experiences I have around dependency are more about things that feel
less of a clear boundary and more entangled. And those can be
really bad in a way too, because it can be a space of abuse or
things not being good. But also I feel like interdependence suggests that something can be paid back.
DANI: Dependency is that entanglement that doesn't presuppose
contrast with independence.

In other words, dependencies refuse to be compartmentalized, predictable, measurable, or neatly reciprocatable, unlike the way interdependence was imagined and interpreted in the practice of the care collectives that those I spoke to were part of. Here, I would like to note that Sam's, Sara's, and Da-ni's critiques are not necessarily about the idea of interdependency itself or how it is defined by disability justice activists, but how it is understood and enacted within their collectives. On the contrary, their understanding of interdependency and dependency, they assert, was rooted in and emerged from their learning of disability justice activism.

Dependency is understood as messily transgressing and leaking through time-space boundaries. Dependency was described during my interviews as a sticky, oozy, glue-like substance leaking out of our bodyminds, reaching out and sticking to others. It is not only what we each embody, but it simul-taneously and inherently exists between people to constantly blur the divide separating and containing each bodymind. Thus, dependency arises 24/7, whether it is met and responded to with care by collective members or not. It seems like as long as a body lives, it has dependency, which at times be-comes needs. Therefore, those I interviewed asserted that dependency is a more accurate way to represent disabled people's experiences. Insisting on highlighting and reclaiming the idiosyncratic dependency that disabled people embody and experience, they were wary of and even resisted diving into the universalist notion that "everyone is dependent." Although dependency is the truth and nature of all lives, it was also emphasized that "everyone is dependent *in different ways and degrees* [emphasis added]." Continuing the sentence, Dani asserted, "[Dependency] puts everybody in the same kind of positioning, knowing that everybody's got some shit different. It's like difference without separation." By illuminating the differences among us, they nod to the reality of ableist social context shaping and amplifying disabled people's dependency as unusual, non-normative, and a burden. Simultaneously, though, they refuse to flatten the unique experiences and bodyminds of disabled people and their lives. Many of the people I talked to began to name dependency as *crip wisdom*, the idea introduced by disability justice artist group Sins Invalid to emphasize the unique insights and wisdom that disabled, sick, Deaf, neurodiverse, and Mad people, and many others living with disabling conditions, nurture and put forward.[53]

Dani articulated dependency as desirable in the opening quote of this section, when they suggested:

> Sometimes we posit need as something you don't have, that you want to have. . . . We would say, "I can't walk," rather than, "I walk in half block spurts, and then I sit down on my walker." You know? I would prefer to think of "how can I *add* my walker to your march?" as opposed to "how did your march forget about my walker?"

Sam brought up the following:

> [Dependency is] something disabled people really show [to] the world, and it's one of our powers to show what the generative wealth of need and dependency is.

In fact, many described being entangled with each other in their messy dependencies as an unavoidable element of socializing and simply being friends with one another as disabled people. This unavoidability is especially strong in the given society, where people's needs for personal care attendance are rarely met by the state. To be friends or in an intimate care collective together in the current political climate, therefore, entails co-experiencing and co-struggling against ableist incidents happening at the intersection with other forms of social oppression. Depending on one another for care needs is a necessity for people to be in a shared space and time to interact and relate. Every member I talked to shared the desire for their care collectives to be about being entangled in a messy, hard, and scary space *together*, instead of expecting it to be exclusively clean, reciprocal, respectful, and comfortable all the time or letting others go through it alone. They were shifting the emphasis of their collectives toward sharing an abundance of dependent moments together—to struggle and find joy through one another. Ruby said,

> The thing I have learnt about interdependence in the care collectives is that it's not . . . a particularly easy thing to practice. . . . It's not all about harmony or balance. . . . It is very much being actually in the struggle. . . . There's times where people's different access needs and their personalities [rub against each other]. . . . There are opportunities for a lot of clash and conflict. But to create an interdependent society, an interdependent culture, an interdependent community, an interdependent family is [about being in] struggle to be in constant dialogue . . . and supporting one another. . . . It's a process.

Messy Dependency

I offer an idea of wildness and mess as possible strategies for forging
queer trajectories and states of being in a world that is bent
(so to speak) on cleaning up and taming unruly jungles and
wildernesses. . . . Mess opens up other stories that do not yield to
the calls for temperance, cleanliness, and measured behavior. Mess,
then, is not an impediment to living but a way of being in the
world.—Martin F. Manalansan iv, "Messy Mismeasures"

Being in conversations and tracing the narratives about care collective experiences with those who were part of them were our way of retracing and reaffirming that dependency is the fabric of care collectives and means of our being together. Dependency—alongside care needs and the desire to meet the needs that emerge from the fabric of dependency—was the root of why we came together in respective collectives, chose to co-struggle, and collectively committed to be in uncomfortable spaces of exploring and experimenting to meet our care needs and desires together. To live and care for each other by centering our dependency is messy, and mess is the ground they continue to nurture.

Mess, on one layer, is a reality of disabled people's lives as they survive and thrive in a society full of ableism and intersecting oppressions that pose constant obstacles to doing so. Acknowledging, relating, and reclaiming each other's dependencies and their messy nature and then co-navigating life through them is what disabled friends have been doing always and already, as members of care collectives have taught me. What I would like to capture here is, therefore, how the messy dependency that the collective members I interviewed were grappling with is a means of living together. Simultaneously, this collective endeavor is an enactment of a portal to re-imagine and transgress how society is set up, how care is structured, and how our everyday lives are constructed around the hegemonic enforcement of independence.

Critical anthropologist Martin F. Manalansan IV followed the lives of migrant queer people who navigate precarious living in New York City and theorized their living space. In the opening quote of this section and the following, Manalansan explains that messiness or being mismeasured is a fabulous rupture from which the radically queer and unruly future can emerge:

> Mismeasures are messy engagements that are performed in order to move, live, and survive. Mismeasures are those that thrive in spaces of the wild and the undomesticated. They are about impossible lives made livable through various fabulous and creative narratives that are spun and woven by minoritarian subjects. In other words, the failure or refusal to domesticate, clean up, temper, and tame the unpredictable and immeasurable lives of queer immigrants also contains a possible escape hatch or alternative from the strictures of oppressive evaluative frames, however temporary and momentary they may be. . . . "queer metrics" or the "mismeasurable" can become the basis for envisioning and forging possible futures. Wildness and mess are tactics that either go against or at least coexist with the modern normative inclination to clean, to temper, to count and be counted, to be visible, to be valued and to value any phenomena on the basis of standardized units and scales, and to refuse the con-comitant compulsion to clean, tame, and domesticate.[54]

The concepts of mess and mismeasure are developed against the backdrop of Western (neo)colonial and neoliberal politics, where measurement has been the crucial tool for control and oppression. To measure, in this context, means to clearly categorize individuals by reducing their complex person-hood and tempering their dynamic natures. To be messy is, therefore, si-multaneously a resistance against the neocolonial setup and a means to explore queer migrant futurity, as much as such transgression attracts the acute risk of being pushed out of state protection and services or put under excessive state surveillance and violence.[55]

Dependency is one way such a "mess" manifests and materializes in dis-ability communities. Disability communities' unique experiences and critical insights in dependency constitute crip wisdom, especially in contrast to how independence is hegemonic. Being measurable by neatly fitting into the state's image of docile, deserving disabled citizen is made a necessity for disabled people to receive public healthcare services or supplemental income, no matter how inadequate those services may be and how they are a medium for the state and industry to extend their control over disabled people's lives.[56] How care has been set up as well is based on such premises as how people's care needs, and hence dependency, are made neatly measurable, compartmentalizable, and quantifiable to be met by checkbox care tasks.

One thing that becomes increasingly clear is that dependency is way messier than how care is set up and deployed to contain and manage dependency in the U.S. public healthcare assemblage. To live and fully embrace interdependency and dependency in the status quo is more wild, complicated, and rich than collective members initially imagined. In care collectives, members began to question the ways that long-term care has been set up in the larger society, as they noticed how they were accustomed to structuring care in the normalized manner, which needed to be fundamentally disrupted. Messiness and the unruly and wild nature of dependency swamped how interdependency was translated and practiced in care collectives. At the time when those I interviewed were participating in care collectives, they were, therefore, in the middle of the collective engagement of trial and error to grasp our dependencies' messy transgressive nature, their overwhelming massiveness, and their potential. In reality, enacting collective care was full of uncomfortable messes, which members narrated as challenges. Such challenges are not a mere challenge but simultaneously a resistance against the neoliberal, quantified care that is meant to tame messy dependency. The challenges were the result of living against the forces of the status quo where care, care needs, and labor are normalized and standardized and opposite of how we were practicing care. We were, in other words, in the middle of adjusting our imagination to rethink and embrace our dependencies together and through care.

Attempts and efforts to live a more disability-centric life through interdependent care collectives, against the current of the status quo, are destined to be a mess. Although the idea and practice of interdependency and messy dependency are distinguished in the preceding sections, I see all the challenges and desires that those care collective members faced as examples and snapshots of them enacting messy dependency. Interdependency is an integral part of messy dependency and vice versa as I understand it. In practicing interdependency, collective members have been endeavoring together to connect to their bodyminds to acknowledge what they need, to learn how to ask for help, and to come to a collective understanding of dependencies as more massive than how the care structure is framed and thus more transgressive of personal boundaries than they had expected. Interdependency, after all, is community wisdom and a principle of disability justice that has lifted up many lives (including mine), and it is certainly not ready to be simply dismissed or replaced by another idea like messy dependency. Thus, I argue that both claims of interdependency and messy dependency are rooted in the desire to put forward more disability-centered ways to live and connect with one another, and to reimagine how society can be set up and how we can live without leaving anyone behind in unwanted isolation. The collective commitment to explore interdependency as well as the desire for messy dependency are part of one journey to reclaim the dependencies we each embody and to turn such experiences and insights not into shameful things to hide and fix but into crip wisdom.[57]

Crip wisdom on in/ter/dependency certainly includes disability communities' critical analyses of how their dependencies are partly socially constructed and amplified. The U.S. disability rights movements continue to assert how the dependency of disabled people is (1) the result of an inaccessible and exclusionary society that forces disabled people to rely on others to conduct their daily living, and (2) weaponized to justify and further enforce violent ableist treatments that disabled people face.[58] Building on this critical wisdom, disability justice activists have further asserted that everyone is dependent by explaining that independence is myth. Further, disability justice activists' embracing of interdependency is a move to illuminate crip wisdom to redefine and reinterpret the larger society—that everyone depends on others.[59]

My contribution to this crip wisdom on in/ter/dependency with messy dependency is regarding how those I talked to *desired* to be entangled in each other's messy dependency. They are reclaiming dependency not as negative, something to avoid, or to universalize, but as the rich and unique wisdom and even resource that disability communities hold and can show to the world. Sam described need and dependency as the community's generative wealth. Dani offered an example by asking how their walker and hence disability and dependency on others (including assistive devices) can add to and further enrich the protest march, while such elements are often automatically thought of as a hindrance. Instead, they asserted that it is a way to apply queer and crip politics on desiring to their dependencies.[60] Additionally, such a shift and foreground of dependency inherently entails resistance. Acknowledging and embracing their dependency as a messy, unruly, and wild element that transgresses boundaries, time/space borders, rationality, and logics dovetails with a move toward transgressing the mundane custom of categorizing and de/valuing disabled people against the measurement of independence. Dependency leaks everywhere, every time, and defies the independence-based situating of people into the human-dehuman spectrum.

The root of how these care collective members came to articulate challenges and yearn to rethink and reclaim dependency was in asserting people's value regardless of their abilities and capacities to contribute to the collectives. One of the challenges continuously manifested in care collectives was resistance toward the idea of interdependency being the new measure to assess collective members, based on their capacity, ability, and productivity to work toward the reciprocal care practices or to make their relationships harmonious and without conflict. It is a collective challenge to promise to offer care regardless of a person's productivity, capacity, ability, and likability. Another promise is to keep expanding collectives to make the circle of care bigger. Members I talked to shared their collectives' efforts to refrain from forcing someone to engage in care tasks but instead to work on expanding the collective to enlarge its entanglement. They also continue to work not to hold care hostage when a member "acts out" but to provide care while engaging in collective accountability and healing. Ultimately, to collectively embrace our own and each other's messy dependency is to make sure to not leave anyone in (unwanted) isolation and reimagine ways to relate with one another by centering our dependencies.[61]

State Responsibility and a Silver Lining

I have tried having my access [care] needs met in a caregiving collective where disabled queer friends of color and our allies tried to provide mutual aid to each other, out of a spirit of creating a system outside of the state, and in order to practice what we thought disability justice meant. The reality is that I need at least fifteen hours of attendant support a day, and my level of access needs is too high for unpaid people to provide consistently and reliably. The difference in vulnerability and power also can create an environment where abuse can happen very easily. I think the caregiving collective model is something to keep experimenting with and working on. And I also know my life depends on Medicaid funded attendant services and that a caregiving collective will never be enough to keep me out of a nursing home.—Stacey Milbern, "Reflections as Congress Debates Our Futures"

Stacey Park Milbern, a leading disability justice activist who recently became our ancestor, reflected on the interdependent care collective she was part of and articulated its limits that she experienced.[62] As much as she underlined the significance of interdependent care collectives, she also pointed out the complex reality that care needs can involve more than what a small group of people can meet satisfyingly. Milbern's perspective suggests that it takes lots of people power to compensate for the inaccessible and exclusionary ableist setups in order for disabled people to navigate them and also to meet different degrees of care needs that other collective members embody. In the reality where collective members tend to engage in care circulation while they attend to other competing responsibilities, an expansive collective is required to meet all care needs satisfyingly. Such expanding of collective simultaneously comes with and requires significant coordination and communication in order to balance the need to meet the care tasks, the safety of all who are involved, and the circulation of care for all who are part of it without anyone feeling the urge to tame, minimize, or put aside their dependencies and care needs. Medicaid and other forms of structural care are developed in the first place as a way to integrate care needs and responsibility into the fabric of society, which is, thus, what came to be turned into the business opportunities of the care industrial complex and far from social responsibility shared by people equally and compensated accordingly.

As Milbern argued, it is crucial to continue fighting for the improvement or even fundamental abolition of existing care structures to dream and rebuild a more justice-based one.[63] She continuously asserted that we cannot let the government off the hook, particularly in the current U.S. context where the majority of disabled people's care needs, and especially those with lower incomes, are primarily met through public healthcare programs (e.g., Medicaid). Further, care collectives should never be used as an excuse for the government to downsize public healthcare programs or as a tactic to further enforce the individualization of care responsibility. Simultaneously, though, Patty Berne's articulation (at the beginning of this chapter) of how public healthcare programs are deployed as a mechanism to extend the state's control into the lives of disabled people is also crucial for consideration. State-sponsored care rarely meets the needs of disabled people (whether through their exclusion from public supports or the downsizing of services to those who are already enrolled).

Finally, beyond the public healthcare assemblage, what does it mean for people to collectively desire to be entangled in each other's messy dependency in the current sociopolitical context? In the neoliberal society, our lives (in quality and length) are said to be determined by our success or failure to access resources and to compete in the free market independently.[64] In this context, what does it mean for people to desire being entangled in each other's messy dependencies, which is the opposite of what neoliberal political society values and demands? It sounds like to have such desires means desiring collective failure in the political economy, where its consequences include constant debilitation or slow death. What would society be like if people prioritized being entangled in each other's dependencies and collectively failed to live up to neoliberal aspirations? A collective slow suicide, or a silver lining, or a portal to something else? I respond to these questions in the next chapter as I bring up and write about bed activism engaged by sick and disabled people of color. When sick and disabled people (of color) are too sick, fatigued, pained, depressed, debilitated, and incapable, whether and what can such a moment activate? Can there be more than slow death, constant debilitation, and disposability?

5

Bed Activism

When People of Color Are Sick, Disabled, and Incapable

[It is] important [to pay attention to] minuscule movements,
glimmers of hope, scraps of food, the interrupted dreams of freedom
found in those spaces deemed devoid of full human life. . . . Why are
formations of the oppressed deemed liberatory only if they resist
hegemony and/or exhibit the full agency of the oppressed? What
deformations of freedom become possible in the absence of resistance
and agency?
—**Alexander G. Weheliye,** *Habeas Viscus: Racializing Assemblages,*
Biopolitics, and Black Feminist Theories of the Human

At a dimly lit bar in Manhattan, I was hanging out with Trina Rose, a New York City–based disability artist, after a disability cultural event.[1] We were in the midst of a vibrant conversation, discussing various topics—from the event we had just attended and her artworks to disability studies. One particular moment from the evening has stayed with me until today. She had had a traumatic medical consult not long ago for knee pain she was experiencing. Her doctor was pressuring her into surgery (which she later found out was not needed), and her occupational therapy sessions were only making the pain worse. It was in the moment when she was filled with profound pain and surrounded by the ableism inflicted by the medical industrial complex that she turned to disability studies litera-ture. I remember her telling me that she began reading works in disability studies with a hope to distract herself from the pain. I pictured her grasping at straws (i.e., disability studies) to avoid drowning in the sea of pain and daily cruelty of the medical industrial complex. However, during her reading, she found out that many of the disability studies works to which she turned merely retraced ableist realities, including the violence of the medical industrial complex, which she had known intimately and was living in that moment. That scholarship further reminded her of the depressing able-ist realities that pushed her deeper into her desperation. That evening as we were talking, she wondered aloud if and where she could find disability studies which would help her to live.

It has been almost a decade since that conversation, and many details are blurry. Yet I continue asking myself how I can engage in disability studies that help us—disabled people—to live. *Bed activism* is the focus in this chapter. By exploring what bed activism is and the intervention it brings on multiple scales, I reiterate and conclude what I have discussed throughout this book. I write about bed activism here like a torch shining from a bed and showing us where to go or how to be. Being passed down from one bed dweller to another, bed activism, and its torchlike presence, helps people to keep on living together. With this book, I hope to join the forces of disability studies, culture, and activism that help us live our rich and complex lives.

Broadly, I define bed activism as resistance and visioning as well as bed-centered critique of social oppressions emerging from people's bed spaces—and particularly the beds of disabled and sick people. It encompasses both the active and inactive moments unfolding on beds. Examples of bed activism happening in more active moments include when people engage in social movement building on the internet by writing blog posts or op-eds, calling and writing to politicians, or practicing self-care and community care from their beds, whether by making arts or making love (as a form of care as well as a form of resistance, especially when their lovemaking is stigmatized). Bed activism happening in more inactive moments includes when people spend time on beds enduring pain, fatigue, depression, or other bodymind conditions. Many bed dwellers describe even those seemingly inactive moments as entailing transient bits of nurturing and informing aspects.[2] Those inactive moments, for example, give them more insight and knowledge into their bodyminds or the bodymind in general, how their well-being is shaped in relation to the surrounding world, and the power of dream and imagination to sustain oneself. Those continuous and at times indistinguishable moments of in/activeness taking place in beds thus powerfully inform bed activists' visions for what kind of society they want to live in as well as how to relate to and care for one another in sustainable ways—all of which contribute toward bed-born wisdom.[3] Additionally, I am including critical analyses of violence and oppressions taking place in bed spaces as part of the resistance, visioning, and wisdom of bed activism. Such analysis can be about confinement happening through beds at institutions including prisons, migrant detention centers, psychiatric and other hospitals, and residential institutions for people with disabilities; beds as a symbol to encompass domesticity and domestic violence, which could take place on beds and anywhere read as private; or the ways in which beds are manufactured and discarded, and (exploitative) labor and environmental injustices that may accompany the process.

By bed activism and activists, therefore, I am not referring to *anyone's* time spent in bed (i.e., the CEO of a megacorporation spending days in bed, while his corporation exploits workers by making them work nonstop). Instead, by claiming that my focus is analysis, resistance, and vision emerging in beds, I highlight bed time spent by those whose oppressions and marginalization as well as their transformative visions are deeply tied to bed; and I call any form of knowledge, wisdom, dream, and care being nurtured in their beds as bed activism. They could be disabled, sick, chronically pained, debilitated, dying people who find their beds to be a space of safety and a holder and witnesser of their daily experiences. They could be (disabled) people who are incarcerated and whose lives intimately center on beds. Their lives may also be commodified based on a number of beds their fleshes occupy.[4] They could be (disabled) women and gender-nonconforming femme people who find beds to be a symbol of domestic violence and restrictiveness of domesticity. They could be people who are overworked to produce beds for affluent people and nations, or people who are becoming disabled, as discarded beds from affluent nations and neighborhoods are trashed in their neighborhoods and exacerbating environmental injustice. And they may be these people who are simultaneously activating beds as a site of pleasure, desire, intimacy, un/rest, dream, privacy, love, and much more in the middle of surrounding violence.

Bed activism or bed life has been written about and discussed by sick and disabled people over time.[5] Sometimes it is called crip bed time, or sick life, or sometimes the experiences are embodied and lived without a name. I am using the term *bed activism* to address all of these, as well as the time spent not only in bed, but also on the couch, in the bathtub, on the sidewalk, or in a subway seat, as sick and disabled people rest there and shift the space into more than a resting space and instead a space of connecting, dreaming, nurturing, struggling and resisting, loving, and much, much more (as much as such space is saturated with intersecting social oppressions and violence, which I touch on in the following sections). Bed activism offers a liminary space that nurtures crip wisdom emerging in the middle of pain, fear, anger, and oppression as well as love, joy, and peacefulness—a mixture of all of them emerging and occupying beds. And in the term *crip wisdom*, I am including unique wisdom emerging from the everyday lives of disabled, Mad, neurodiverse, Deaf, sick, injured, traumatized, dying, and debilitated people.[6]

I officially started writing about bed activism in the middle of the U.S. upsurge against the election of Donald Trump. It was a time when an ever-growing number of direct actions and other forms of physical protests visibly emerged across the nation. The sheer number of protests and energy taking over the nation was mesmerizing to say the least. It was also exhausting at the same time. It was overwhelming for those who do not have a wealth of energy to be present at those protests as much as they may have wished. Indeed, what was echoed across disability and other communities at the time was how the accessibility and inclusion of people coming from various backgrounds were not necessarily planned for or centered, as the urgency to act took priority.[7] In other words, urgency and the sense of crisis were repeatedly brought up as if they justify and excuse the exclusionary practices observed in some protests. This context made me ask who can occupy these direct-action protests and be present, heard, and valued? Who were imagined as activists and visionaries for the better world, when those protests were being organized? And, eventually, who is welcomed and included in the more-just world these protesters were fighting for and dreaming of?[8] The moments we occupy our beds, what they mean to each of us, and what they activate always drew my attention. Thus, my personal experiences of being excluded from some direct actions gave critical insights in terms of diversifying activism, while also I am granted much privilege to participate in yet other forms of activism. Initially, therefore, I turned to bed activism as a site to reimagine or expand social justice work and to illuminate bed-born wisdom as crucial insights that disability and sick (also neurodiverse, Mad, and more) communities can offer to larger social justice activist circles.

I believe that it is wisdom born out of the bed—which is often automatically unnoticed and considered valueless in mainstream society—that can give crucial analyses of and insights into the violence of the status quo as well as the normalization and hierarchization of protests and other activist work. It is a wisdom and gift that disability and sick communities can offer to the world. Additionally, writing about bed activism is crucial in order not to erase the lives igniting in beds, critical to uplifting fellow bed dwellers and their insights, and to keep us connected and alive together. How can we assert, then, bed activists' activism and vision as world-changing and world-making, when lying in beds is automatically dismissed as outside the purview of what are considered social change and revolutionary works? What are the ways to express and animate the nuances and richness of disabled and sick people's lives, when it is considered that there is rarely a sign of life because they do not fit in the normalized notion of liveliness and vitality? What are the unique social transformations that bed activism puts forward both in terms of *how* resistance is done (i.e., the process) and what is visionable? In other words, I am putting forward interventions that bed activism enables in relation to how activism is imagined and gets done, and also what we are capable of dreaming and envisioning that would not be possible without tapping into bed-born wisdom.

Contextualizing in the larger political arena, bed activism can be considered a by-product as well as an intervention into the capitalism that deeply shapes our lives. The neoliberal political economy, indeed, has come to fundamentally dictate our value system and virtues, determining what our aspirations, behaviors, and shames will be.[9] For example, we are expected to be productive either by laboring to contribute to capitalist wealth accumulation or by letting our oppressed and debilitated status become commodifiable and extractable.[10] This expectation draws a sharp divide between who is deemed useful, and thus valued, and who is not in the larger society. In other words, people's value to society is largely evaluated based on the time we spend *out* of bed by laboring for the capitalist and neoliberal economic system. Additionally, people, particularly from marginalized communities, are evaluated and exploited for their extractability and disposability. People—or more precisely their flesh—who fill up the beds of private institutions such as residential homes, migrant detention centers, or prisons, for example, are commodified for occupying beds.[11] In disability justice activist Leah Lakshmi Piepzna-Samarasinha's words, "Capitalism says that disabled, tired bodies that spend too much time in bed are useless. Anyone who cannot labor to create wealth for owners is useless. People are valued only for the wealth they labor to build for capitalism; crips are useless to capitalism."[12] And also, bed activists I have learned from and feature in this chapter include those who are in the spaces or cracks between those two commodification schemes, as they are sometimes exploited as workers, sometimes as the targets of care, rehabilitation, and other medical industrial complex mechanisms of debilitation economies, and sometimes ostracized from both.

Bed activism, in other words, is emerging from the margins or from outside of a productivity-centered social formation. It is a story hidden, ignored, shamed, and deeply interwoven with the dependencies and needs of sick and disabled people that are registered as *social burdens* in the hegemonic view. It is an antithesis to everything demanded and set up as a virtue in the capitalist worldview and the U.S. doctrine of independence. My motivation to write about bed activism precisely lies in its invisiblized, tabooed, and shamed nature. When I spend my time in bed for days or weeks for my neurological and stress-induced migraines and nausea, I am often in pain, panicking, and very lonely and sad for not living the life people expect or demand of me. As a migrant whose legal rights to stay in this nation have deeply hinged on my capacity to work, not working is not an option. Reading about how disabled and sick people, especially sick and disabled people of color, weave their rich lives from their beds was a revelation. It made me aware that my personal experience is political, and just knowing about the existence of others who are igniting, weaving, and living their bed stories from their beds made me feel less isolated and more connected, and helped me learn to be unapologetic for being who I am.[13]

Such a revelation is very personal, and it may seem minuscule compared to general perceptions of activism for social change.[14] Whereas direct action, for example, operates by centering the power of the masses to directly confront and distract the establishment, the impact of bed activism I am illuminating here seems subtle. The bed activists I feature in this chapter use the methods of art and storytelling, and their objectives seem to involve acknowledging and valuing each other's existence and putting forth the wisdom, visions, and creative imaginations bubbling from bed to bed. Bed activism's effects entail, but are not limited to, forging connections and relationships among those who strive to survive and thrive in their beds, and confirmation that the personal is indeed crucial and political.

Bed activism is constantly growing and extending its synapses, whether in person; through blogs, YouTube videos, and social network sites; or in dreams, stories, and imaginations. Therefore, this chapter covers merely one aspect of bed activism. I will not, for instance, conduct in-depth and expansive analyses of confinement and other violence taking place in beds, although it is a crucial topic that scholars and activists are engaging in and needs far more analysis.[15] Instead, the focus of this chapter is how bed activists put forward bed dwellers' existence itself as the resistance, and how bed activists offer unique insights against the backdrop of how independence undergirds hegemonic society and many mainstream activists' efforts. Also asserted is the pulse of collectivity that is an undercurrent to bed activism, as people relate in various ways from emails to meeting in their dreams. Such relationality and collectivity illuminate the reality that rich lives continue while bed dwellers stay in bed because of the constant debilitation inflicted by the violent status quo and otherwise. In terms of resistance, bed activism shows a different paradigm with which to engage in resistance and visioning for social change, whether via embodying it or through the subtle and nuanced ways it relationally activates one bed dweller and another. Using the key theories I have introduced throughout this book as the backdrop, I will demonstrate unique contributions that bed activism makes. Therefore, what follows is structured into sections to zoom into different aspects of bed activism by weaving them with summaries of chapters covered in this book in a similar format to a conclusion chapter, instead of using more firm structures observable in other chapters.

To unfold bed activism, I am relying on the words and artworks of sick and disabled cultural workers who spin and weave their art from their beds based on their crip (and also queer, people of color, poor and working class, migrant, among other) wisdom in the last decade and so. Johanna Hedva, through their individual and collective works, contemplated the activism afforded to sick people. Challenging how politics are understood or defined as taking place in *public*, they carve space to archive sick people's resistance and visioning with "Sick Woman Theory."[16] Leah Lakshmi Piepzna-Samaransinha, in her blog post, then chapter "So Much Time Spent in Bed:

A Letter to Gloria Anzaldúa on Chronic Illness, Coatlicue, and Creativity," engaged in conversations with queer Chicana writer and activist Gloria Anzaldúa in her bed and in her dream to explore what it is like for queer people of color to experience impairments and claim disability while living as artists.[17] Lastly, in her book *Kindling: Writings on the Body*, Aurora Levins Morales traced the historical background of environmental injustices inflicted by the United States on Puerto Rico that induced many of her disabilities and the sickness she lives with today.[18] She leads a revolution from her bed by teaching us that visions and maps for the revolution are already written in our bodies. All of these artworks and writings, thus, deeply reflect the interacting disability, sick, and Mad wisdom as well as queer, race- and ethnicity-rooted, migrant, poor and working-class communities' rich insights. Although this chapter is woven with the words of these particular cultural worker-activists, my thoughts are also shaped by the writings and artworks of Patty Berne and other Sins Invalid artists, Stacey Park Milbern, Susan Wendell, Ellen Samuels, Jennifer Brea, Carolyn Lazard, and Park McArthur, who have illuminated the realities of living with pain and pleasure, boredom and desire—all while occupying their beds.[19]

I am intentionally putting forward the wisdom emerging at the intersection of critical disability and race thoughts in this chapter with a hope to add critical race, disability, and feminist nuances for one last time to the discussions on capacity and debility I engaged in this book. One way that ableism collides with racism, xenophobia, neocolonialism, cisheteropatriarchy, and other forms of intersecting violence is through labor extortion and by situating Black, Indigenous, people of color primarily as laborers who are expected—and coerced—to capacitate themselves to enter an often physically demanding, violent, and harsh labor force.[20] Ableism also manifests in a way so that their intellectual abilities and capacities are constantly dismissed or purposefully framed as inferior.[21] Racial (and also settler colonialist, neocolonialist, and ableist) capitalism has in turn further inscribed the capacity-based racialization of such populations. And yet conversely, one's incapability to enter the labor force is quickly interpreted as an individual responsibility based on abundant racial and migrant stereotypes (e.g., being seen as lazy) by dismissing the historical and sociopolitical structure of their dispossessions.[22] This capacity-based conceptualization of people of color sweepingly pushes aside the disabling conditions they live with at the state bureaucratic level or further marginalizes those living with more visible disabilities and complex care needs who are deemed unable to labor.[23] While I further tease out these points in earlier chapters, I focus on bed activism conducted by sick and disabled people of color in this chapter to complicate the notion of capacity and durability overtly attached to people of color and to reconceptualize and reimagine with nuance the moments of weakness and inactivity experienced by them as a form of resistance and visioning. As Piepzna-Samarasinha eloquently summarized, "How do we claim this body broken beautiful as not a liability but a gift? [O]ur bodies seen as tough, monster, angry, seductive, incompetent—how can we admit weakness, vulnerability, interdependence[?] . . . Queer people of color never say we are disabled if we have any choice about it. We come from families who believe in being tough, in sucking it up."[24] I am certainly not going to be able to address here in its entirety this complex and rich inquiry Piepzna-Samarasinha put forward. I am including this quotation, nonetheless, to depict the backdrop and context that directs me to feature the words and artworks of bed activists who center race and other intersecting identities and related social in/justice nuances in their critical and aesthetic works.

Finally, I cannot emphasize enough that bed life is not exclusively rosy all the time. It is often accompanied by excruciating pain, fatigue, depression, and other visceral bodymind conditions that are often considered negative and that people wish to live without. In other words, pain is real, fatigue can be frustrating, and depression may feel like a never-ending void. And social oppressions cause or exacerbate such conditions.[25] Furthermore, social oppression is a big reason why bed activists (are forced to) stay in bed. Not only are they lacking care assistants to support them to get out of their beds, the protests they want to join may not have any access measures. In short, bed activism is filed with an entanglement of pain, fatigue, depression, debilitation, dream, pleasure, anger, relief, love, humor, frustration, visioning, brain fog, and much more visceral experiences without a name.[26] Many bed activists, including those I feature in this chapter, explain that their words and art are woven together in the middle of entanglement. The following excerpt from Morales's writing shows the raw feelings and experiences pouring out of her bed and that she wrote for the first time after her stroke. Emphasizing the extra time it took her to write it, she wrote:

> nothing has prepared her
> to do nothing
> but be[27]

She continues to note the feeling of disorientation while she was unable to be in the writing-spirit and writing-self that were familiar to her before her stroke. Feminist disability studies scholar Susan Wendell also described her insights:

> Pain can interfere with imagination, perception, thinking, or feeling. Brain states caused by illnesses or the drugs used to treat them can dull the mind or create such restlessness of mind that focus,

even enough focus to read, may be impossible. . . . I have experienced all these forms of diminished consciousness at one time or another. Nevertheless, I have also found that it is possible to *be both very ill and intensely alive.* Consciousness can be more focused during illness, awareness heightened, even when the realm of action has shrunk to a room, a chair, or a bed.[28]

I recognize and explore in the following how bed activism has complex ties to the surrounding social oppressions that keep these activists in bed, and our bodyminds do embody various degrees of in/capacities and limits too. And yet I still push us not to let go of a glimpse of the joy, humor, dreams, and visions that nonetheless occupy our lives and bed time. I write to pass down the bed-born wisdom to other bed dwellers and further describe the importance of illuminating those moments.

Ontological Resistance

One way to begin untangling the resistive nature of bed activism is to tap into how it occupies the margins or even the cracks of the capitalist and neoliberal forces that exploit not only people's labor capacities but also debilities. More precisely, bed dwellers are opening up, exploring, and nurturing different paradigms or ways to be, rather than the value attached to economic-centric way of being. Bed activism is developed by bed dwellers who are incapable of being or refuse to be part of such a culture of values and disrupt and transgress it instead. The wisdom they assert from their beds, I argue, embodies critiques of such structural exploitation and offers a different value system based on people's existence, which I call *ontological resistance*, instead of on their abilities and capacities to live closely aligned with social norm and capitalist demands. Bed-born activism and wisdom, as I interpret it, is raw, embodied, and rooted in our being and not necessarily and solely in our doing. I offer the term to signal and emphasize *existence* or the nature of being itself as a key area. By using the term *ontological resistance*, I am echoing the statement "To exist is to resist," which appears on a poster by Sins Invalid.[29] Sins Invalid is a disability justice art performance-activism organization that has been a leading force of the disability justice movement. Here, they used this statement to show their supports for and solidarity with the ongoing struggles and resistances in Palestine.[30] The statement describes how people's existence itself, and the fact that they continue living within the oppressive society that wishes otherwise, is already resistance. This notion of "To exist is to resist" can certainly be materialized into a wide range of tangible ways to exercise resistance. Right above the statement on the Sins Invalid poster, for example, it states, "Disability

Justice means resisting together from solitary cells to open-air prisons" to note that solidarity is one way that such resistance materializes. The statement can be further expanded to mean that marginalized people's existence, visibility, analyses, vision, and dreams emerging from them are transformative, revolutionary, resistance, and resilience. I want to emphasize that existence and state of living always and already contain infinitive wild potentials and possibilities to enact resistance in a greater number of ways than political economy, for instance, can contain and appropriate. Thus, I am keeping its potential and possibility open here, without prescribing or providing examples, to resist allowing this potential to be quickly turned into potential to act and hence vacuumed into functionality- and productivity-based measurement and valuing.

Debilitation or incapability to work and capacity to labor are areas where the neoliberal synapses extend to commodify people's debilitation and capacitation. Care is a case in point. It has been deployed as a mechanism to maintain and further enforce social stratification. Through care, the neoliberal political economy exercises its tactics to use one's capacities and debilities as the unit of evaluation, manipulation, and exploitation. In this book, such moments of care injustice are unfolded—how care becomes the social setup where people, particularly in marginalized communities, are constantly debilitated and further marginalized.

As the privatization of medical welfare (i.e., Medicaid) accelerates, with managed care, reconfiguration of which disabled individuals are allowed to enroll and receive care intensifies based on their degree of debilitation and the financial values attached to their debilities. Under the neoliberal turn of welfare programs for single mothers and families in need (implementation of Temporary Assistance for Needy Families [TANF] under the Personal Responsibility and Work Opportunity Reconciliation Act of 1996) and the flourishing of the global neoliberal migration force that sped up care labor migration, care labor was further pushed to be the responsibility of lower-income women of color. These changes occurred in an overlapping period with the spread of Medicaid managed-care programs. Care has been the site where gendered, racial, neocolonial and migration, and crip economies interact, which is simultaneously intensified by neoliberal political forces to reevaluate and exploit those already marginalized populations into further marginalization.

How can we engage in resistance in this context? How can we engage in valuing each other as we are instead of what we can do (i.e., ability) or how much we can do (i.e., capacity), by resisting being commodified and profited from in the political economy? Especially in the context where the deployment of capacity- and debility-based evaluation and exploitation functions as a tactic to further enforce racism, cisheteropatriarchy, neocolonialism, and ableism, resistance and counternarratives by marginalized communities often followed similar tactics. In history, many of them have relied on showing their *true* productivity and contribution to the larger society as well as how they are *normal*, hence capable and not disabled.[31] How can we, then, engage in resistance that does not hinge on proving one's worth based on one's abilities and capacities?

Furthermore, one consequence of such exploitation in the current neoliberal public healthcare assemblage is how care is becoming necropolitical. The common theorization that occupies care studies—in both feminist and disability studies approaches—often assumes that either the care providers or care receivers exclusively take the sacrifices (e.g., harsh working conditions or low-quality care) on behalf of or in advancement of the other. In reality, and particularly under the public healthcare structure, I theorize that both those who are situated as care workers and care recipients experience mutual and constant debilitation under the name of care through overlapping and separate, and also mutually constructed, mechanisms. One is through harsh working conditions and the other is through low-quality and at times dangerous care, although this juxtaposition is not meant to equalize the experiences they are subjected to but to highlight the interwoven nature of the exploitative mechanisms they are implicated in (see Chapters 1 and 2 for more). The well-being of both populations is thus deprioritized under the shade of flourishing care economy—particularly that of the care industry complex, which subcontracts governmental projects.

On this backdrop, Johanna Hedva's work captures the powerful and nuanced forces emerging from beds.[32] From the standpoint, sit-point, or lie-down-point of being sick and in their bed, Hedva spun Sick Woman Theory.[33] Their writing on Sick Woman Theory began as they sat on their bed while being in pain and sick, listening to a Black Lives Matter march outside their window. They raised their fist in solidarity with the march and further drifted into contemplation on how to build solidarity and be part of the movement from their bed. In other words, they asked, "What modes of protest are afforded to sick people?"[34] Given the exclusionary sociopolitical context, they asserted that "Sick Woman Theory is for those who were never meant to survive but did . . . for those who are faced with their vulnerability and unbearable fragility, every day, and so have to fight for their experience to be not only honored, but first made visible."[35] I read their work as also asking what kind of protest would open up *because of and by centering* sick and disabled people who are insisting not only on surviving but on engaging in social change from their beds or on asserting that their survival is resistance and vision on its own. One example they point out is embracing the potential of liberation which emerges *because* they are outside of the state's care. They describe one objective of the Sick Woman Theory as "resist[ing] the notion that one needs to be legitimated by an institution, so that they can try to fix you. You don't need to be fixed, my queens—it's the world that needs the fixing."[36] For Hedva, liberational potential comes from a degree of release from the compulsory able-bodiedness and able-mindedness within which the medical industrial complex is invested and that are a tool of state control.[37]

Bed activism provides a window to rethink people's value beyond and against the commodification of their capacity and debility. Through developments in Sick Woman Theory, Hedva and other bed dwellers are turning their beds into a space where people can be valued as who they are, regardless of their productivity and financial value as assigned by the capitalist structure. Further, their intimate knowledge of being vulnerable, fragile, and precarious is recognized as a defiant alternative to the virtues of independence and individualism enforced in the United States and elsewhere. Hedva offers this alternative by honoring and prioritizing what their bodymind tells them and what they need. To put their well-being first is a defiant act, they argue, against the backdrop of how people's bodyminds are expected to modify themselves in order to fit into the neoliberal formation. Such modification can happen by aspiring them to become ideal citizens or turning them into subjects of exploitation and disposability, including being cured (unnecessarily) by the medical industrial complex or criminalized under the carceral logics, for instance.[38]

Disability justice activist and artist Leah Lakshmi Piepzna-Samarasinha has also emphasized how bed activism is simultaneously a critique of the productivity-based valuing of people and a materialization of other and more nurturing ways to be: "It is so difficult to write both what sucks about disability . . . and the joy of this body at the same time. The joy of this body comes from . . . the hard beauty of this life, built around all the time I must spend resting. The bed is the *nepantla place of opening*."[39] She continued,

[Bed time] is not logical, rational, clock time, punch-the-clock time. . . . Our bodies can't work like that, so they dream instead. Steal time for dreams, poetry, world changing, on that thin edge of barbwire. We dream a way through the teeth of the dragon of whitecapitalist-patriarchal amerika.[40]

More than a defiant space, bed activism also shows how people continue to weave rich lives, whereas the theorization of neoliberalism and social oppression often stops its analysis at stating how marginalized populations are put to debilitation or slow death.[41] What is rarely discussed or even acknowledged is how the lives of those who are constantly debilitated by the current neoliberal social oppressions continue on. Both Hedva's and

Piepzna-Samarasinha's (and others') writings hold layered realities including painful portrayals of the cruel consequences of living outside of the state's care or without the benefits of conforming to capitalist demands, and acknowledging how state supports (e.g., Medicaid) are crucial and needed for the survival of many disabled and sick people. Among these layers, they also capture the rich and colorful lives emerging from beds and the ambiguity that a bed holds.

One of the wisdoms of disability communities and studies is, I believe, acknowledging and honoring the complex and rich lives of those who are deemed as injured, disabled, sickened, maddened, or debilitated. To be categorized as such often reduces one's life to victimhood, if the life is ever recognized at all. It can even become *crucial* for people to be strategically categorized into debilitated victim status in order to pursue compensation as well as social change of the violent status quo that caused their debilitation in the first place. When their debilitation is the result and evidence of social oppressions interwoven in the public healthcare structure and otherwise, and when their pity- or anger-inducing victimhood and the corresponding affect are leveraged to mobilize politicians and incite the masses for social change activism, what does it mean to claim that their lives are rich and to shed light on how they are navigating lives full of community and other interpersonal care? It is a political question. Given this backdrop, how can we complicate lives that are put to constant debilitation? Can those who are debilitated experience joy and capacitating vibrancy, and live happily, and can they express and write about it if the social conditions they are subjected to, in fact, continually push them toward debilitation and slow death?

These are some of the questions I have endeavored to address throughout this book, and they are deeply implicated in bed activism as well. In reality, people's lives and their daily experiences are way more nuanced, contradictory, complex, and rich than a theory can contain or explain comprehensively—they are a mixture of debilitation and joy, and they are more than just slow death and co-capacitation. Care is an example. It surprises us by forging non-normative and unexpected connections and relations between people (and nonhuman beings too) in the middle of the violent status quo. It extends its synapses to glue person to person into sometimes painful and sometimes nurturing collectivity.

While acknowledging the hostile and violent status quo manifesting under the name of care, this book also sheds light on the lives continuing under this constant debilitation, through the affective collectivity forged in the daily engagements of long-term care by those who are situated as care recipients and workers. In other words, repetition of encounters and care practices can be a portal for developing and nurturing affective and haptic connections, although this kind of connection is often overlooked in theorization of human connection and relation. As much as care-based exploitation and oppression can be exercised in the hands of care partners (i.e., care workers and recipients) as structural injustices trickle down to the moments of their encounters, care can also offer a space to forge capacitative connections and interdependence between those situated as care workers and care recipients at the interpersonal level as they encounter and co-experience daily lives with and through one another. Those interpersonal connections, particularly within the industry-run U.S. neoliberal public healthcare assemblage, where personal relationship is prohibited, can disrupt the assemblage from within.

Similarly, bed activists I trace in this chapter and others describe beds as a dreaming place or *nepantla*, in-between-ness (to draw from Piepzna-Samarasinha's quote in the previous section) in the middle of intersecting oppressions. The examples I have offered so far in terms of what bed activism asserts and activates, including the shift in how we value time spent in bed, or stating that existence is resistance, do not necessarily entail the same kind of visibility and force that direct action, for example, is considered to assert. The impacts of bed activism may not be as readily measurable in a way that activism is often expected to be (e.g., bringing about policy change).[42] Also, while direct action—including how it attracts the media, and how it is reported by the media—can reach millions of people worldwide immediately, attention given to bed activism may differ in quantity and quality. And yet I refuse to dismiss the force and power of bed activism. As the phrase "To exist is to resist" demonstrates, keeping on living and existing entails power on its own, particularly against the context of necropolitics where certain marginalized populations are put to debilitation or slow, acute, and premature death.[43] And this does not mean to dismiss questions on quality or livability of life as surrounding environments do shape and impact them, especially under constant state violence and oppression. And yet what I am trying to assert here is that as oppression and marginalization materialize at various scales and temporalities, so should the fight to resist them and to live otherwise.

Bed activism or time spent in beds, in the theorization of necropolitical neoliberalism, can be interpreted as one way that slow death and debilitation manifest or the consequences of such. Bed activism, indeed, occupies a precarious and ambiguous space. Black studies scholar Alexander G. Weheliye has theorized that the profound violence that Black communities face disregards their humanity and agency by diminishing them to flesh. In the middle of theorizing cruel anti-Black racism, though, Weheliye has also gathered and illuminated many almost invisible moments of resistance that are rarely recognized as such, which is articulated in the quote that opened this chapter.[44] Articulating the narrow and limited way that resistance is recognized in the larger society, Weheliye has pushed us to reimagine resistance. Similarly, to call bed time as activism is profoundly an act of acknowledging that rich lives continue on in the bed. It is to recognize the agency of bed dwellers at moments when such agency rarely resembles what is recognized as agency in mainstream society or activism. It is to value the insights and visions bubbling from bed spaces even when the time in bed does not yield any product that is visible and tangible (e.g., writing a blog post), or even when people do not reflect on their inactive moments in bed to articulate them and turn them into a kind of crip wisdom that is comprehensible to others. The works of those artists whose works center the time they spend in bed are ways not to let those lives be overlooked and devalued. Writing and talking about bed activism is itself a way to visiblize and value the richness of time spent in bed, no matter how it may be registered as unproductive in the hegemonic society or unpleasant it may feel. It is a subtle gesture to defy the larger society's demands and expectations.

Subtle activism could deceive us with its magnitude. Knowing about bed activism and that there are people who value bed time could help others to live. To loop back to the opening story about Trina Rose in this chapter, what significance she may have had from reading disability studies scholarship that helps her to live. Such impact is not simply comparable to the impacts that larger social protests assert, and yet such impact is too important to let go. Indeed, what is asserted with the focus on rich lives continuing on in and out of beds in the middle of violent juncture of social oppressions and neoliberal political economy is that our lives and existence are more than what can be vacuumed into these dominant social formations. As much as I argued throughout this book that it is not only people's labor capacity but also debilitation that are exploited in the current political formation, our lives are more than that. We are part of multiple assemblages.[45] This means that one can be simultaneously part of the U.S. neoliberal public healthcare assemblage and part of assemblages of undercommons that are disrupting the former assemblage from within, which I further lay out in Chapter 3. To acknowledge that rich, nuanced, and complex lives continue on for those who are disabled, sickened, and debilitated is, therefore, to acknowledge them as more than objects to be compartmentalizable into oppressive socioeconomic forces.

Pulse of Collectivity

What the bed witnesses cannot be vacuumed clearly into a single notion of either debilitation or capacitation of the bed dweller. Bed is a nuanced space full of ambiguity. It yields unanticipated connections across time and space, whether in person or virtual, with living people, dead people, imaginary people, or more-than-human creatures and spirits—all taking place in beds. As much as bed activism seems like an individual endeavor on one level, it is deeply collective as well. One of the significances of bed activism as well as an objective of this activism I learned from the readings of the activist artists featured in this chapter is forging connections and relationships among bed dwellers from their beds. Connecting and relating can happen not only through being physically in the same space at the same time. As I brought up earlier, for me, readings the writings of bed dwellers and knowing that there are other disabled and sick people of color leading their rich lives from their beds made me feel less alone and more connected, while physically being in my bed alone. We connect, relate, and transgress isolation in multiple ways.

Bed is a space that is more than furniture that holds a body. It is a shifting space with so much happening, whether what emerges there may or may not be recognizable to others or easily explainable. Piepzna-Samarasinha, for example, described her bed as nepantla—"place of opening"— where she encounters Gloria Anzaldúa as the two connect across living/dead spaces and past/present time: "What I know is that Gloria Anzaldúa and I meet in bed. Not like you think. Maybe like you think. . . . It's sexy. And it's just life. Gloria and I meet in bed, in the chronically ill sickbed heaped with pillows where we both spend so much time."[46] Owning the time spent in bed, which is to reclaim crip and sick time, she continues on to describe that it is by reading Anzaldúa's work in her bed that she launched into conversations with Anzaldúa. She asked her for advice on how to be a disabled, queer artist of color and sustain a career in the highly demanding art world. By resting in a bed and defying "punch the clock time," she curved space and time to move between her dream, hardships of the art world, the words of Anzaldúa, and their conversations. She is, in other words, not alone in her bed, regardless of what an outsider may observe.

Disability justice activist and writer Aurora Levins Morales also wrote about forging relationships to situate oneself and one's experiences in the wider web of people who have gone through, who are going through, or who will go through bed activism, whether they are alive today, were alive a century ago, or have not yet been born. Bed activism is inherently collective, as the writings of Morales teach:

It is a political, . . . a deep, ecological sense of the web in which my flesh is caught, where the profound isolation of chronic illness forces me to extend my awareness beyond individual suffering, beyond the chronic pain of my muscles and joints. . . . All over the world women sick in bed are thinking about these things. . . . All over the world people whose bodies tremble and mutate, . . . who sweat and cramp and can't remember what they were saying, are making connections.[47]

The writings by Piepzna-Samarasinha and Morales signify that personal experiences of bed life are inherently political and collective. The internet is certainly one place where those with access to it connect actively with one another, such as the Sick Woman Theory Tumblr pages created by Hedva.[48] The distribution of writings and other artworks on bed activism, whether in blogs, letters, or published books, is another way connections are forged. It may be a conversation one has in their dream and knowing that bed activists exist that validates that we are not alone and connected to those bed dwellers in multiple ways—sensually, imaginably, physically, cognitively, and otherwise.

Visions Embodied within Sick and Disabled Bodyminds

Our bodyminds archive and accumulate wisdom about ourselves and our relationships to the surrounding world—yet another point I read through writings by bed activists. To rest in bed and to build bed activism often involve directing our gazes inward. Bed dwellers spread their roots inward, deeper within, while navigating the disabling and sickening world from their beds from time to time. In Aurora Levins Morales's words,

> what takes me to the core, to the place of new insight is listening with all my being to the voice of my flesh. And going in, going deeper, allowing the pain, there is the moment when I come clear: My body and your bodies make a map we can follow. . . . What our bodies, my mother's and yours and mine, *require in order to thrive, is what the world requires.* If there is a map to get there, it can be found in the atlas of our skin and bone and blood . . .[49]

Part of going deeper inward is to find clarity in our bodyminds, their needs and desires, when such voices or perspectives are often overshadowed by what society demands of us and how it disciplines our bodyminds.[50] It also involves accessing its intimate knowledge on the world to reunderstand and reexamine society through the perspectives of our bodyminds. Going inward can be about observing and reflecting on how different bodyminds are de/valued, how needs of certain bodyminds are trivialized or ignored, and how dependency is loathed. What our bodyminds need, to repeat Morales's words, is what the world needs. Bodyminds, these bed activists insist, are full of knowledge. A vision for social change and a dream of what kind of world we need in order to allow everyone to be part of it without leaving anyone behind are also already and always in our bodyminds, as Morales explained.

More specifically, the bodies Morales narrated repeatedly in her book are those of two Caribbean women—her mother and herself—living and having lived with cancer as well as environmental illness inflicted by the environmental injustices endured in Puerto Rico and inflicted under U.S. imperialism. She articulated in her book *Kindling: Writings on the Body* how such disabling and sickening conditions are not solely the embodied conditions of bodyminds but are at times constructed or exacerbated by violence inflicted within the sociopolitical context.[51] In other words, she wrote about debilitated bodyminds that occupy beds. She specifically centered such bodyminds and lives as a site that offers critical analyses of the violent status quo and history as well as visions of how to live in more sustainable and just ways to lift up one another: "When I can hold the truth of my flesh as one protesting voice in a multitude, a witness and opponent to what greed has wrought, awareness becomes bearable…. As my aching body and the storm-wracked body of the world tumble and spin around me, I enter the clear eye at the heart of all this wild uprooting, the place our sick bodies have brought us to . . . where transformation begins."[52] Crucially, though the vision expressed by these three activist-artists is articulated in words and book chapters and blogs, it does not need to be. I am sure that most bed-born wisdom is not translatable into words. Visions can emerge in our dreams, hallucinations, music that our bodyminds make, or gut feelings that may not be articulatable but only are feelable and haptic.

Bed activism is a portal where the knowledge archived in and emerging from bodyminds is centered as the starting point and core, not only to envision another world but also to reimagine and diversify resistance for social change. Throughout this book, I attended to the process of resistance making and the micro activism in the everyday lives of disabled people—particularly through the circulation of care. Messy dependency, and in particular disabled queer folks' shared desire to be entangled in each other's messy dependency, is a theme and area where I tease out this micro activism's macro potential. The notion of messy dependency reflects and illuminates the significance of reclaiming the dependencies' messiness as crip wisdom, while independence is a societal virtue and norm enforced for people to perform. Additionally, the idea of messy dependency is a reminder that it is messy and not-so-straightforward to live our vision, and particularly to resist, transgress, and change the force and flow of the status quo. It can be hard, scary, agitating, and uncomfortable at times to endeavor living our visions collectively. To situate the knowledge emerging from disabled and sick bodyminds and their beds to diversify activism is, for me, to endeavor to envision how care already is and should be further recognized as a foundation for social change—no matter the scale on which it is carried out.

One of the things this tracing of bed activism shows is that protests and resistance can emerge anywhere and anytime, across macro and micro levels. Direct action is often considered the hallmark of protest and activism, given that it involves a large number of people taking up a public space to deliver and demand their messages. Such a format is energized, broadcasted, or recognized as protest.[53] It is direct action that has brought changes and justice over the course of history. Records of the civil rights movement taught us at the visceral level the power of being present in public en masse and in front of armed police. Photos and stories of the disability rights movement expanded our imaginations and visions of who we are and what we can become.[54] The actual presence and visibility of many people in a public space has its own power.

Disability rights activist communities have historically worked to make direct action accessible and inclusive to diverse groups of people. Many activists and scholars have pointed out how (mutual) care has been always present and instrumental to enable such direct action, though it is often overlooked.[55] The "Save the Medicaid" rally I opened Chapter 1 with depicts how accessibility is integrated and centered in the rally organized by disability communities in solidarity with other communities. It had a Communication Access Realtime Translation (CART) captioner and American Sign Language interpreters, and it was organized in a wheelchair-accessible space. Simultaneously, multiple interpersonal and spontaneous care webs at the rally site emerged so that all the participants could be together at the space. Additional access measures could include having quiet resting space for those who are overwhelmed by the protest to take a break, chairs for people to sit down, on-site care supporters to attend to rally participants for their spontaneous care needs, a healing justice team for those who are experiencing extra vulnerability due to the presence of police, and earplugs to mitigate the overwhelming noise from speakers.[56] How about digital participation for those who live far away or those who cannot be in the middle of the city because of its pollution? How can we expand and increase virtual and other entry points to such protests? What would meaningful participation and access be like for those who cannot be there in person because they are incarcerated, whether at prisons, detention centers, or mass residential institutions for disabled people? How about sick and disabled people who are experiencing pain, fatigue, depression, or other bodymind conditions and cannot participate in protests in person or even digitally at the moment, or have no access to people who can assist them to get out of bed and onto the streets? Also, care workers who attend sick and disabled people cannot drop their duties spontaneously to join protests. Not only the material conditions of protest but also the temporality of urgency and expectations for speedy turnaround shape the norm of protests. Many cannot join because they cannot take time off from their work last minute or have no time off at all. For others, keeping up with the speed of a march, for example, is simply not an option, especially for many disabled and sick people. Such urgency and speedy turnaround also often means a nonstop work schedule for protest organizers—which can compromise the sustainability of the activism, including the well-being of organizers. Johanna Hedva contemplated this in/visibility in activist spaces, asking: "who is allowed in to the public space, . . . *who's in charge* of the public. . . . *who's in charge of who gets in*. . . . [W]e must contend with the fact that many whom these protests are for, are not able to participate in them—which means they are not able to be visible as political activists."[57]

Simultaneously, protests are constructed through countless moments of micro resistance and visioning as well.[58] Disability activism and studies offer expertise regarding recognizing and illuminating such moments. What I am putting forward with bed activism, then, follows in the footsteps or wheel traces of disability activists' and scholars' strategies to insert a critical disability twist into how we imagine and engage in the notion of participation.[59] One reason I turned to bed activism is how it shows a fundamentally different paradigm approach to protests. To quote Hedva: "Sick Woman Theory is an insistence that most modes of political protest are *internalized, lived, embodied, suffering, and no doubt invisible*."[60] Here, Hedva has reiterated what other bed activists have also asserted: that activism, development of vision, and other-world-making take place beyond public space, as protests are often imagined to be. Instead, they argue that protests are embodied and hence not necessarily visible. They are woven through our existences. Also, by stating that vulnerability is the fundamental truth of bodyminds, Hedva demands that the surrounding society be re-formed by centering the vulnerable nature of one another. Bed-born wisdom and vision for the world, therefore, must begin with the vulnerability of our bodyminds and their dependency on one another.[61] The map is drawn through connections among ourselves that are tied with our care for one another. Our existences— regardless of capacity and ability—are the compasses directing us where we need to go, the *nepantla*, the opening space and emerging point. What if we start activism and protest from the place of dependencies and out of care for one another? How might our demand change, if we truly value one another based on our existence and not based on our ability to use big words and jargon? Who can be visible and present then, and whose insights and visions born out of their bodyminds are taken seriously?

Conclusion

As much as my wild dream and messy writings on bed activism are nowhere near concludable, I write bed activism as a disability strategy in the middle of the neoliberal political economy. It is an intervention to reimagine our lives by centering our needs and dependencies.

This is not to say that bed life is always revolutionary and pleasant. As I stated in the introduction to this chapter, bed is also a site where oppressions manifest and materialize. It is a site of multiplicity. Many are tied to bed (literally and figuratively) and bed becomes a site for the financialization of people.[62] People are forced onto bed under the carceral archipelago, whether at prisons, detention centers, psychiatric hospitals, or institutions for people with intellectual and developmental disabilities as well as for senior people.[63] How people have different access to beds as well is a sign of who are valued or devalued (e.g., the divide between those who have access to hospital beds to receive quality medical care and those who do not).[64]

And yet, bed time is more than that too. It is not singularly or exclusively a space of oppression or resistance. Therefore, in this chapter I spotlight the one layer of complex bed life by highlighting the reality that rich lives continue on within the context of the status quo, which too often means constant debilitation to many. Bed observes so many struggles and injustices, and it is critical to untangle it and recognize it. Similarly, it is also injustice to overlook resistance and visioning emerging from beds, as micro as they may be, in the middle of oppression. Thus, to illuminate the potentials of bed time—bed activism—is only an opening to critically contemplate the lives circulating around, in, and through beds that need to continue to be told.

Bed activism entails the potential to offer a space to vision a world where needs are considered sacred and dependencies are desired and considered *generative*, as they bring people together to be entangled with each other.[65] As much as bed activism can be read as a critique of the current violent status quo or even some of the mainstream activism I have witnessed since the U.S. election in 2016, bed activism is also a way to open up our imagination and diversify what is legitimated and normalized as a valid and effective protest. It is an activism that entails different methods, objectives, effects, and affects. It is a way to rethink activism as happening in an "internalized, lived, [and] embodied" manner, to reiterate Hedva's words.

Bed activism is a crip middle finger to all the forces that establish the boundaries between those who are recognized as the *useful disabled* and those as the *unuseful*. It is a way for people to connect and possibly be entangled in one another's bed life, while the larger society dismisses them as disposable and burdensome, and yet to continue weaving their lives together to make them as colorful as they can be. Certainly, on the one hand, my descriptions of bed activism can be read as dreamy, unrealistic, or too abstract. I believe, though, on the other hand, that knowing that our bed times entail collective, shared, and nurturing aspects; knowing that there are people sharing and shaping bed lives with you; and believing that you are worthy as you are can help us to live—to return to the conversation I had with Trina Rose regarding a disability studies that would help us to live, with which I opened this chapter.

Bed activism is about sharing and reinstating that the personal is political, particularly for sick and disabled people who cannot keeping up with (or refuse to keep up with) capitalist demands and thus are considered *disposable* or who may be trying to make a living in the political economy while simultaneously accumulating more impairments, fatigue, depression, and debilitative conditions. Finally, while my focus in this chapter was to think of bed activism and its significance from a more micro, personal, and interpersonal place, Hedva seems to have a grand view on the potentiality of bed activism: "The most anti-capitalist protest is to care for another and to care for yourself. . . . Because, once we are all ill and confined to the bed, . . . prioritizing the care and love of our sick, pained, expensive, sensitive, fantastic bodies, and there is no one left to go to work, perhaps then, finally, capitalism will screech to its much-needed, long-overdue, and motherfucking glorious halt."[66] In this quote, Hedva offered a glimpse of a dependency-centered world where people's messy dependencies are recognized, are taken seriously, and take center stage. Hedva has opened up our imagination to the possibility of people collectively prioritizing being entangled in each other's messy dependency, and not to leave anyone in isolation. What if we all reclaim our messy dependencies and prioritize our collective care? As much as Hedva's work often includes cautious notes on how difficult it is to *live* our vision, dream, and politics, this invitation for wild imagination opens us up to a glimpse of their bed activism life.

The significance of bed activism is not fully knowable or capturable because it is continuously unfolding. My focus is primarily on the significance of bed activism at a personal level—how it helps disabled individuals to live—and this significance cannot be measured neatly or reduced into micro or macro scales, as one's life is always and already micro and macro simultaneously, given that it is full of potential to interrupt and redirect the macro. Hedva's call to care for oneself and others as anticapitalist protest has captured this micro-cum-macro potential and significance of bed activism as well as the political intervention it asserts. The personal is, always and already, political, as I have traced regarding the concept of care throughout this book.

I have attempted to show how care complicates and also brings up crip-licious moments in our lives—particularly the lives of those whom inter-secting social oppressions and political economy constantly debilitate.[67] Care is commodified in the current political economy and situated as a modality for constant debilitation. It also brightens up our everyday lives by connecting people in unexpected ways. Through care, people's capacities and debilities are manipulated and exploited as well as regained and re-claimed collectively. We live in a time and space where many are put under this constant debilitation. Migrants are detained and dehumanized at the U.S.-Mexican border and elsewhere. White supremacists use guns to com-mit mass murder based on supremacist ideologies, while *psychiatric disabil-ity* is the term used to scapegoat this supremacist violent ideology and to reassert brutal sanist stereotypes of psychiatric disability. Anti-Black racism forces Black families to have difficult conversations with their children on what to do during an encounter with cops. Asian Americans are constantly attacked as if COVID were caused by them. Social welfare to support and uplift disabled people continuously disappoints. Environmental injustices are getting more dire, pushing marginalized populations further to take all the associated risks and losses. Indigenous communities are repeatedly on the front lines to continue attending to and protecting the earth. State-sponsored care is forever used as a tactic of state violence to divide people who matter and people who do not.

And yet care is a survival strategy, a visioning and enactment of other-world-making activated by marginalized and debilitated communities in the moment of impossibility. People are daring to care for one another in the careless world, whether from bed or elsewhere, by committing to be entangled in each other's messy dependencies.

Postscript

What about COVID?

finished writing this book before the COVID-19 global pandemic.[1] As the book manuscript was reviewed, I was repeatedly asked, "But what about COVID?" What about COVID. We are still deep in this COVID pandemic. I am too busy, too exhausted, and too focused on the collective survival of us all and have not had a chance to pause to feel or think about COVID—let along analyze it. As of May 2021 in the United States, vaccines has been (unequally) distributed to many, and the Centers for Disease Control (CDC) announced that people who are vaccinated can "resume activities that [they] are doing prior to the pandemic . . . without wearing a mask or staying 6 feet apart."[2]

We are, nonetheless, far from being over the pandemic (will we ever be?), as most of the world's population continues to live in close proximity to COVID and resist becoming the death toll. This includes the United States, certainly, which continues to be submerged in COVID-intensified and -caused inequality (e.g., being differently risked to contracting COVID or different in/access to medical care and vaccines). All I have been doing is making sure my family, friends, neighbors, students, community members, and strangers survive this pandemic—and then I get crushed from the exhaustion of surviving, and then I get up and survive again. It is like I have been going on and on in survival mode so that my emotions and despair of the reality will not catch up to me. What is written in this postscript is, therefore, disorganized, messy, and somewhat intimate notes. Recording messy realities as mess and scribbling all over the place the overwhelming thoughts and feelings that are part of living in an ableist society are all core processes of disability activism-, culture-, and scholarship-making and nurturing.[3] It is our resistance against the ableism that is infused in mainstream notions of *professionalism*—including the enforced standards of building knowledge in logical, rational, and/or autonomous ways. This oppressive world is disorienting by nature, and disorientation is the ground on which disabled people operate by coming together to be entangled in each other's dependency-rich life.[4]

How does approaching care as analysis (as a site of analysis and an analytical tool) provide an entry point to the question of "What about COVID?" On one hand, the COVID pandemic continues to intensify the existing social oppressions and divisions between who is meant to survive and who is made out to be disposable. The COVID pandemic is like a storm that intensifies and speeds up historically developed logics of oppression. Indeed, the COVID pandemic and its timeline should not be thought of as distinguishable from ongoing racism, xenophobia, and global (neocolonial) injustices against which communities came together to form movements such as Black Lives Matter, protests against anti–Asian American hate crimes, various forms of mutual aid emerging all over the world to care one another, and continuing uprisings against the occupation of Palestine.[5] The discrimination and inequality observable during the COVID pandemic (e.g., in/access to medical care) and these specific cases of violence (state-sanctioned and otherwise) are intertwined, overlapping, and also distinct ways that interlocking systems of oppression materialize and dictate our proximity to death. On the other hand, simultaneously, all the wisdom of disability and intersecting marginalized communities who are always and already surviving crisis after crisis without supports from the government, public, and private entities but with each other have been illuminated. People have been thirsty to adapt such wisdom, as they formed mutual-aid grocery runs for neighbors and learned to navigate their worlds from their bed spaces, without necessarily knowing and acknowledging the historical roots of these practices.[6]

COVID cannot be reduced to an apolitical biomedical disease that affects anyone and everyone equally. It has intensified and has been intertwined with and indistinguishably become sociopolitical matter where people are differently situated to bear COVID-related risks at the intersections of social oppressions and privileges they are granted. Who is risked living in closer proximity to COVID (or having COVID within them) or who is considered as a risk itself; who can keep social distance or be forced to be in close proximity with others; who is prioritized for medical care; who has access to personal protective equipment (PPE) and vaccines; who is historically and continues to be outside the purview of governmental responsibilities to care?

Care is one way to think through these provocations. What I wrote in this book is happening in front of you and me, to us, to our loved ones in a more explicit manner, so much so that we cannot look away. Necropolitical care is made bare and hence more visible, feelable, imaginable, and increasingly being lived at this moment. It is manifesting in more crystallized, more intense, hyperfast death (instead of slow death). Those who are situated as care workers and care recipients are situated (or forced) to live with or be risks by being in close contact at residential homes and other care facilities or during their daily long-term-care routines happening at their homes, while their vulnerability is simultaneously distinct and intertwined. Disabled people, who are often seen as homogeneous united communities, are differently risked with COVID depending on where they are located sociopolitically and geographically. Some are placed in crowded facilities including residential institutions, migrant detention centers, prisons, and psychiatric hospitals and are experiencing disproportionately higher chances of contracting COVID and becoming part of its death toll—and often forgotten. Another group of disabled people (especially those with white-collar jobs) are cynically noticing that all the accommodations to work from home (e.g., Zoom meetings) that they have been fighting for but have been constantly denied were magically implemented overnight, when nondisabled people needed them too to keep the economy going. And yet another set of disabled people continue working as essential workers or have lost their jobs (which is a lifeline, when government does not recognize their care needs or the meeting of their care needs as public duty and does not provide welfare supports).

Essential workers or carers for our most fundamental and basic needs are expected to risk their lives and well-being by showing up to work in person. Meanwhile their wages, work benefits, and access to PPE and how they are treated in society for being Amazon storage workers, grocery store employees, construction workers, agricultural workers, janitors at various institutions (e.g., hospitals, residential homes), and care attendants do not reflect the magnitude of the life-making work they do. They are situated (and forced) to capacitate themselves to labor for others' lives, while being designated with all risks as if their lives are disposable. This reality shows how care (as people are situated as the carers for our basic needs) is again instrumental to recognize how the line of who is to be cared for and who is (forced) to care is drawn. It demonstrates how care is used to make economically (and otherwise) marginalized people even more marginalized.

This analysis is intertwined with an examination of to whom care is available and what kind of care. During the COVID pandemic, care priority was drawn clearly in our faces and being broadcasted through press conferences of politicians—to whom will ventilators be allocated, and who will have access to hospital beds or any space at all in hospitals? Care rationing has been made visible as it specifies that, in the case of scarce medical supplies such as ventilators, people with disabilities (from those with intellectual and developmental disabilities that are considered *severe* to those with physical disabilities who need long-term care) will not be provided with lifesaving equipment.[7] There have been numerous stories about how the medical industrial complex withheld medicines for lupus to treat COVID, when there was misinformation that the medicine can shorten the course of COVID that has been proven wrong; meanwhile lupus is known to affect women of color more disproportionately and hence its research and treatment has historically been deprioritized.[8] While such an ableist eugenic pulse has been alive in discrete ways over the long term, the COVID pandemic brought it into the light.[9] Here, again, care becomes the measurement to see which people are valued and which people are not as they are differently situated in the spectrum of care priorities.

Additionally, such care analysis illuminates how the COVID pandemic shows that the U.S. obsession with independence and individual rights is never individual or independent but profoundly nested in collective responsibility and risk bearing—which is to talk about dependency. While many declared that not wearing a mask is exercising their right to individual freedom against governmental orders (or they never believed in COVID or took it seriously), what was lacking in their social imagination, or fundamentally disregarded, was that wearing a mask is not only about protecting the wearer but the people around them as well, because they may be carrying and spreading COVID asymptomatically. In other words, following CDC guidelines (i.e., wearing a mask, social distancing, and sanitizing one's hands) to keep safe from COVID is not enough, if others around you do not follow them as well. My safety deeply depends on you as much as yours depends on me. This is so, while risk was not equally distributed based on a person's work situation (e.g., being an essential worker), living conditions (e.g., living in closed confinement), and care needs (e.g., needing care workers to attend long-term-care needs). Thus, such conditions are deeply shaped by one's class, race, disability, gender, and migration status (among other factors), as I laid out throughout this book. Not only was risk borne or forced on people disproportionately, but also dependency on others to secure one's safety was experienced in varying degrees. For instance, disabled people engage in intimate long-term-care tasks with (different) care workers day to day, and their safety from COVID profoundly depends on the precautions that their care workers are able and willing to take, when not maintaining social distance (to engage in care) is a requirement to live. And when disabled and other people are forced to live in confining spaces—from prisons and migration detention centers to residential facilities for elderly and disabled people, among others—their safety is, again, deeply compromised or even violated and thus depends on the people around them. An individual's decision is not solely personal, since the collective society must live with the consequences, or as a collective dictate the consequences that the individual must face. At the same time, though, it is the collective of people (e.g., neighbors, friends, and strangers) that helps the individual to survive as well.

Crip wisdom or wisdom emerging from the daily lives of disabled, neurodiverse, sick, Mad, Deaf, and otherwise crip people has sustained our lives and taught us how to navigate the world from beds and other spaces that we call our homes. The already-set-up network that disability and other intersecting marginalized communities have developed and nurtured over time has allowed us to smoothly check in with one another to assess what is needed to survive in this pandemic together, to pass crucial information, and to circulate resources such as food, masks, and hand sanitizer. Their knowledge on how to avoid infection and boost immunity with basic household items we already have or can afford gave us tangible ways to create our own survival tools. And their long-term experience in navigating the world and transforming the status quo from their bed spaces gave us various entry points to continue fighting against life-taking social oppressions intensified by the pandemic.

Already set-up and running Facebook groups specifically for sick and disabled people, for instance, have been vital spaces for people of different locales not only to share information but also to continue forming nurturing relationships to sustain one another materially and emotionally. Such networks, for example, allowed people to come together to start a campaign, Crip Fund, to raise money from those who have it and to distribute it to trans, queer, poor and working-class, Black, Indigenous, and disabled people of color who need it.[10] Additionally, the existing networks allowed this information to circulate quickly to both raise and distribute funds. Such networks have been a way for people to check in with each other, create documents and spreadsheets (i.e., Google Docs and Google Sheets) based on what people need, and organize grocery runs and emotional check-ins in different locales. Some, like Disability Justice Culture Club, created survival bags with homemade hand sanitizer and face masks made with affordable items and household items that people already had.[11] Then they distributed them to people experiencing houselessness and others who needed them. People living with immunocompromising conditions for decades shared deep wisdom on which household food items like garlic help to keep our immunity boosted.[12] Still others shared their experiences on collective survival by explaining how to create mutual-aid groups.[13]

Disabled people—particularly trans, queer, gender-nonconforming, migrant, poor and working-class, Black, Indigenous, and disabled people of color—have profound expertise on how to navigate life collectively with what they already have or can make on their own and how to run the world from their kitchen, couch, bed, bathtub, or whatever they call their home. This was particularly true when they were ostracized from structures of care, whether set up by governments, families, or private entities. Their creative and caring ways to navigate their collective lives was evident at the height of the Black Lives Matter protests and revolutions, for instance. The COVID pandemic forced many to rethink how to change the world from various sites in additions to the streets—something that disability and sick communities (along with other marginalized communities) have always worked on.[14] "26 Ways to Be in the Struggle, beyond the Streets," written by activists from various communities, is one example; the booklet is full of ideas on how to make protests and revolutions accessible, inclusive, and sustainable and how to offer multiple entry points for people with various needs, desires, and world-changing visions.[15] Bed space has been a dream-making and life-making space to many disabled and sick people where bed-born wisdom is nurtured and bed activism is activated. This is true even though beds are also spaces of confinement or even spaces that many are denied access to (e.g., beds became scarce property at hospitals to which many did not have access).[16] These networks of homegrown knowledge and bed-born wisdom and activism are all examples of what can emerge when we come together by centering our vulnerabilities, needs, and dependencies on one another as sacred and generative wealth we each carry—the themes woven together in this book.[17]

Additionally, these examples of crip wisdom are coming out of disabled people's experiences of making world and living rich lives, while they are often situated outside of state protection and margins of capitalist investment and formation (or when state protection actually functions as surveillance and control). What I repeatedly observed during this pandemic is how so many disabled people demonstrated what I read as emotional immunity or shielding, while navigating their daily lives through pandemic anxiety and mess. They continuously have said that crises have been always and already part of their everyday realities of living in this ableist status quo without state supports. To loop us back to the introduction of this book, navigating care crises was not necessarily a unique event during Superstorm Sandy or the COVID pandemic but infused in the mundane everyday lives of those who are situated as care recipients and care workers. Much matter-of-factness and cynical humor has been exchanged within disability communities as we watched nondisabled people panic because of the discomfort of unknowing, without any tools and knowledge about how to navigate life during a pandemic. This certainly does not cancel out the number of deaths and COVID-intensified and -caused oppressions that disabled people faced. It simply shows the depth of crip wisdom of disabled people, which has been nurturing them way before the COVID pandemic started and enabled them to navigate their rich lives while simultaneously being embedded in the cruel sociopolitical formation that we call the status quo.

My thoughts are all over the place. The mess is the ground where disability communities operate as much as it is a symptom of being exhausted and being in survival mode for such a long time under the COVID pandemic. While my thoughts shared here are for those who are *living* during the COVID pandemic, I am also thinking about the deceased and how we are living with the dead and their spirits and ghosts. How do we circulate care with the dead? How do dead people continue to care for us? How do we celebrate and enrich the death and life of dead people? How are they continuously entangled and interdependent with us?

Surviving is exhausting, and it is in this exhaustion that we care, dream, and relate. Being disabled is not worse than death but the beginning of crip wisdom and entering into messy entanglements with each other's dependencies with care, while we come to crip wisdom from wildly different paths. It is by living that we explore this terrain. By living and existing, we already embody the potential to collectively realize other-world-making, enjoy crip-licious moments in the middle of hardship, and turn over the oppressive status quo which at the same time makes us not want to continue living in it. It is my hope that *Just Care* offers a glimpse of care that helps us live and want to live by collectively relating, dreaming, and visioning—so that one day we can together dream a vision that we currently do not know how to dream.

x,

A.

Notes

INTRODUCTION

1. In addition to the list of content warnings provided for this book, this chapter includes mentions of death due to power failure, care-based violence, armed conflict, and police brutality.

2. I use the term *care* instead of *assistance* and *attendance*, whose use has been advocated by the Independent Living Movement and more commonly used in disability communities. I further describe those terms and my choices later in this chapter under the section titled "Caring." Pseudonyms are used throughout the book to maintain confidentiality.

3. Smith, "The Institutional Bias."

4. I use the term *migrant* throughout this book to encompass both immigration and migration. My use of the term *migration* instead of immigration is intended to resist the political and historical drawing of national borders that lay ground for xenophobia and migration injustices.

5. Erdos, "Hurricane Sandy"; Wiley, "After Sandy."

6. Keller, "Mapping Hurricane Sandy's."

7. Daniel, "Who Died"; Keller, "Mapping Hurricane Sandy's."

8. Fine, *Caring Society?*; Flanders, "Can 'Caring across Generations'"; Folbre, *For Love and Money*; Tronto, *Caring Democracy*.

9. Fine, *Caring Society?*; Flanders, "Can 'Caring across Generations'"; Folbre, *For Love and Money*; Tronto, *Caring Democracy*.

10. Folbre, *For Love and Money*; Tronto, *Caring Democracy*.

11. Michener, *Fragmented Democracy*; Olson, *Politics of Medicaid*; Quadagno, "Transformation of Medicaid."

12. Glenn, *Forced to Care*; Guevarra, *Marketing Dreams*; Kelly, *Disability Politics*; Malatino, *Trans Care*; Michener, *Fragmented Democracy*; Nadasen, Mittelstadt, and Chappell, *Welfare in the United States*; Olson, *Politics of Medicaid*.

13. Fineman, *Autonomy Myth*; Kittay, *Love's Labor*; McKenzie, "Autonomy and Automatons"; Nedelsky, *Law's Relations*; Stoljar, "Informed Consent"; Spade, "Solidarity Not Charity."

14. Gossett, Stanley, and Burton, "Known Unknowns"; Piepzna-Samarasinha, *Care Work*; Spade, "Solidarity Not Charity."

15. Cohen and Jackson, "Ask a Feminist"; Gossett, Stanley, and Burton, "Known Unknowns"; Green, "Coronavirus"; Ferguson, *One-Dimensional Queer*; Milbern, "Reflections as Congress Debates"; Mingus, "Access Intimacy"; Nelson, *Body and Soul*; Park, Jimenez, and Hoekstra, "Decolonizing the US Health System"; Piepzna-Samarasinha, *Care Work*; Sins Invalid, *Skin, Tooth, and Bone*; Spade, "Solidarity Not Charity."

16. I use the term *bodymind* throughout this book, instead of thinking of body and mind separately. Here, I am following Margaret Price's conceptualization of bodymind to resist the idea of body as separate from mind, and advocate instead to think how they are interconnected and mutually constructive (Price, "Bodymind Problem").

17. The term *crip wisdom* has been developed and used during Sins Invalid's annual performance, *Birthing, Dying, Becoming Crip Wisdom*. The term is used widely in disability communities to signal wisdom emerging, being nurtured, and put forward by those who are disabled, sick, Mad, neurodiverse, Deaf, or traumatized, or have any other disabling conditions. See Sins Invalid, *Skin, Tooth, and Bone*; Piepzna-Samarasinha, *Care Work*.

18. Berne, "Disability Justice"; Sins Invalid, *Skin, Tooth, and Bone*. See also Mingus, "Access Intimacy"; Piepzna-Samarasinha, *Care Work*; Milbern, "Reflections as Congress Debates"; Piepzna-Samarasinha and Wong, *#StaceyTaughtUs*.

19. María Puig de la Bellacasa's *Matter of Care: Speculative Ethics in More Than Human Worlds* is one of the crucial texts to expand care scholarships beyond the realm of human-centered analyses. A widely cited definition of care by Berenice Fisher and Joan Tronto also expands the understanding of who is the actor of care or subjects of being cared for to nonhuman entities. Also see Fineman, *Autonomy Myth*; Kittay, *Love's Labor*; McKenzie, "Autonomy and Automatons"; Nedelsky, *Law's Relations*; Puig de la Bellacasa, *Matter of Care*; Stoljar, "Informed Consent"; and Tronto, *Moral Boundary*, in their theorization of care as inherently relational.

20. Sharpe, *In the Wake*, 139.

21. Tronto, *Moral Boundary*, 103.

22. See, for example, Milbern, "Reflections as Congress Debates"; Mingus, "Access Intimacy"; Piepzna-Samarasinha, *Care Work*; Sins Invalid, *Skin, Tooth, and Bone*.

23. Daly, "Care Policies," 34.

24. Kelly, *Disability Politics*; Thomas, *Sociologies of Disability*; Watson et al., "(Inter) dependence, Needs."

25. Fisher and Kang, "Reinventing Dirty Work"; Tronto, *Caring Democracy*.

26. Hayman, "Independent Living History"; Kelly, *Disability Politics*; Morris, *Independent Lives* and "Independent Living and Community Care"; Shakespeare, "Social Relations."

27. Kelly, *Disability Politics*, 29.

28. Glancing at care scholarship and even care-related activism, therefore, my initial observation highlighted the divide between how feminist and disability studies as well as feminist and disability rights movements engaged in the topic of care and associated care-based oppressions. Christine Kelly articulates this tension. Kelly describes "academic debates about care which is built on Independent Living critiques, and occur

most often and directly between disability scholars and activists on the one hand, and feminist care researchers aiming to revalue gendered forms of labour on the other. . . . The earliest and ongoing conversations between feminists and disability scholars (often also feminists) are characterized by silence on the part of the former, or hostility on both parts." Kelly, *Disability Politics*, 6–32; also see Thomas, *Sociologies of Disability*; Shakespeare, "Social Relations"; Watson et al., "(Inter)dependence, Needs."

29. This specific focus is observable in many activist works for just care too. It can be at the sites of historic Independent Living Movement and domestic workers' unionization work. Or at the height of domestic worker uprisings in the 2000s to demand basic rights for domestic workers, alongside with agricultural workers, who were historically excluded from the Department of Labor's fundamental labor protection policies. Such uprisings were met with vocalized and mobilized upsets and agitation of disability rights organizations, who feared that workers' basic rights such as paid sick days and compensation for overtime work under unincreased public healthcare budgets meant discontinuation of their long-term care in their own homes and reinstitutionalization. Even within such agitated moments and the history of aforementioned care-related activism, I would like to note that there have always been many disabled people who were in solidarity and fought alongside care workers, as well as care workers who joined disability rights movements. Or within the care justice movement frontier, there have been national campaigns such as Caring Across Generations, who "have been building a movement of all ages and backgrounds to transform the way we care." The campaign has been bringing together communities of domestic workers, senior people, and disabled people to rethink how care is practiced in the contemporary United States and to fight for more-just ways to engage in care. See Kelly, *Disability Politics*; Nadasen, *Household Workers Unite*; Caring Across Generations, "About."

30. Kittay, *Love's Labor*.

31. Erevelles, *Disability and Difference*. Also see Bailey and Mobley, "Work in the Intersections"; Fritsch, "Intimate Assemblages"; Glenn, *Forced to Care*; Kafer, *Feminist, Queer, Crip*; Kelly, *Disability Politics*; Kittay, *Love's Labor*; Schalk and Kim, "Integrating Race"; Piepzna-Samarasinha, *Care Work*.

32. I am building specifically on work by Nirmala Erevelles. Erevelles, *Disability and Difference*.

33. Folbre, *For Love and Money*.

34. Donovan, "Home Care Work"; Erevelles, *Disability and Difference*; Glenn, *Forced to Care*; Haley, *No Mercy Here*; Michener, *Fragmented Democracy*.

35. Duffy, *Making Care Count*; Folbre, *For Love and Money*; Glenn, *Forced to Care*; Meyer, *Care Work: Gender Labor*; Tronto, *Moral Boundary, Caring Democracy*, and "There Is an Alternative."

36. Bailey and Mobley, "Work in the Intersections"; Mitchell and Snyder, *Biopolitics of Disability*.

37. Bailey and Mobley, "Work in the Intersections"; Boris and Klein, *Caring for America*; Glenn, *Forced to Care*; Guevarra, *Marketing Dreams*; Haley, *No Mercy Here*; Nadasen, Mittelstadt, and Chappell, *Welfare in the United States*.

U.S. public healthcare programs such as Medicaid have inherently been the indicator of who is considered worthy of such social protections and who is not, though the protections they provide may not be of the desired quality and in fact may be disguised as state surveillance or at times violence. See Michener, *Fragmented Democracy*; Olson, *Politics of Medicaid*; Quadagno, "Transformation of Medicaid"; Sins Invalid, *Skin, Tooth, and Bone*.

Controversies over Medicaid expansion under the Affordable Care Act, particularly in the South, for example, highlight the role of white supremacy in determining whose care needs are prioritized as public matters and whose are turned into individual responsibility or a burden to society. Within these controversies, lower-income Black men are used as the scapegoat for strong opposition toward Medicaid expansion in Southern states, as their enrollment in public healthcare programs and their well-being are deemed not to matter and therefore to be unworthy of taxpayer money, which funds Medicaid. See Artiga, Stephens, and Lyons, "Advancing Opportunities"; Bouie, "Mississippi's Race."

38. While eligibility for such welfare, like Temporary Assistance for Needy Families, specifies that the support is for *families*, such welfare programs have historically targeted their supports more specifically for *single mothers*. Therefore, I use the term *single mothers* to describe the enrollees and beneficiaries of the welfare, though such programs may include fathers and other care givers. See Gordon, *Pitied but Not Entitled*; Nadasen, Mittelstadt, and Chappell, *Welfare in the United States*.

39. Fine, *Caring Society?*; Malatino, *Trans Care*; Piepzna-Samarasinha, *Care Work*; Manalansan, "Messy Mismeasures"; Tronto, *Moral Boundary*.

40. Aizura, "Communizing Care"; Gossett, Stanley, and Burton, "Known Unknowns"; Hoffman, *Hospital Time*; Malatino, "Tough Breaks" and *Trans Care*; Manalansan, "Messy Mismeasures."

41. Chang, *Disposable Domestics*; Cranford, *Home Care Fault Lines*; Erevelles, *Disability and Difference*; Flores-González et al., *Immigrant Women Workers*; Francisco-Menchavez, *Labor of Care*; Guevarra, *Marketing Dreams*; Parreñas, *Servants of Globalization*; Yeates, "Global Care Chains."

42. Under Medicaid, for example, non–U.S. citizen, migrant people are granted emergency care. This means that they need to be in life-threatening condition in order for the public healthcare supports to kick in. Additionally, there are many cases where those who sought emergency care supports are later funneled into medical deportation. See Park, Jimenez, and Hoekstra, "Decolonizing the US Health System."

43. Guevarra, *Marketing Dreams*; Vora, *Life Support*.

44. Narayan, "Colonialism and Its Others," 135.

45. Erevelles, *Disability and Difference*; Kelly, *Disability Politics*; Kittay, *Love's Labor*; Morris, "Independent Living"; Shakespeare, "Social Relations."

46. Berne, "Disability Justice"; Nishida, "Abuse"; Powers and Oschwald, *Violence and Abuse*.

47. Bailey and Mobley, "Work in the Intersections"; Miles, "Strong Black Women."

48. Fabricant and Fine, *Changing Politics*, 4.

49. See, for example, Brown, *Neo-Liberalism*; Foucault, *Society Must Be Defended*; Giroux, *Neoliberalism's War*; Harvey, *Brief History*.

50. Shaviro, "'Bitter Necessity'" [emphasis added].

51. Glenn, *Forced to Care*; Harvey, *Brief History*; Naidoo, "Entrenching International Inequality."

52. Goodley, Lawthom, and Runswick-Cole, "Dis/Ability and Austerity."

53. Harvey, *Brief History*, 65 [emphasis added].

54. *Mutual Aid: Building Solidarity during This Crisis (and the Next)* by Dean Spade highlights this point with examples from historical social change movements.

55. Nelson, *Body and Soul*.

56. See, for example, Gillett, *Grassroots History*; Gossett, Stanley, and Burton, "Known Unknowns"; Hoffman, *Hospital Time*; Spade, "Solidarity Not Charity."

57. Ferguson, *One-Dimensional Queer*; Gossett, Stanley, and Burton, "Known Unknowns"; Lewis, "Trans History," 57–90.
58. Cambiando Vidas, "Cambiando Vidas."
59. Park, Jimenez, and Hoekstra, "Decolonizing the US Health System"; also see Cambiando Vidas, "Cambiando Vidas."
60. Green, "Coronavirus"; McArthur and Zavitsanos, "Other Forms"; Milbern, "Reflections as Congress Debates"; Mingus, "Access Intimacy"; Piepzna-Samarasinha, *Care Work*; Sins Invalid, *Skin, Tooth, and Bone*.
61. I thank disability studies scholar Liat Ben-Moshe for pointing this out during our personal conversations.
62. Baker, "Seeing 'Black Lives Matter.'"
63. Pham, "Principles of Pride."
64. Organized Communities Against Deportations, "Campaigns."
65. See Chapter 4 of this book for this point.
66. Sins Invalid, *Skin, Tooth, and Bone*.
67. S. Margaret, personal communication, 2016; Piepzna-Samarasinha, *Care Work*. Furthermore, such activism and philosophy were always and already engaged in and enacted by disabled folks occupying multiple marginalized identities and communities without using the term *disability justice* (e.g., the decades-long activism by Leroy F. Moore Jr. to bring racial, class, and disability activism together; Moore, "Tearing Down").
68. Gossett, Stanley, and Burton, "Known Unknowns"; Milbern, "Reflections as Congress Debates"; Mingus, "Access Intimacy"; Nelson, *Body and Soul*; Park, Jimenez, and Hoekstra, "Decolonizing the US Health System"; Piepzna-Samarasinha, *Care Work*; Sins Invalid, *Skin, Tooth, and Bone*; Spade, "Solidarity Not Charity."
69. hooks, "Theory as Liberatory Practice"; Morales, "Genealogies of Empowerment," 26.
70. Morales, "Genealogies of Empowerment," 26.
71. See hooks, "Theory as Liberatory Practice"; Morales, "Genealogies of Empowerment," 26.
72. Espiritu, *Home Bound*; Mbembe, "Necropolitics" and *Necropolitics*; Berlant, "Slow Death"; Puar, "CODA" and *Right to Maim*; Lorde, *Sister Outsider*; Harney and Moten, *Undercommons*; Manalansan, "Messy Mismeasures"; Morales, *Kindling*; Piepzna-Samarasinha, *Care Work*; Hedva, "Sick Woman Theory."
73. Massumi, "Autonomy of Affect" and *Ontopower*.
74. Clough, "Affective Turn"; Deleuze and Guattari, *Anti-Oedipus*, *A Thousand Plateaus*; Fox, *Body*; Lara et al., "Affect and Subjectivity"; Livingston, *Debility and the Moral Imagination*; Massumi, *Politics of Affect*; Puar, *Right to Maim*; Spinoza, *Ethics*.
75. Miserandino, "Spoon Theory."
76. Deleuze, *Spinoza*, 48–49; see also Spinoza, *Ethics*, III, D3.
77. Greg and Gregory, "Inventory of Shimmers."
78. Fox, *Body*; Massumi, *Politics of Affect*; Puar, *Right to Maim*.
79. Massumi, *Pleasures of Philosophy*, xvi; *Politics of Affect*, 48, emphasis in the original; *Ontopower*, 4.
80. See Fritsch, "Gradations of Debility"; Livingston, *Debility and the Moral Imagination*; Puar, "CODA" and *Right to Maim*.
81. For example, see the special issue on "Affect, Subjectivity, and Politics" in *Subjectivity*'s 10th edition. Also see Million, "Felt Theory"; Ajo, Ben-Moshe, and Hilton, "Mad Futures"; Gorman, "Quagmires of Affect"; Chen, *Animacies*.

82. Ajo, Ben-Moshe, and Hilton, "Mad Futures"; Gorman, "Quagmires of Affect."
83. Gorman, "Quagmires of Affect."
84. Clough, "Affective Turn"; Fox, *Body*; Lara et al., "Affect and Subjectivity"; Massumi, *Politics of Affect*; Puar, *Right to Maim*; Zola, "Bringing Our Bodies."
85. See, for example, Ashley and Billies, "Effective Capacity"; Lara, "Wine's Time"; Lara et al., "Affect and Subjectivity"; Liebert, "Beside-the-Mind"; Liu, "Toward a Queer Psychology"; Nishida, "Relating through Differences."
86. See, for example, Brown, "Like Festering Wounds."
87. See, for example, Pickens, *Black Madness*; Silentmiaow, "In My Language."
88. See Erevelles, *Disability and Difference*; Baggs, "Holding Onto My Humanity"; Silentmiaow, "In My Language"; Sequenzia and Grace, *Typed Words Loud Voice*; also see Brown, Ashkenazy, and Onaiwu, *All the Weight*, for more on neurodiversity, intersectional ableism, and resistance in general.
89. See, for example, Baggs, "Holding Onto My Humanity"; Clare, *Brilliant Imperfection*; Goodley and Rapley, "How Do You Understand." Eli Clare (*Brilliant Imperfection*), among others, has addressed that this privileging of cognitive function has also been used within disability rights communities, as many with physical disabilities tactically highlight their cognitive competencies to argue for their worth and deservedness to take part in mainstream society.
90. Schalk, *Bodyminds Reimagined*.
91. Price, "Bodymind Problem."
92. See, for example, Brown, Ashkenazy, and Onaiwu, *All the Weight*; Sequenzia and Grace, *Typed Words Loud Voices*. Further, I believe that disability studies is an area that can further complicate and expand affect theory. Price's conceptualization of bodymind to denote the idea of body is separate from mind is one (Price, "Bodymind Problem"). Tanja Ajo, Liat Ben-Moshe, and Leon J. Hilton ("Mad Futures") organized a whole issue in *American Quarterly* to point out the overlap on topics that both affect theorists and Mad and disability studies scholars engage with, as much as the issue also articulates ableist and sanist notions embedded within scholarships written with affect theories (e.g., Verlinden, "On Affect Theory's Hidden Histories"). Spoon theory, which emerged from the daily experiences of living with the chronic illness and fatigue of lupus, is another area where disability community wisdom can offer critical analysis to the affect theory. See Miserandino, "Spoon Theory."
93. Miserandino, "Spoon Theory."
94. This is a quote from an interview of Eli Clare. See Fritsch, "Resisting Easy Answers."
95. See, for example, Bailey and Mobley, "Work in the Intersections"; Ben-Moshe, *Decarcerating Disability*; Erevelles, *Disability and Difference*; Lewis, "Ableism 2020"; Miles, "Strong Black Women"; Minich, "Enabling Whom?"; Puar, *Right to Maim*; Schalk and Kim, "Integrating Race."
96. Erevelles, *Disability and Difference*; Grech, "Disability, Poverty and Development"; Meekosha, "Decolonizing Disability"; Morales, *Kindling*; Puar, *Right to Maim*; Soldatic, "Transnational Sphere of Justice"; Soldatic and Grech, "Transnationalising Disability Studies."
97. Puar, *Right to Maim*, 65.
98. McArthur and Zavitsanos, "Other Forms of Conviviality," note 4.
99. See, for example, Brown, Ashkenazy, and Onaiwu, *All the Weight*; Gibson, "Grounding Movements"; Lewis, "Honoring Arnaldo Rios-Soto"; Moore, Gray-Garcia, and Thrower, "Black and Blue"; Sins Invalid, *Skin, Tooth, and Bone*.

100. Berne, "Disability Justice"; Sins Invalid, *Skin, Tooth, and Bone.*

101. Statistics show that more than half of those who are harmed or killed by police have some kind of disability including psychiatric disabilities (Sins Invalid, *Skin, Tooth, and Bone*). Also, many police officers regularly describe certain behaviors and attitudes that are read as disruptive, offensive, erratic, or "off" as the reason why they engaged in violent actions against civilians in order to "manage, control, and contain" them. Sometimes disability is named (e.g., "she is being mad") or implicated to justify their violence. It is as if disability at the intersection of one's race, gender, and sexuality (among other markers) warrant a person's killing. See Krip Hop Nation and 5th battalion ent., *Broken Bodies*; Lewis, "Honoring Arnaldo Rios-Soto"; Moore, Gray-Garcia, and Thrower, "Black and Blue"; Sins Invalid, *Skin, Tooth, and Bone*; Thrower and Moore, *Where Is Hope*; Altiraifi, "Grounding Movements"; Ben-Moshe, *Decarcerating Disability*; Ware, "Disabled: Not a Burden."

102. Altiraifi, "Grounding Movements"; Lewis, "Ableism 2020."

103. See, for example, Baynton, "Disability and the Justification."

104. Kim, *Curative Violence*; Milbern and Piepzna-Samarasinha, "Disability Justice Activists Look"; Nishida, "Understanding Political Development"; Piepzna-Samarasinha, *Care Work*; Sins Invalid, *Skin, Tooth, and Bone.*

105. Clare, *Brilliant Imperfection*, 26.

106. Metzl, *Protest Psychosis*; Nishida and Ostrove, "Power as Control"; Washington, *Medical Apartheid.*

107. Such a notion is certainly getting more complicated under the current neoliberal political economy, where disabled populations are commodified through various mechanisms (see Hughes, "Disabled People as Counterfeit Citizens"; Roulstone, "Personal Independence Payments"; McRuer, *Crip Times*). Also see Harney and Moten, *Undercommons.*

108. Here, my move to focus on the rich lives that continue on for those who are disabled, debilitated, or injured is certainly not a strategy to overlook, justify, or trivialize the violence inflicted in this oppressive status quo and throughout the history. Thus by "rich life," I am not arguing for a singular notion of life full of positivity, but acknowledging the nuanced, complex, and complicated everyday lives that are full of ambiguity and nonetheless continue on.

109. Piepzna-Samarasinha, *Care Work*; Sins Invalid, *Birthing, Dying.*

110. See, for example, Nishida, "Relating through Differences."

111. Kafer, *Feminist, Queer, Crip*; McRuer, *Crip Theory*; Sandahl, "Queering the Crip."

112. Thomas, *Sociologies of Disability.*

113. With the term *ableism*, I encompass *sanism* (hierarchy-making and de/valuing of people based on their psychiatric differences, whether perceived and diagnosed or otherwise, measured and constructed on ideas such as sanity, competency, and more); *audism* (hierarchy-making and de/valuing of people based on their auditory abilities and capacities, whether perceived and diagnosed or otherwise, that place supremacy on those who can hear in a socially standardized way); and *healthism* (excessive value and privilege attached to the state of being healthy and degrading those who are incapable [or perceived as incapable] of maintaining such status); and other forms of disability-related stigma that construct ability- and capacity-based supremacy and dispossession that negatively affects disabled people or those who are perceived as disabled. I use the term *ableism* with the recognition that it happens in dynamic interactions with other

forms of -isms (e.g., racism). See Sins Invalid, *Skin, Tooth, and Bone*; Fat Rose, "What Is Fat Rose?"; Stoll, "Fat Is a Social Justice Issue."

114. hooks, "Theory as Liberatory Practice"; Morales, "Genealogies of Empowerment."

115. How many participants researchers generally recruit is deeply shaped by the methodology they employ and disciplinary standards, and thus is an area of controversy. I conducted focus groups, individual interviews, and participant observations with these numbers of people because that was how many people could be recruited over the three-month recruitment period; also, the decision was rooted in my training in life story interview methods, theoretical and interdisciplinary work, and feminist disability studies. Care is a topic that is profoundly considered private and involves intimate layers of people's lives. Therefore, while I distributed flyers widely, talked to many gatekeepers in both disability and care worker circles, and volunteered at events hosted by care agencies to recruit people, I also felt that it was extremely important for me not to cross the line by talking to individuals to *convince* them to participate in this research. Instead, I communicated my intention to a group and waited to see if individuals would come talk to me and were curious to join this research project. Also, life story interviewing, theoretical and interdisciplinary approaches to scholarly works, and feminist and disability studies all taught me that an individual's story is personal *and* political and tells us so much about the larger society. My methodological approach to this research project is not one of positivist or even mainstream ways that constructivism is used where expectation often lies in having a certain number of participants or hours of interviews to find commonality. Instead, I treat each person's story as homemade theory, to use a term offered by Aurora Levins Morales, which shows us *one* aspect of how society shapes an individual's life and vice versa, similar to how academic-made theory interprets and explains one way to understand the topic under focus. See Morales, "Genealogies of Empowerment."

116. In comparison to general focus group research where researchers are instantly taken as the authority and *knower*, the focus groups I conducted had a more distinct sense of participants' urge to *teach* me. I reflect such atmospheres in the ways they talked to me and carried themselves. I assume that this is partially attributable to my subjectivity as a young-looking, feminine cis woman who migrated from Northeast Asia and who speaks English as her second language with an accent—all of these denote the (cultural) understanding of naivety, particularly in contrast to focus group participants who are older and who have lived in the United States for most if not all of their lifetime.

117. Conversations (i.e., focus groups and individual interviews) with those who receive and provide long-term care under Medicaid were recorded, transcribed, and analyzed with content analysis, which is a process I used to organize and group the transcriptions in order to understand key theses that those I talked to shared with me individually and collectively. When I hung out and pitched in with care tasks during participant observation, I also took notes during and after the time spent with care partners. Those notes are included throughout this book so that we can have shared scenes of care practices as I trace and theorize care. All of these recordings were done with the permission of those I talked to (and approved by the university institutional review board who checked the ethicality of this research). Also, all those I talked to and who contributed to this research were paid for their time and for consulting on this research with their expertise. See Braun and Clarke, "Using Thematic Analysis"; Patton, *Qualitative Research*.

118. Similar to the conversations I had in focus groups and individual interviews, those conversations were recorded, transcribed, and analyzed with the permissions of those I talked to (and approved by the university ethics board).

CHAPTER 1

1. In addition to the list of content warnings provided for this book, this chapter includes mentions of settler colonialism; imperialism; slavery; anti-Black sexism, racism, and criminalization; forced institutionalization; eugenics; and care-based violence including death.

2. Save Medicaid and other healthcare-related activism has been active since the beginning of the Trump administration in 2017 as the administration worked to repeal and replace the Patient Protection and Affordable Care Act (also known as Obamacare). This opening sketch illustrates the rally against the Medicaid cap introduced as part of the American Health Care Act to replace the Affordable Care Act. The cap would have limited the Medicaid funding that each state receives from the federal government (which is the main budget for Medicaid along with the funds from state governments) and would have gradually ended the Medicaid expansion that the Affordable Care Act enabled. This not only would have affected current beneficiaries who could have lost necessary medical and health care, but also would have closed doors to those who would need such supports in the near future. Forcing the cap would be absurd when senior citizens who require long-term care are only increasing drastically, and when the medical and healthcare needs of children and disabled people are certainly not going away. It is as if the safety net is shrinking for those who needs public health supports.

3. Wong, "My Medicaid, My Life," para. 2.

4. See, for example, Robinson, *Black Marxism*; Leong, "Racial Capitalism"; McRuer, *Crip Times*.

5. Glenn, *Forced to Care*; Tronto, *Caring Democracy*.

6. Espiritu, *Home Bound*, 47.

7. Kaiser Family Foundation, "Date Note."

8. The U.S. Department of Labor's Fair Labor Standards Act of 1938 originally exempted domestic workers (including domestic care workers) from the minimum wage and overtime protection guaranteed to other workers (agricultural workers were exempted as well). This continued even under the amendment in 1974 and until the recent amendment that became effective in 2015. With the 2015 ruling, domestic workers including care workers are now guaranteed minimum wage and overtime protection (even though some participants in this research told me about ways that undocumented migrant workers are hired at less than minimum wage in the care structure). The data and narratives offered by Medicaid recipients and care workers were collected in 2013, prior to the final ruling. See U.S. Department of Labor, *Fact Sheet*.

9. Additionally, works by Kateřina Kolářová and others illustrate how affluent people from the Global North who require long-term care go to the nations of the Global South to receive such care. It is another example of how care is subcontracted across national borders, while in this case those with long-term-care needs move instead of those who are becoming care workers. See Kolářová, "'Grandpa Lives.'"

10. See also Oliver, *Politics of Disablement*; Shakespeare, *Help*; Vasey, *Rough Guide*.

11. See, for example, Erevelles, *Disability and Difference*; Fritsch, "Intimate Assemblages"; Glenn, *Forced to Care*; Kelly, *Disability Politics and Care*; Kittay, *Love's Labor*; Watson et al., "(Inter)Dependence."

12. Aizura, "Communizing Care"; Malatino, *Trans Care*; Manalansan, "Queering the Chain"; Piepzna-Samarasinha, *Care Work*.

13. Newer scholarships on care increasingly address the racialized, queer, and transnational nature of care work in addition to the gendered aspect. See, for example, Glenn, *Forced to Care*; Guevarra, *Marketing Dreams*; Manalansan, "Queering the Chain"; Parreñas, *Servants of Globalization*; Vora, *Life Support*.

14. Care crisis is also attributed to a devastating lack and high turnover of care laborers and hence incapacity to meet the needs of an increasing number of people needing long-term care. Glenn, *Forced to Care*; Fine, *Caring Society*; Folbre, "Nursebots to the Rescue?" and *For Love and Money*.

15. Berkin, *Revolutionary Mothers*; Chang, *Disposable Domestics*; Duffy, *Making Care Count*; Glenn, *Forced to Care*; Parreñas, *Servants of Globalization*.

16. Glenn, *Forced to Care*; Malatino, *Trans Care*; Manalansan, "Queering the Chain"; Nadasen, Mittelstadt, and Chappell, *Welfare in the United States*; Francisco-Menchavez, *Labor of Care*.

17. Boris and Klein, *Caring for America*.; Duffy, *Making Care Count*; Glenn, *Forced to Care*; Nadasen, Mittelstadt, and Chappell, *Welfare in the United States*; Parreñas, *Servants of Globalization*.

18. I would also like to note that more men of lower income are entering care work, especially working at residential homes for disabled people, compared to white men. Baines, "Staying with People."

19. Puar, "CODA" 155 [emphasis added].

20. Mitchell and Snyder, *Biopolitics of Disability*, 40 [emphasis added]; see also Deleuze, "Postscript on Control Societies"; Foucault, *Society Must Be Defended*; Shaviro, "'Bitter Necessity.'"

21. Fritsch, "Gradations of Debility"; Puar, "CODA"; Shildrick, "Why Should Our Bodies."

22. As the organization of society and its political economy is said to have transitioned from disciplinary to neoliberal and control society, the target of control also has changed from individual and mass (e.g., a group of workers) to dividual, as argued by Deleuze (also see Foucault, *Birth of Biopolitics*). I am foregrounding the political economy of neoliberal control society in this chapter to shed light on the ways that control of the population or individuals is increasingly targeting different parts or layers of an individual rather than the individual as a whole. Such parts can be their DNA information, or the layers can be from their capacity—actual and constructed—to thrive in the free market and to exercise their financial power through accumulating and spending. Thus, instead of a number of cookie-cutter, molded workers who engage in the same work together uniformly, workers nowadays are modulated and individualized to compete against one another. In Deleuze's words, "We're no longer dealing with a duality of mass and individual. Individuals become 'dividuals,' and masses become samples, data, markets, or 'banks.'" Steven Shaviro further elaborates this point: "Our identities are multiple, and they are continually being decomposed and recomposed, on various levels, through the modulation of numerous parameters . . . [such as] my medical record and the databases that track my Visa card use. . . . Each of these identifies me separately, for particular purposes" ("'Bitter Necessity,'" 10–12). I am using this dividual-based framework to claim that today's Medicaid operates based exclusively on dividuals and not individuals. The concept of *dividual* is originally used in a rather neutral way: that everyone is turned into a dividual as they are regulated through their passwords and fingerprints that allow

people to have different levels of access to information-technology databases (which are the new currency). Further, quoting Foucault, Shaviro points out the characteristic of neoliberal and control society as that "the neoliberal regime cannot be explained in terms of the disciplinary society and its 'normative mechanisms,'" and thus "there is an optimization of systems of difference, in which the field is left open to fluctuating processes," and "in which there is an environmental type of intervention instead of the internal subjugation of individuals." Further, "both [neoliberal and control society] accounts see the multiplication of differences, and the continuing 'optimization,' or 'modulation' of loose, 'fluctuating processes' as a practice of control." My interest is therefore in how dividuals are differently capacitated and debilitated in relation to their race, gender, geopolitical origin, and disability status as well as based on the profitability of such capacity and debility in the free market guided by the neoliberal and control society. How do those markers on a bodymind signify the person's capability and debility, and in return, through the mechanism of the U.S. public healthcare assemblage, how are they further enhanced as bodies are affected, reconfigure, and adjust to new roles, new encounters, new events, and new milieus? See Deleuze, "Postscript on Control Societies," 180; Foucault, *Birth of Biopolitics*; Shaviro, "'Bitter Necessity,'" 6–7.

23. Folbre, *For Love and Money*; Glenn, *Forced to Care*; Kelly, *Disability Politics and Care*; Shakespeare, "Social Relations of Care"; Tronto, *Caring Democracy*.

24. Centers for Medicare and Medicaid Services, "Eligibility"; I am including denizens and not only U.S. citizens, since Medicaid covers medical needs of non–U.S. citizens in a very limited way. If a non–U.S. citizen acquires emergency medical needs that are life threatening, they can receive medical care funded by Medicaid. This also means that they cannot visit medical institutions until their medical and health situations worsen to the point of life-or-death. See Park, Jimenez, and Hoekstra, "Decolonizing the US Health System."

25. Skowronski, "State-by-State Guide."

26. As of April 2020, Alabama, Florida, Georgia, Kansas, Missouri, Mississippi, North Carolina, Oklahoma, South Carolina, South Dakota, Tennessee, Texas, Wisconsin, and Wyoming have not adapted the Medicaid expansion. See Kaiser Family Foundation, "Status of State Medicaid."

27. One in 7 adults, ages 19–64; 2 in 5 children; 5 in 8 nursing home residents; 1 in 3 individuals with disabilities; and 1 in 5 Medicare beneficiaries received Medicaid services and supports as of October 2019. See Kaiser Family Foundation, "Medicaid in the United States." The U.S. budget can be divided into mandatory spending (about 65 percent of the total budget), discretionary spending (almost 30 percent), and interest and federal debt (6 percent). See National Priorities Project, "Federal Spending." While Medicaid is an assistance program for low-income people, Medicare is an insurance program, regardless of their income, for people over sixty-five years old, younger disabled people, and those who receive dialysis. See U.S. Department of Health and Human Services, "What Is the Difference."

28. Rudowitz, Orgera, and Hinton, "Medicaid Financing."

29. Rudowitz, Orgera, and Hinton, "Medicaid Financing"; Kaiser Family Foundation, "Medicaid in the United States."

30. Paradise, "Medicaid Moving Forward"; Kaiser Family Foundation, "Five Key Facts"; Rehabilitation Research and Training Center on Disability Statistics and Demographics, "Annual Disability Statistics"; U.S. Census Bureau, "Nearly 1 in 5."

31. Kaiser Family Foundation, "Medicaid in the United States."

32. Kaiser Family Foundation, "Medicaid State Fact Sheets."

33. Many of them also take up additional care administration from other entities; Hinton, Rudowitz, Stolyar, and Singer, "10 Things to Know."

34. Bernstein, "Advocates Say" and "Medicaid Shift Fuels Rush"; Michener, *Fragmented Democracy*.

35. See, for example, Park, Jimenez, and Hoekstra, "Decolonizing the US Health System."

36. Michener, *Fragmented Democracy*.

37. Henschel, "Judge Stripped." A Social Security judge was stripped of disability cases in 2016 for using sexist and racist terms to describe those who came in front of him to request services. It is one example of how stereotypes can determine which people are considered as deserving public supports. I unfold this point further in the next chapter.

38. See also Katz, *Poverty and Policy*, *In the Shadow*, and *Undeserving Poor*; Patterson, *America's Struggle*; Pimpare, "A People's History"; Trattner, *From Poor Law*.

39. Michener, *Fragmented Democracy*, 34.

40. Michener, *Fragmented Democracy*, 9.

41. Olson, *Politics of Medicaid*. Medicaid long-term care (which is the focus in this book) is often portrayed as white middle class medical welfare. Medicaid is both at large and within long-term-care programs still filled disproportionately with people of color from the lower class. Nonetheless, political scientist Laura Katz Olson explains that an unexpectedly large portion of white, formerly middle class (and mostly elderly) people are in the long-term-care program because of the program's more relaxed financial criteria for eligibility. Additionally, because of the high costs of long-term care in general (whether provided in nursing homes or at people's own homes), it is relatively easy for middle-class people to use up their savings on long-term care and to enter the eligibility pool. Olson further explains that fear and anxiety over the high costs of outsourcing long-term care and its demanding nature for their family members drive this population and their family members to be powerful lobbyists for Medicaid long-term-care programs. This is said to be a reason why Medicaid long-term-care programs have avoided fundamental reforms, compared with other programs under Medicaid. See Olson, *Politics of Medicaid*. See also National Center for Health Statistics, "Table P-11."

42. Ehrenreich and Hochschild, *Global Woman*; Guevarra, *Marketing Dreams*; Manalansan, "Queering the Chain"; Parreñas, *Servants of Globalization*; Yeates, "Global Care Chains."

43. Guevarra, *Marketing Dreams*; Lindquist, Xiang, and Yeoh, "Opening the Black Box"; Manalansan, "Queering the Chain"; Yeates, "Global Care Chains."

44. Folbre, *For Love and Money*; Guevarra, *Marketing Dreams*; Parreñas, *Servants of Globalization*.

45. See, for example, Banks, "Black Women's Labor Market"; Donovan, "Home Care Work"; Dunbar-Ortiz, *Indigenous People's History*; Guevarra, *Marketing Dreams*; Haley, *No Mercy Here*; Vora, *Life Support*.

46. Phillips, "Agencement/Assemblage," cited in Puar, "I Would Rather," 57.

47. Guevarra, *Marketing Dreams*; Hinton, Rudowitz, Stolyar, and Singer, "10 Things to Know"; Lindquist, Xiang, and Yeoh, "Opening the Black Box."

48. While managed care was implemented and became popular in private sectors since the late 1920s, it was not until the 1990s that the program was more widely implemented in public healthcare programs. As the managed-care plan was turned into

formal Medicare options under the Medicare Advantage program, it has spread widely across Medicaid as well. See National Council on Disability, *Chapter 1*.

49. Elflein, *Total Medicaid Expenditure.*

50. Centers for Medicare and Medicaid Services, "National Health Expenditure."

51. Nga and Weiner, "An Overview of Long-Term Services."

52. Center for Medicare and Medicaid Services, "Managed Care" [emphasis added].

53. See, for example, Hinton, Rudowitz, Stolyar, and Singer, "10 Things to Know"; Polson, "Caring Precariat." Examples of day-to-day operations that are handled by care industries include the following: "negotiate payment rates and sign contracts with various long-term care providers, and work with only those providers in their network [under the organizations' managed long-term-care plans]. [Their managed long-term-care plans] determine the level and intensity of services for each individual in each care setting." See Healthcare Education Project, "Managed Long-Term Care," 9.

54. Kaiser Family Foundation, "Medicaid and Managed Care." These waivers and policies include State plan authority (section 1932[a]) and waiver authorities (section 1915[a] and [b] and section 1115). The number of states that use managed long-term services and supports programs increased from eight in 2004 to sixteen in 2012 and twenty-six in 2014; the number is only increasing (Centers for Medicare and Medicaid Services, "Managed Care," "Section 1115 Demonstrations").

55. Hinton, Rudowitz, Stolyar, and Singer, "10 Things to Know"; Kaiser Family Foundation, "Medicaid and Managed Care"; Centers for Medicare and Medicaid Services, "Managed Care"; National Conference of State Legislatures, *Managed Care.* As of 2019, thirty-nine states plus Washington, D.C., implement managed care for some portion of their care provision. Degree of implementation varies, and in/voluntary enrollments in managed care differ from state to state and program to program as well. See Hinton, Rudowitz, Stolyar, and Singer, "10 Things to Know." Even when it is stated as "voluntary," though, applicants of Medicaid are opted in to managed care as a default, unless they actively take steps to opt out such enrollment in the case of New York State. See New York State Department of Health, "Access NY Health."

56. Hinton, Rudowitz, Stolyar, and Singer, "10 Things to Know."

57. Hinton, Rudowitz, Stolyar, and Singer, "10 Things to Know."

58. Regardless of the hopeful and forceful push for managed care by governments and industries, critiques of and concerns about managed care have been shared. These include, for example, the fact that the wholesale of Medicaid services is not compatible with the disabled population, whose needs and care requirements are unique from individual to individual. See Olson, *Politics of Medicaid.* Thus, in the rapid development of public healthcare privatization, people have pointed out that there are not enough regulatory policies or data on how care industries are running public healthcare services. As I lay out more throughout this chapter, in the swift transition of administrative authorities to industries, a number of devastating changes have been enforced without clear records being collected and examined at the governmental level.

59. McCann, "States with the Most"; Kaiser Family Foundation, "Medicaid State Fact Sheets."

60. Bernstein, "Advocates Say Managed-Care."

61. Some of the first jobs that newly inaugurated New York governor Andrew Cuomo initiated in 2011 were with the Medicaid Redesign Team. Since that time, the team has implemented the Medicaid Global Cap to limit the Medicaid budget, which makes up 25 percent of New York State's public spending and serves 5 million people as of 2014 (1

in 4 New Yorkers). This cap is pushed regardless of the steady increase of Medicaid enrollees in New York State by 25 percent between 2007 and 2012 (from 4,106,785 in 2007
to 5,097,920 in 2012). See Cuomo, "Governor Cuomo"; New York State Department of
Health, "Medicaid Enrollees."

62. McCann, "States with the Most"; Kaiser Family Foundation, "Medicaid State
Fact Sheets."

63. Bernstein, "Pitfalls Seen," para. 5.

64. Debra Lipson, Maria Dominiak, Michelle Soper, and Brianna Ensslin describe
how the New York State per-capita is calculated: "New York … [is] using sophisticated
risk-adjustment approaches to set [Medicaid Long Term Services and Supports] program
rates. [New York State has] linked functional assessment data with managed care plan
encounter data and have developed risk-adjustment models to better reflect the varying
risk of individuals enrolled in different managed care plans. Both states have found that
functional data, particularly ADLs [activities of daily living] and IADLs [instrumental activities of daily living], along with certain neurological diagnosis codes (e.g., Alzheimer's
disease/dementia, Parkinson's disease, and paralysis including hemiplegia, paraplegia,
and quadriplegia) significantly improves the predictability of expected costs." See Lipson, Dominiak, Soper, and Ensslin, *Developing Capitation Rates*, 4.

65. McCann, "States with the Most"; Kaiser Family Foundation, "Medicaid State
Fact Sheets."

66. Harris-Kojetin et al., *Long-Term Care Services*.

67. U.S. Census Bureau, "Annual Services," cited in Polson, "Caring Precariat"; Di-
Napoli, "Medicaid in New York." The latter numbers on New York State's Medicaid
managed-care spending are based on Medicaid managed-care premium payments.

68. Also see Mitchell and Snyder, *Biopolitics of Disability*. At a disability studies conference in New York City, Jasbir Puar explained the point as a response to Rosemarie
Garland-Thomson's question on whether there is a space for disabled people to inhabit
this world. Puar stated that disabled and/or injured bodies are *needed* in this neoliberal
political economy. Bringing up examples of medical industries' reliance on disabled
bodyminds as well as a number of armed conflicts occurring around the world, including the Israeli occupation of Palestine, which continues to create disabled and injured
people, she emphasized that disabled and injured bodyminds are not going away anytime soon.

69. Medicaid Matters New York and Elder Law Attorneys, New York Chapter, *Mis-
managed Care*.

70. Managed care is set up to provide the same rate per capita to every member of a
plan regardless of their needs and the costs of their care. This is to balance out the *risk*
among enrollees assigned to the plan by redistributing the funds not used by those with
less care needs (hence care costs remain lower) for the care for those who require more
complex care (hence the costs of care can be higher). This report, though, shows that
in reality some care agencies offer care mostly to those whose costs of care are less to
increase their revenues. See Medicaid Matters New York and Elder Law Attorneys, New
York Chapter, *Mis-managed Care*.

71. Medicaid Matters New York and Elder Law Attorneys, New York Chapter, *Mis-
managed Care*.

72. Bernstein, "Lives Upended," para. 8.

73. Overwhelming numbers of service cuts laid out in articles include Medicaid enrollees who once worked as care workers for their entire adult lives who then became
disabled, since their bodyminds cannot endure the intense physical labor of providing

long-term care anymore. Additionally, effects of drastic service cuts include devastating consequences such as severe injury of a blind elderly man who fell off his bed one morning after his personal care service was terminated by an agency, and an enrollee who passed away two weeks after her care was cut. See Bernstein, "Pitfalls Seen."

74. Bernstein, "Advocates Say," para. 3 [emphasis added].

75. Bernstein, "Medicaid Shift Fuels Rush."

76. Bernstein, "Medicaid Shift Fuels Rush."

77. Bernstein, "Pitfalls Seen."

78. National Center for Health Statistics, "Table P-11."

79. Olson, *Politics of Medicaid.*

80. Olson, *Politics of Medicaid.*

81. New York State Department of Health, *Transitional Cases.*

82. Chen, *Animacies*; Gorman, "Quagmires of Affect."

83. National Center for Health Statistics, "Table P-11."

84. Bernstein, "Medicaid Home Care."

85. Tronto, "There Is an Alternative."

86. Garland-Thomson, "Feminist Disability Studies."

87. Mohanty, *Feminism without Borders.*

88. PHI, "Workforce Data Center."

89. Scales, "It's Time to Care"; U.S. Census Bureau, "Annual Services."

90. Scales, "It's Time to Care."

91. PHI, "FACTS 5" and "Projected Growth."

92. Glenn, *Forced to Care*, 7.

93. Banks, "Black Women's Labor Market"; Chang, *Disposable Domestics*; Donovan, "Home Care Work"; Duffy, *Making Care Count.*

94. Nadasen, Mittelstadt, and Chappell, *Welfare in the United States.* Further, migration and gender justice activist Grace Chang describes the mutually implicative natures of reforms on welfare programs for single mothers and immigration as they happened in the 1990s and on. See Chang, *Disposable Domestics.*

95. U.S. Bureau of Labor Statistics, "Labor Force."

96. Parreñas, *Servants of Globalization.*

97. Hardt and Negri, *Empire*: Flores-González et al., *Immigrant Women Workers*; Folbre, *For Love and Money*; Glenn, *Forced to Care*; Lindquist, Xiang, and Yeoh, "Opening the Black Box"; Parreñas, *Servants of Globalization*; Yeates, "Global Care Chains."

98. Glenn, *Forced to Care.*

99. Chang, *Disposable Domestics*; Parreñas, *Servants of Globalization*; Vora, *Life Support.*

100. Lowe, *Immigrant Acts*, 359.

101. Harvey, *Brief History*; Parreñas, *Servants of Globalization*; Vora, *Life Support.*

102. Guevarra, *Marketing Dreams*, 24.

103. Choy, *Empire of Care.*

104. Francisco-Menchavez, *Labor of Care*, 2–18; Guevarra, *Marketing Dreams*; Folbre, "Nursebots to the Rescue?" and *For Love and Money*; Parreñas, *Servants of Globalization.* The 1946 Bell Trade Act, for example, included permission for U.S. corporations to have the same level of privilege and rights afforded to Filipino businesses, which Guevarra describes as devaluated Filipino currency, and led to the trade deficit against the United States. See Guevarra, *Marketing Dreams.*

105. Additionally, the U.S. Immigration and Nationality Act of 1965 is said to have caused the rapid increase in skilled migrants to the United States from Asian nations.

Guevarra explains: "The legislation was strategic: in 1965 the [United States] was facing its first national nursing shortage, prompting the US labor secretary to waive the labor certification requirement for foreign nurses and to allow them to come to the United States even if they did not have prearranged employment." See Ong and Azores, "Migration and Incorporation," cited in Guevarra, *Marketing Dreams*, 30.

Further, feminist sociologist Rhacel Salazar Parreñas explains that the relatively better labor protection offered in the United States compared to other nations attracts more workers who long to be employed in the states. See Parreñas, *Servants of Globalization*.

106. See also Boyd and Pickoff, *Gendering Migration*.

107. See also Durano, "Women in International."

108. See also Glazer, "Nurse Immigration."

109. Folbre, "Nursebots to the Rescue?," 356, cited in Bach, "International Migration."

110. Lindquist, Xiang, and Yeoh, "Opening the Black Box."

111. See, for example, Vora, *Life Support*.

112. Filipino nurses, for example, are often associated with an image of a "necessarily gendered and heterosexual [trope, which signifies] the productive femininity . . . [who offer not only] a much gentler and welcoming 'touch,' [but also . . . a sanitized physical body that may strategically mask their foreignness to the extent that it is 'fit' for public consumption" for marketing purposes. This is in addition to the Americanized nursing education they have gone though. See Guevarra, *Marketing Dreams*, 133–135.

113. Guevarra, *Marketing Dreams*, 138.

114. Guevarra, *Marketing Dreams*.

115. Guevarra, *Marketing Dreams*.

116. Guevarra, *Marketing Dreams*; Vora, *Life Support*.

117. Boris and Klein, *Caring for America*, 13.

118. Glenn, *Forced to Care*; Nadasen, Mittelstadt, and Chappell, *Welfare in the United States*.

119. Haley, 2016; Nadasen, Mittelstadt, and Chappell, *Welfare in the United States*; Molina, "Medicalizing the Mexican."

120. See, for example, Haley, *No Mercy Here*. Also see Chapter 2.

121. Glenn, *Forced to Care*.

122. Banks, "Black Women's Labor Market"; Boris and Klein, *Caring for America*; Donovan, "Home Care Work"; Nadasen, Mittelstadt, and Chappell, *Welfare in the United States*; Tronto, *Moral Boundary*.

123. See, for example, Bailey and Mobley, "Work in the Intersections."

124. Haley, *No Mercy Here*, 82 [emphasis added].

125. Haley, *No Mercy Here*; also see Bailey and Mobley, "Work in the Intersections."

126. Glenn, *Forced to Care*, 25–26.

127. Glenn, *Forced to Care*, 32–33.

128. Glenn, *Forced to Care*.

129. Sharpe, *In the Wake*.

130. Also see Banks, "Black Women's Labor Market"; Donovan, "Home Care Work."

131. Boris and Klein, *Caring for America*; Nadasen, Mittelstadt, and Chappell, *Welfare in the United States*.

132. Glenn, *Forced to Care*; Nadasen, Mittelstadt, and Chappell, *Welfare in the United States*.

133. Nadasen, Mittelstadt, and Chappell, *Welfare in the United States*.

134. Nadasen, Mittelstadt, and Chappell, *Welfare in the United States*, 33–35 [emphasis added].

135. See, for example, Nadasen, Mittelstadt, and Chappell, *Welfare in the United States*.

136. Glenn, *Forced to Care*; Nadasen, Mittelstadt, and Chappell, *Welfare in the United States*; Soldatic and Meekosha, "Place of Disgust." Linda Gordon also adds to the racial analysis of welfare programs by describing how the fact that the majority of welfare recipients are white people is obscured, and how welfare came to be stigmatized as a tool to specifically stereotype African American single mothers as avoiding work. Thus, welfare has been turned into an indicator of individuals' moral failures used to characterize African American single mothers. See Gordon, *Pitied but Not Entitled*. Thus, TANF completely excluded recent migrants. See Nadasen, Mittelstadt, and Chappell, *Welfare in the United States*.

137. Glenn, *Forced to Care*.

138. Also see Nadasen, Mittelstadt, and Chappell, *Welfare in the United States*.

139. Glenn, *Forced to Care*; Acs and Loprest, *Leaving Welfare*, cited in Glenn, *Forced to Care*; Nadasen, Mittelstadt, and Chappell, *Welfare in the United States*. Also, large numbers of welfare recipients were pushed out of TANF as a form of punishment for minor issues including missing appointments or not filling out forms properly. See Glenn, *Forced to Care*.

140. Glenn, *Forced to Care*. One study shows that although these women worked thirty-five hours in an average week, their average income was a third below the federal poverty line at the time. See Glenn, *Forced to Care*.

141. Glenn, *Forced to Care*, 175.

142. It may also come with the capacity to purchase upward class mobility for themselves and their families, particularly for migrating care workers.

143. Chang, *Disposable Domestics*.

144. See, for example, Kelly, *Disability Politics and Care*; Nadasen, *Household Workers Unite*; Poo, *Age of Dignity*; Shakespeare, "Social Relations of Care."

145. Hochschild, "Global Care Chains," 131.

146. Dodson and Luttrell, "Untenable Choices."

147. Francisco-Menchavez, *Labor of Care*, 4.

148. Dodson and Luttrell, "Untenable Choices."

149. Francisco-Menchavez, *Labor of Care*, 4.

150. Johnson and McRuer, "Cripistemologies."

CHAPTER 2

1. In addition to the list of content warnings provided for this book, this chapter includes mentions of murder of disabled people by their care providers and death.

2. Erevelles, *Disability and Difference*; Fine, *Caring Society*; Kelly, *Disability Politics*; Shakespeare, "Social Relations of Care"; Watson et al., "(Inter)Dependence, Needs."

3. See Chang, *Disposable Domestics*; Daly and Standing, "Introduction"; Erevelles, *Disability and Difference*; Fisher and Kang, "Reinventing Dirty Work"; Glenn, *Forced to Care*.

4. Foregrounding relational analysis also means that I am building on the work of scholars who have been weaving gender and disability studies together to deepen our understandings of how gender and disability (and cisheteropatriarchy and ableism) are enacted together daily. See Erevelles, *Disability and Difference*; Hall, *Feminist Disability Studies*; Kafer, *Feminist, Queer, Crip*; Kelly, *Disability Politics*; Schalk and Kim, "Integrating Race."

5. Chang, *Disposable Domestics*; Fisher and Kang, "Reinventing Dirty Work"; Hardt and Negri, *Empire*.

6. Hardt and Negri, *Empire*; Foucault, *Society Must Be Defended*.

7. Chang, *Disposable Domestics*; Daly and Standing, "Introduction"; Guevarra, *Marketing Dreams*; Giroux, "Reading Hurricane Katrina"; Fisher and Kang, "Reinventing Dirty Work"; Flores-González et al., *Immigrant Women Workers*; Francisco-Menchavez, *Labor of Care*; Hochschild, "Emotional Labour"; Vora, *Life Support*.

8. Puar, *Right to Maim*; Shaviro, "COVID-19 Infections."

9. Mbembe, "Necropolitics" and *Necropolitics*; Berlant, "Slow Death"; Gilmore, *Golden Gulag*; Hong, *Death beyond Disavowal*; Ferguson and Hong, "Sexual and Racial Contradictions"; Puar, *Right to Maim*; Reeve, "Biopolitics and Bare Life."

10. See Bailey and Mobley, "Work in the Intersections"; Piepzna-Samarasinha, *Care Work*; Sins Invalid, *Skin, Tooth, and Bone*.

11. Berlant, "Slow Death"; Duarte, "*Black Earth Rising*"; Ferguson and Hong, "Sexual and Racial Contradictions"; Gilmore, *Golden Gulag*; Hong, *Death beyond Disavowal*; Mbembe, "Necropolitics" and *Necropolitics*; Reeve, "Biopolitics and Bare Life."

12. Hardt and Negri, *Multitude*, 108.

13. Foucault, *Society Must Be Defended*, 241, 246, 247, 253.

14. Abbott, "Conflict over the Grey Areas," 300.

15. See, for example, Chang, *Disposable Domestics*; Piepzna-Samarasinha, *Care Work*.

16. Chang, *Disposable Domestics*; Daly and Standing, "Introduction"; Mol, *Logic of Care*.

17. See, for example, Fine, *Caring Society*; Fisher and Kang, "Reinventing Dirty Work"; Francisco-Menchavez, *Labor of Care*; Guevarra, *Marketing Dreams*; Parreñas, *Servants of Globalization*.

18. Kelly, *Disability Politics*; Shakespeare, "Social Relations of Care."

19. Morris, *Independent Lives* and "Independent Living"; Shakespeare, "Social Relations of Care."

20. A direct-payment policy means that disabled people who require long-term care directly receive the public healthcare funding to recruit, hire, and train their own personal assistants. See Kelly, *Disability Politics and Care*, for more information on this policy. See also Hayman, "Independent Living History"; Morris, *Independent Lives* and "Independent Living"; Shakespeare, "Social Relations of Care."

21. On the one hand, care studies scholars respect and follow the terminologies advocated by independent living and disability rights movements such as consumers in order to empower disabled care receivers. On the other hand, though, they also articulate that it is false to believe that disabled people and especially those who receive their long-term care under public healthcare programs have the ultimate power to dictate their long-term care just like people who privately hire their care workers. See Boris and Klein, *Caring for America*; Kelly, *Disability Politics*.

22. Chang, *Disposable Domestics*; Erevelles, *Disability and Difference*; Fisher and Kang, "Reinventing Dirty Work"; Glenn, *Forced to Care*; Guevarra, *Marketing Dreams*; Hong, *Death beyond Disavowal*; Roulstone, "Personal Independence Payments."

23. Baines, "Staying with People"; Chang, *Disposable Domestics*; Daly and Standing, "Introduction"; Guevarra, *Marketing Dreams*; Vora, *Life Support*; Hochschild, "Emotional Labour"; Flores-González et al., *Immigrant Women Workers*; Fisher and Kang, "Reinventing Dirty Work"; Mohanty, *Feminism without Borders*.

24. See, for example, Chang, *Disposable Domestics*; Daly and Standing, "Introduction"; Erevelles, *Disability and Difference*; Fisher and Kang, "Reinventing Dirty Work."

25. Bernstein, "Advocates Say," "Pitfalls Seen," and "Medicaid Shift Fuels Rush." Under the managed-care programs that were implemented in the majority of the states, care industries receive per-capita—or set funds—from governments for each Medicaid enrollee they provide for. They are also given administrative authority from the state government to decide how much and what kinds of care would be provided and to whom, within the guidelines set by the governments. Please see Chapter 1 for more descriptions of managed care.

26. See, for example, Glenn, *Forced to Care*; Tronto, *Caring Democracy*.

27. Enrollment in Supplemental Security Income (which is managed by the Social Security Administration) automatically determines enrollees' eligibility to Medicaid as well in most of states. This is why Keisha brought up her encounter with Social Security, while she described her application for Medicaid. See Rupp and Riley, "State Medicaid Eligibility."

28. Throughout the book, I use the terms *expert discussion* and *expert* to refer to focus groups and all of research participants.

29. See, for example, Bernstein, "Medicaid Shift Fuels Rush."

30. Michener, *Fragmented Democracy*; Olson, *Politics of Medicaid*; Soldatic, *Disability and Neoliberal State*.

31. See, for example, Bernstein, "Advocates Say" and "Medicaid Shift Fuels Rush." See Chapter 1 for more on this point.

32. Daly and Standing, "Introduction"; Olson, *Politics of Medicaid.*

33. Henschel, "Judge Stripped."

34. Longmore Institute, "Disability Visibility Justice"; O'Toole, *Fading Scars*; Rodríguez-Roldán, "Who Gets to Be"; Schweik, "Lomax's Matrix"; Sins Invalid, *Skin, Tooth, and Bone*; Wright, *Physical Disability.*

35. Please see the work of Premilla Nadasen, Jennifer Mittelstadt, and Marisa Chappell, who describe how such stereotypes are politically developed and spread to deter more women of color from attempting to enter welfare programs. See Nadasen, Mittelstadt, and Chappell, *Welfare in the United States.*

36. Chang, *Disposable Domestics*; Haley, *No Mercy Here*; Michener, *Fragmented Democracy*; Molina, "Medicalizing the Mexican."

37. See, for example, Berne, "Disability Justice."

38. As Supplemental Security Income recipients are automatically eligible for Medicaid in most states, many who receive Medicaid also are enrollees of the program. To receive it, applicants need to prove that the total of things they own values less than $2,000 for a single person and $3,000 for a married couple. Thus, they need to submit medical proof of their disabilities and incapacities (in the case of disabled applicants). Social Security Administration, *Supplemental Security Income (SSI).*

39. This expert discussion was held before the U.S. Congress passed the Achieving a Better Life Experience (ABLE) Act at the end of 2014. This policy allows disabled people and their families to save more than $2,000 under the disabled individuals' names without losing necessary social services such as Medicaid. Though this is major progress for disability communities, as the policy is still in the process of implementation at the time of this manuscript writing and has not yet had any direct effect on disabled people's lives, I am including narratives on the $2,000 limit in this book. See Internal Revenue Service, "ABLE Accounts"; U.S. Department of Health and Human Services, "2017 Poverty Guidelines."

40. "Managed care organizations operate under Article 44 of the Public Health Law and the Insurance Law and must be certified by [the New York State] Department of Health." NY Codes, Rules, and Regulations (Title 10, Part 98) for managed care specifies that managed-care long-term-care plans must be signed off by New York State commissioners (and the superintendent) for its quality strategy. It is crucial to note that the New York State DoH website states that since many of the plans under Medicaid managed care are new, "quality monitoring [is] not as established as those of the traditional plans [Child Health Plus and Family Health Plus]" as of March 2021. This made me wonder about the readiness and thoroughness of quality assurance at the structural level established by the state government. Finally, the individual managed-care organizations that I looked into do have their own quality assurance, which can be reviewed only upon request of enrollees (in the case of Aetna, which provides managed long-term-care plans for people over twenty-one years old in New York City). See New York State Department of Health, MCO's Certified by NYS Department of Health, Chapter II, and Quality Strategy for the New York State Medicaid Managed Care Program; Aetna Better Health of New York, "New York Managed Long-Term Care Program."

41. Bernhardt, McGrath, and DeFilippis, Unregulated Work.

42. These expert discussions were often filled with their observations of an overwhelming number of cases in which a care worker who was fired by a care agency was immediately hired by another agency. With this example, they demonstrated the lack of adequate gatekeeping for care workers.

43. Bernhardt, McGrath, and DeFilippis, Unregulated Work.

44. Bernstein, "Advocates Say" and "Medicaid Shift Fuels Rush."

45. See endnote 8 from Chapter 1 and Bernhardt, McGrath, and DeFilippis, Unregulated Work. Here Alisha also mentioned the recent (at the time of the interview) change in wages for "sleep-in" care work, in which the care worker lives at the enrollee's residence to provide care around the clock. While care workers stay and care for twenty-four hours, eight to ten hours are automatically deducted from the wage calculation, since those hours are considered as care workers' resting and sleeping time. Alisha responds that this does not reflect the reality of care work, since care workers are asked to attend enrollees even in the middle of night (i.e., to get a glass of water) and their sleep is often disrupted.

46. The interview was conducted in 2013, and this number may have changed since then.

47. Bernhardt, McGrath, and DeFilippis, Unregulated Work, 69. Many of those I encountered during the time of this research shared stories of how undocumented migrant people are hired and work as care workers for less than minimum wage.

48. See Bernhardt, McGrath, and DeFilippis, Unregulated Work. This interview was conducted prior to the application of the Fair Labor Standards Act to domestic service under the U.S. Department of Labor, which brings minimum wage and overtime protection among other labor protections to those care workers. See endnote 8 in Chapter 1 and U.S. Department of Labor, Fact Sheet.

49. Hochschild, "Behind Every Great Caregiver."

50. See Ehrenreich and Hochschild, Global Women; Fisher and Kang, "Reinventing Dirty Work"; Lynch et al., Affective Equality.

51. This interview was conducted prior to the application of the Fair Labor Standards Act to domestic service under the U.S. Department of Labor, which brings minimum

wage and overtime protection among other labor protections to those care workers. See endnote 8 in Chapter 1 and U.S. Department of Labor, *Fact Sheet*.

52. Bernhardt, McGrath, and DeFilippis, *Unregulated Work*.

53. Such shifting of responsibility was certainly fueled by the lack of investment by the federal and state governments in medical welfare too. As the "care pimp" metaphor indicates, care agencies as well can be seen on the verge of desperation and ready to engage in every possible way to make revenue. Nonetheless, as the line between the state and business industries gets blurrier and blurrier under the neoliberal political economy, and based on multiple news reports on how much revenue is brought to the agencies and luxurious lives that families of CEOs lead, agencies too need to be held accountable along with the state for their divestment in the well-being of those who are situated as care workers and recipients. See Bernstein, "Pitfalls Seen" and "Medicaid Shift Fuels Rush."

54. Bernhardt, McGrath, and DeFilippis, *Unregulated Work*, 72.

55. According to PHI, 43 percent of home care workers receive their health insurance from Medicaid, Medicare, or other public health coverage. In total, 84 percent of these workers have some kind of health insurance. See PHI, "Workforce Data Center."

56. Mbembe, "Necropolitics," 11–12 [emphasis added].

57. Mbembe, "Necropolitics," 39–40.

58. Berlant, "Slow Death," 754–755; see also Ferguson and Hong, "Sexual and Racial Contradictions"; Gilmore, *Golden Gulag*; Reeve, "Biopolitics and Bare Life."

59. Chang, *Disposable Domestics*; Ferguson and Hong, "Sexual and Racial Contradictions"; Hong, *Death beyond Disavowal*; Puar, *Right to Maim*.

60. See, for example, Daly and Standing, "Introduction."

61. Bernstein, "Medicaid Home Care."

62. Nadasen, *Household Workers Unite*.

63. Vora, *Life Support*.

64. See, for example, Brown, "I Am Not Afraid"; McGuire, *War on Autism*.

CHAPTER 3

1. In addition to the list of content warnings provided for this book, this chapter includes mentions of care-based violence including exploitation of care workers and ableism disguised as care for care recipients including life threatening ableism.

2. Erevelles, *Disability and Difference*, 197.

3. My making of and emphasis on the disability status of Medicaid enrollees or those who are situated as care recipients do not mean that they are the only ones with disabilities or that care workers do not identify as disabled or experience impairments. Please see Chapters 1 and 2 for more discussions on this topic.

4. Throughout my conversations with those who are involved in Medicaid long-term-care programs, many repeatedly told me stories of sudden separations of care workers and enrollees that were facilitated and enforced by care agencies. After working together for various lengths of time, care workers were sometimes suddenly assigned to a new client without any heads-up or consultation. Medicaid enrollees are often confused and upset by this unexpected change and the unavoidable burden of rebuilding care practice routines with the new person, as they each need to learn how to co-conduct care routines together. Care workers also find this sudden change disturbing, as they are also often not told why it is happening or given information on the new client. Both care

workers and enrollees interpret this sudden separation and change in care partners as some kind of penalty or punishment imposed on them by care agencies (e.g., for forging connections with each other).

5. Harney and Moten, *Undercommons*.

6. I am using the term *preconscious* as I conceptualize affective collectivity based on affect theory, which theorizes human (and nonhuman) relations. Brian Massumi's seminal writing on affect lays out the relationship between affect and emotion by conceptualizing affect as the force that a body registers or is affected by as much as it is the force that a body emits based on its existence. Such being affected and affecting occurs preconsciously, while the force comes to be recognized and interpreted as emotion (e.g., interpreting the force as a threat or joy, for example). Although Massumi later reconceptualized the divide as much less clear-cut and in a way conflated two concepts (affect and emotion), I still find the conceptual divide helpful to understand the sensual, outside-of-cognitive relationality that people grow and develop in their daily lives. Additionally, by emphasizing the preconscious bodily and bodymind activation, I am not arguing that it is without influences of social stratification or suggest the moment as a purely biological reaction. Indeed, the affective collectivity I conceptualize here is itself a product of encounters fostered in oppressive healthcare structure. See Massumi, "Autonomy of Affect"; Gorman, "Quagmires of Affect."

7. One example of this cognition-based theorization of human relation takes place in social psychology, whose canonical schools of research include *intergroup relationships*, which situates people's cognitive capacity as key for the development of any human connections such as solidarity and friendships (e.g., group processes and intergroup relations). See Hogg and Abrams, "Editorial."

8. Baggs, "Holding onto My Humanity."

9. See also Fineman, *Autonomy Myth*; Kittay, *Love's Labor*; McKenzie, "Autonomy and Automatons"; Nedelsky, *Law's Relations*; Stoljar, "Informed Consent"; and Tronto, *Caring Democracy*. These authors write eloquently about relational ontology of people, which practices of care illuminate.

10. Harney and Moten, *Undercommons*.

11. See, for example, Berlant, "Slow Death"; Fritsch, "Gradations of Debility"; Livingston, *Debility and the Moral Imagination*; Puar, "CODA" and *Right to Maim*.

12. Cacho, *Social Death*; da Silva, "No-Bodies"; Gilmore, *Golden Gulag*; Mbembe, "Necropolitics."

13. Here, I am using the notion of slow death, described by Lauren Berlant. The concept of slow death illuminates the phenomenon in which people's labor toward a better life or sustaining their daily lives loses its boundaries and merges with their constant debilitation, which pushes them toward premature death. Highlighting the exploitative and debilitative nature of labor under neoliberalism—particularly the labor and lives of marginalized populations—Berlant has described how people are living while slowly dying, as we weather and deteriorate in the political economy. Please read Chapters 1 and 2, where I use the concept to illustrate the current state of the U.S. public healthcare assemblage. See Berlant, "Slow Death."

14. Berlant, "Slow Death"; Mbembe, "Necropolitics."

15. Brown, "Neo-liberalism and the End"; Puar, *Right to Maim*.

16. Hong, *Death beyond Disavowal*, 7.

17. Ferguson and Hong, "Sexual and Racial Contradictions," 1063.

18. Although I noted this point toward the beginning of this chapter, I would like to reemphasize that my intention is not to suggest that those who are marginalized must reach this point of resistance, resilience, and even revolution. It is not a way to recategorize *good* and *bad* disabled people. See Rodriguez-Roldán, "Who Gets to Be."

19. Hogg and Abrams, "Editorial"; Slife, "Taking Practice Seriously."

20. Watermeyer, *Toward a Contextual Psychology*. This standardization and valuing of humans based on a specific cognitive function has been constructed and used as a mechanism of state violence and is traceable back to (settler) colonialism, chattel slavery, and more. At the intersection of ableism, racism, and colonization, *Western* cognitive function was set up as a marker of civilization and justified discrimination against Indigenous people and people of color as *uncivilized* and thus needing to be disciplined by the West during the colonial era and even afterward. See Wynter, "Unsettling the Coloniality," as well as Chen, *Animacies*; Clare, *Brilliant Imperfection*; Erevelles, *Disability and Difference*; Harney and Moten, *Undercommons*; Price, *Mad at School*; Sins Invalid, *Skin, Tooth and Bone*; Wynter, "Unsettling the Coloniality"; Wynter and McKittrick, "Unparalleled Catastrophe."

21. There are certainly others who write about the relationality forged in the care practices. My work is built on their works. See Fritsch, "Intimate Assemblages"; Gibson, Carnevale, and King, "'This Is My Way'"; Shildrick and Price, "Deleuzian Connections." See also the concept of *access intimacy*, developed by disability justice activist Mia Mingus as an example of an affective way that care-based relationships are built. See Mingus, "Access Intimacy: The Missing Link."

22. Silentmiaow, "In My Language"; Baggs, "Why We Should Listen."

23. See, for example, Erevelles, *Disability and Difference*; Sequenzia and Grace, *Typed Words Loud Voices*.

24. Their past experiences in care practices, such as the unfortunately common incidents of stealing (which happens to both recipients and providers), condition them to be cautious of their new care partners. Regina, a young disabled Black woman who is a Medicaid enrollee, explains, "They stole from me. . . . It was a strain on our relationship. . . . It made it hard to look for someone [new]." Also see Chapter 2 for more on this point.

25. The roles of care provider and recipient as well as populations who (are pressured to) take on such roles are constructed in the assemblage of U.S. public healthcare. Thus, the assemblage is affected by multiple interacting social injustices such as global migration injustices, neocolonialism, white supremacy, cisheteropatriarchy, ableism, and classism, among others. In this context, innate differences among people's capacities to live independently in a given society and the need for others' support to do so are further amplified and solidified; thus, a division is created between the roles of care provider and care recipient. I do, however, argue in the previous chapter that such divisions are often blurred, particularly as care workers are subjected to harsh working conditions over the time and as they debilitate. See Chapters 1 and 2 for further descriptions of the U.S. public healthcare assemblage.

26. Although Maria shared this example as her frustration of how the agency micromanaged her relationship with her care partner (i.e., care worker), it can also be read as a safeguard for care workers given that the agency intervenes in the negotiation instead of leaving it up to the care partners. In this case, though, it is the Medicaid enrollee who bears the inconvenience due to the limit of Medicaid long-term care, as she continued inhabiting the house, which is not fully cleaned up to her standards.

27. This conflict is one layer of reality: how marginalized communities and individuals are put in a false dichotomy and antagonistic positions, regardless of how such an encounter can potentially foster solidarity, as they are entangled in each other's oppressive experiences.

28. Care routines consist of activities of daily living (ADLs) and instrumental activities of daily living (IADLs) such as eating, bathing, dressing, and managing finances. In the cases of Medicaid enrollees I talked to, first, their care routines are determined as social workers are sent to them to assess their care needs. Second, enrollees and care workers are assigned and given a slip of paper that includes a list of care activities. Next to each activity is a box to check when the task is performed and space for additional notes. Using the paper as a guide, care workers and enrollees engage in care practices.

29. Park McArthur and Constantina Zavitsanos also made notes on such co-conducting motions during care routines. See McArthur and Zavitsanos, "Other Forms."

30. Venn, "Individuation, Relationality, Affect," 156.

31. As English is a second language to both me and Sophia, the interview involved a lot of communication through body language. In a way, we spontaneously developed our own ways to communicate through a mixture of Spanglish, Japanglish, and body language.

32. This quote came out during the focus group with disabled people who receive Medicaid long-term-care services. This narrative specifically came from Anton, a middle-aged descendant of Latino migrants with learning disabilities. Unlike other participants of the focus group, he was the only one who needed long-term-care services but was not receiving them at the time of the interview. He attributed the lack of services to the lack of supports to help him to fill out paperwork, which is extremely difficult for him because of his multiple learning disabilities.

33. See, for example, Blackman, "Embodying Affect"; Wearing, Gunaratnam, and Gedalof, "Frailty and Debility."

34. See, for example, Clough, "Affective Turn."

35. Harney and Moten, *Undercommons*; Miserandino, "Spoon Theory"; Mingus, "Access Intimacy: The Missing Link" and "Access Intimacy, Interdependence and Disability Justice."

36. Lorde, *Sister Outsider*, 56 [emphasis added].

37. In the realm of affect theories, various scholars have articulated that as well. For instance, in media studies scholar Lisa Blackman's words, "The body is not bounded by the skin . . . but rather our bodies always extend and connect to other bodies . . . and to practices, techniques, technologies and objects which produce different kinds of bodies." As political philosopher Gilles Deleuze explains, "Existing bodies do not encounter one another *in the order* in which their relations combine. . . . [E]xisting bodies, being themselves composed of extensive parts, meet *bit by bit*. So parts of one of the bodies may be determined to take on a new relation imposed by some law while losing that relation through which they belonged to the body." Thus, while attention is given to *body* in affect studies, I replace it with *bodymind* to assert disability studies' insight that body and mind are interwoven and mutually affective. See Blackman, *Embodying Affect*, 170; Deleuze, *Expressionism in Philosophy*, 237 (emphasis in original); Ajo, Ben-Moshe, and Hilton, "Mad Futures"; Price, "Bodymind Problem."

38. See, for example, Wearing, Gunaratnam, and Gedalof, "Frailty and Debility."

39. Gorman, "Quagmires of Affect," 309.

40. Here, I am building on critical psychologist Brent D. Slife's insight that "practices are the individual's main way of relating, with beliefs and values secondary to, and serving the relation we have, with others." Also shaping my writing on affective bodyminds is Rachel da Silveira Gorman's articulation of "affect as the experience of the intensification of ideology, in which the diversifying complexes mediating social relations vanish into the appearance of unmediated essence." It is my intention, then, to theorize affective collectivity without losing the mediation Gorman points out, and I lay this out in previous chapters in terms of the U.S. public healthcare assemblage. See Slife, "Taking Practice Seriously," 158; Gorman, "Quagmires of Affect," 311.

41. Feminist theorist Donna Haraway notes the following on recursive encounters or rituals as a key portal for bodies to connect and relate:

All the actors become who they are in the dance of relating, not from scratch, not ex nihilo, but full of the patterns of their sometimes-joined, sometimes-separate heritages both before and lateral to this encounter. . . . [W]ho they are is in constant becoming in these rituals. Greeting rituals are flexible and dynamic, rearranging pace and elements within the repertoire that the partners already share or can cobble together. . . . [A] greeting ritual [i]s a kind of embodied communication, which takes place in entwined, semiotic, overlapping, somatic patterning over time, not as discrete, denotative signals emitted by individuals. An embodied communication is more like a dance than a word. The flow of entangled meaningful bodies in time—whether jerky and nervous or flaming and flowing, whether both partners move in harmony or painfully out of synch or something else altogether—is communication about relationship, the relationship itself, and the means of reshaping relationship and so its enacters.

See Haraway, *When Species Meet*, 126.

42. And in Julian Henriques's words, "Affect revolves round repetition. Repetition can cause affective attachment . . . In addition, affect can also cause repetition." See Henriques, "Vibrations of Affect," 77.

43. See, for example, Sequenzia and Grace, *Typed Words Loud Voices*.

44. McCarthy and Prokhovnik, "Embodied Relationality," 18–19.

45. Deleuze, *Spinoza*, 19, 27, 28 (emphasis in original). Also see Deleuze, *Expressionism in Philosophy*.

46. Manalansan, "Messy Mismeasures."

47. Curti and Moreno, "Institutional Borders," 414.

48. Flores-González et al., *Immigrant Women Workers*; Folbre, "Nursebots to the Rescue?" and *For Love and Money*; Glenn, *Forced to Care*; Lowe, *Immigrant Acts*.

49. Bernstein, "Pitfalls Seen," "Medicaid Shift Fuels Rush," and "Lives Upended"; Polson, "Caring Precariat"; Polson, DeFilippis, and Bernhardt, "Working without Laws."

50. See, for example, Fritsch, "Intimate Assemblages"; Mitchell and Snyder, *Biopolitics of Disability*; Puar, "CODA."

51. Ehrenreich and Hochschild, *Global Woman*; Erevelles, *Disability and Difference*; Flores-González et al., *Immigrant Women Workers*; Folbre, *For Love and Money*; Glenn, *Forced to Care*.

52. Spinoza, *Ethics*.

53. Spinoza, *Ethics*, I, P11, Alter.

54. Spinoza, *Ethics*, IV, P37, Schol.

55. Critical geographer Susan Ruddick elaborates on this power emerging through connection by calling it "the task of freedom":

The expansion of our capacity to act is at once *relational*, produced by mutually reinforcing collaborations, and the outcome of a complex interplay of affect and reason. It is through this interplay that we move from a passive experience of joy to an active understanding of the nature of the associations that empower.

See Ruddick, "Politics of Affect," 26 [emphasis added].
56. DeLanda, *A New Philosophy*.
57. Fox and Alldred, "Sexuality-Assemblage."
58. Harney and Moten, *Undercommons*, 26.
59. Halberstam, "Wild Beyond," 6.
60. Harney and Moten, *Undercommons*.
61. According to critical disability studies scholars Dan Goodley, Rebecca Lawthom, and Katherine Runswick-Cole, "One of the most significant contributions of critical disability studies has been the dislodging and deconstruction of *the fantasy of ableist human one-ness*. Disability demands mutuality, support and interdependence." Reassessing and revaluing a state of dependency that is overtly associated with disabled people and thus stigmatized, this quote captures the reality that humans—regardless of disability status—are inherently dependent beings and maneuver the world in relation with their surroundings. See Goodley, Lawthom, and Cole, "Posthuman Disability Studies," 353 [emphasis added]; Chandler, "Cripping Community"; Fritsch, "Intimate Assemblages"; Gibson, Carnevale, and King, "'This Is My Way'"; Ruddick, "Politics of Affect," 26.
62. See, for example, Butler, *Precarious Life*.
63. Mingus, "Access Intimacy, The Missing Link," "Access Intimacy, Interdependence."

CHAPTER 4

1. In addition to the list of content warnings provided for this book, this chapter includes mentions of institutionalization, eugenics, suicide, and care-based violence.
2. Creating Collective Access, *Creating Collective Access*; Dandy Shots, "Loree's Care Collective"; Duguay, "Repeat after Me"; McArthur and Zavitsanos, "Other Forms of Conviviality"; Milbern, "Reflections as Congress Debates"; Piepzna-Samarasinha, *Care Work*; Sweeney, "Young, Hot, Queer and Crip."
3. Piepzna-Samarasinha, *Care Work*; Dandy Shots, "Loree's Care Collective."
4. Duguay, "Repeat after Me"; Milbern, "Reflections as Congress Debates"; Piepzna-Samarasinha, *Care Work*; Sins Invalid, *Skin, Tooth, and Bone*.
5. Sins Invalid, *Skin, Tooth, and Bone*. The ten principles put together by Sins Invalid (a leading disability justice activist and performance art organization) are "intersectionality, leadership of those most impacted, anti-capitalist politics, cross-movement solidarity, recognizing wholeness, sustainability, commitment to cross-disability solidarity, interdependence, collective access, and collective liberation." See Sins Invalid, *Skin, Tooth, and Bone*, 22–27.
6. Piepzna-Samarasinha, *Care Work*; Sins Invalid, *Skin, Tooth, and Bone*. While those activists did the labor of articulating and putting forward activism of disability justice, elements that make up this activism have been practiced by activists and community

members since long before that. Also see Abdelhadi, "Addressing the Criminalization of Disability"; Cowing, "Occupied Land"; Timmons, "Towards a Trans Feminist."

7. Nishida, "Understanding Political Development"; Piepzna-Samarasinha, *Care Work*; Sins Invalid, *Skin, Tooth, and Bone*. Also by naming these communities, my intention is not to say that people from these communities are equally represented in disability justice activism. Many of those who are considered as people who coined and nurtured the work of disability justice do not necessarily (or at least publicly) identify as Indigenous people. There are increasing numbers of writings by Indigenous disabled activists on disability justice and articulations by them on how what Indigenous communities have been doing is inherently disability justice (or at least overlaps with its principles). See Cowing, "Occupied Land"; Driskill, "Anti-Colonial Disability"; LaDuke, *All Our Relations*.

8. Sins Invalid, *Skin, Tooth, and Bone*, 25 [emphasis added].

9. Mingus, "Access Intimacy, Interdependence and Disability Justice," para 33.

10. Mingus, "Access Intimacy: The Missing Link," "Access Intimacy, Interdependence and Disability Justice."

11. Gossett, Stanley, and Burton, "Known Unknowns"; Lewis, "Trans History"; Malatino, "Tough Breaks" and *Trans Care*; Nelson, *Body and Soul*; Park, Jimenez, and Hoekstra, "Decolonizing the US Health System"; Spade, "Solidarity Not Charity." See the Introduction on more elaborated descriptions of various community care.

12. Johnson, Mitchell, and Nuriddin, "Syllabus"; Lewis, "Trans History"; Skloot, *Immortal Life*; Washington, *Medical Apartheid*.

13. Nelson, *Body and Soul*.

14. Ferguson, *One-Dimensional Queer*; Gossett, Stanley, and Burton, "Known Unknowns"; Lewis, "Trans History"; Malatino, "Tough Breaks" and *Trans Care*.

15. Ferguson, *One-Dimensional Queer*; Gossett, Stanley, and Burton, "Known Unknowns"; Lewis, "Trans History."

16. Park, Jimenez, and Hoekstra, "Decolonizing the US Health System."

17. See, for example, Nishida, "Understanding Political Development."

18. Butler, *Precarious Life*. Analyzing the post-9/11 United States through the nation's heightened vulnerability, Judith Butler writes: "The dislocation from First World privilege, however temporary, offers a chance to start to imagine a world in which that violence might be minimized, in which an inevitable interdependency becomes acknowledged as the basis for global political community." Butler further continues:

I confess to not knowing how to theorize that interdependency. I would suggest, however, that both our political and ethical responsibilities are rooted in the recognition that radical forms of self-sufficiency and unbridled sovereignty are, by definition, disrupted by the larger global processes of which they are a part, that no final control can be secured, and that final control is not, cannot be, an ultimate value.

Not only Butler but many others have often suggested interdependence as an alternative or even antidote to the neoliberal formation. And yet how interdependency manifests and materializes in people's everyday life is rarely given attention and focus. See Butler, *Precarious Life*, xii–xiii.

19. Hedva, "sick woman theory: an interview." See also Piepzna-Samarasinha, *Care Work*; Aizura, "Communizing Care," and McArthur and Zavitsanos, "Other Forms of Conviviality," for discussions on similar challenges.

20. Manalansan, "Messy Mismeasures."

21. For more on methodologies and methods, see the Introduction.

22. Fineman, *Autonomy Myth*; Kittay, *Love's Labor*; McKenzie, "Autonomy and Automatons"; Nedelsky, *Law's Relations*; Puig de la Bellacasa, *Matter of Care*; Stoljar, "Informed Consent"; and Tronto, *Moral Boundary* and *Caring Democracy*.

23. Kelly, *Disability Politics and Care*; Kittay, *Love's Labor*; Morris, *Independent Lives* and "Independent Living"; Shakespeare, "Social Relations of Care."

24. Brown, "I Am Not Afraid"; Kelly, *Disability Politics and Care*; Kittay, *Love's Labor*; Morris, *Independent Lives* and "Independent Living"; Shakespeare, "Social Relations of Care."

25. Kelly, *Disability Politics and Care*; Morris, *Independent Lives* and "Independent Living"; Shakespeare, "Social Relations of Care."

26. Fineman, *Autonomy Myth*; Kittay, *Love's Labor*; McKenzie, "Autonomy and Automatons"; Nedelsky, *Law's Relations*; Puig de la Bellacasa, *Matter of Care*; Stoljar, "Informed Consent"; and Tronto, *Moral Boundary* and *Caring Democracy*.

27. Altiraifi, "Grounding Movements"; Genzlinger, "Mel Baggs"; Gibson, "Grounding Movements"; Lewis, "Ableism 2020."

28. Baggs, "Holding onto My Humanity."

29. Silentmiaow, "In My Language"; Genzlinger, "Mel Baggs." Also, critical race theorist Sylvia Wynter, for instance, has expanded on the entangled nature between the histories of Renaissance and colonization since the fifteenth century to understand the making of MAN (i.e., human) and Others. Wynter describes how the normal-abnormal and rational-irrational and hence human-other divides are developed and enacted in the force of racism, settler colonialism, and classism as secular knowledge building (i.e., physical science and then bioscience) took over the theocentric framework under the Renaissance. Simultaneously, a new racist and colonialist hierarchy of human is established to take over the previous one constructed within the Judeo-Christian framework under the projects of colonization. See Wynter, "Unsettling the Coloniality"; Wynter and McKittrick, "Unparalleled Catastrophe."

30. Erevelles, *Disability and Difference*.

31. Kittay, *Love's Labor*, 4 and 131 [emphasis added].

32. This reflects and speaks to Lewis's definition of ableism. See Lewis, "Ableism 2020." One place such a human-dehuman spectrum is clearly exercised in the United States is in its immigration policy and its use of the notion of *Public Charge* under the Immigration and Nationality Act to actively prevent disabled migrants (and any migrants who are considered as unfit according to the U.S. ideal) from entering the nation. See Jacobs, "Tortured Choice"; Hung and Perez, "Trump's New Wall."

33. Goodley, Lawthom, and Cole, "Dis/Ability and Austerity"; Kelly, *Disability Politics and Care*; Kittay, *Love's Labor*; Malatino, *Trans Care*; McArthur and Zavitsanos, "Other Forms of Conviviality."

34. Fabricant and Fine, *Changing Politics of Education*; Harvey, *Brief History*. There has been an increase in literature that critically analyzes the commodification of self-care and flourishment of the self-care industry as a mechanism to further enhance the neoliberal regime and control. See Kim and Schalk, "Resistance, Care."

35. Goodley, Lawthom, and Cole, "Dis/Ability and Austerity."

36. Lewis, "Ableism 2020"; Ben-Moshe, *Decarcerating Disability*.

37. Kelly, *Disability Politics and Care*; Kittay, *Love's Labor*; McArthur and Zavitsanos, "Other Forms of Conviviality"; Morris, *Independent Lives* and "Independent Living"; Shakespeare, "Social Relations of Care."

38. Lewis, "Ableism 2020." For instance, cisgender (white middle-class) women were historically diagnosed with psychiatric disability for not obeying gendered expectations of docility, while their failure and inability to be financially independent was rarely seen as a sign of disability. This example shows that concepts of disability and ableism are inherently shaped by sexist notions of which ability and capacity are to be considered as standards and norms and against which disability is constructed. See Metzl, *Protest Psychosis*; Nishida and Ostrove, "Power as Control."

39. See, for example, Gibson, Carnevale, and King, "'This Is My Way.'"

40. Fleischer and Zames, *Disability Rights Movement*; Kelly, *Disability Politics and Care*; Morris, *Independent Lives* and "Independent Living"; Shakespeare, "Social Relations of Care."

41. Such heavy investment in independence by the disability rights movement in the United States has been well articulated and critiqued by transnational feminist and other disability studies scholars of the Global South. See Erevelles, *Disability and Difference*; Kim, *Curative Violence*.

42. Kelly, *Disability Politics and Care*; Morris, *Independent Lives* and "Independent Living"; Shakespeare, "Social Relations of Care"; Vermont Center for Independent Living, *Independent Living Movement*.

43. Kelly, *Disability Politics and Care*; Morris, *Independent Lives* and "Independent Living"; Shakespeare, "Social Relations of Care."

44. Kelly, *Disability Politics and Care*.

45. See, for example, Mingus, "Access Intimacy: The Missing Link" and "Access Intimacy, Interdependence and Disability Justice."

46. Mingus, "Access Intimacy: The Missing Link" and "Access Intimacy, Interdependence and Disability Justice"; Nishida, "Understanding Political Development." In other words, disabled people experience and analyze the misinterpretation or infusion of the virtue of independence with ableism, particularly in the arena of rehabilitation. Physical therapist and disability studies scholar Barbara E. Gibson and her colleagues, for example, describe how disabled individuals are measured against an unachievable standard of independence, and their rehabilitation training is aimed mostly (if not entirely) toward the goal of independence—doing everything on their own without asking for assistance. In everyday life, who conducts their activities of daily living absolutely independently? Instead of pouring all of one's rehabilitation training and energy into the goal of independence (to do it all oneself), what are other opportunities toward which this rehabilitation training and energy could go? Why is it that disabled people are forced to adhere to the U.S. ideology of independence without consideration of its pitfalls and instead of society shifting its values (e.g., independency) to make itself more inclusive and liberatory to all? See Gibson, Carnevale, and King, "'This Is My Way.'"

47. See, for example, Duguay, "Repeat after Me"; Milbern, "Reflections as Congress Debates"; Piepzna-Samarasinha, *Care Work*; Sins Invalid, *Skin, Tooth, and Bone*.

48. Trnka and Trundle, *Competing Responsibilities*.

49. Trnka and Trundle, *Competing Responsibilities*.

50. For instance, in Lewis's definition of ableism, ability to perform and fit into the notion of *desirability* is one of the ways for ableism to be enacted. See Lewis, "Ableism 2020"; Reclaim Ugly, "Mission and Values."

51. Here, I am using the term *mental disability* as disability and Mad studies scholar Margaret Price does to denote "impairments of the mind" including but not limited to "psychiatric disability, mental illness, cognitive disability, intellectual disability, mental

health service user (or consumer), neurodiversity, neuroatypical, psychiatric system survivor, crazy, and mad." See Price, "Defining Mental Disability," 298.

52. This is another example Ruby brought up during what followed the preceding quote.

53. Sins Invalid, *Birthing, Dying, Becoming*.

54. Manalansan, "Messy Mismeasures," 496.

55. Manalansan, "Messy Mismeasures."

56. Patty Berne, one of the prominent disability justice activists, defines interdependence as a way to escape the state surveillance that comes with welfare programs. See Berne, "Disability Justice."

57. Green, "Coronavirus"; Sins Invalid, *Skin, Tooth, and Bone*.

58. Morris, *Independent Lives* and "Independent Living"; Shakespeare, "Social Relations of Care."

59. Kittay, *Love's Labor*; McArthur and Zavitsanos, "Other Forms of Conviviality"; and Fineman, *Autonomy Myth* noted different forms of dependencies—one constructed within the given sociopolitical force (i.e., capitalism)—while my position is that those dependencies are not discrete but on a continuum. Although we all embody different levels of dependencies, they are further amplified and intensified by the surrounding forces.

60. Carrie Sandahl, Robert McRuer, and Alison Kafer, among others, have theorized interconnectedness of queer and crip. Here, I am also referencing to McRuer's question of "what might it mean to welcome the disability to come, to desire it?" See Sandahl, "Queering the Crip"; McRuer, *Crip Theory*, 207; Kafer, *Feminist, Queer, Crip*; Johnson and McRuer, "Cripistemologies."

61. This notion of not leaving anyone in (unwanted) isolation is, I believe, inherently a principle of disability justice work. I learned this phrasing first from disability justice activist Sebastian Margaret.

62. We always, always love you, Stacey ♥.

63. Here, I am building the argument also based on what I have learned from the Abolition and Disability Justice Coalition. See Abolition and Disability Justice Coalition; "Abolition and Disability Justice Coalition."

64. Goodley, Lawthom, and Cole, "Dis/Ability and Austerity"; Puar, *Right to Maim*.

CHAPTER 5

1. In addition to the list of content warnings provided for this book, this chapter includes mentions of gun violence and mass murder.

2. Here and throughout this chapter, I trace works of disabled and sick artists and scholars who write about bed-born wisdom and activism. These include works by Joanna Hedva, Aurora Levins Morales, and Leah Lakshmi Piepzna-Samarasinha. Works by the following activists, artists, and scholars have also informed this chapter profoundly: Patty Berne and other Sins Invalid artists, Stacey Park Milbern, Jennifer Brea, Ellen Samuels, Susan Wendell, Carolyn Lazard, and Park McArthur. See Hedva, "Sick Woman Theory"; Morales, *Kindling*; Piepzna-Samarasinha, *Care Work*; Sins Invalid, *Skin, Tooth, and Bone* and *Birthing, Dying, Becoming*; Fat Rose, "Stacey Milbern"; Piepzna-Samarasinha and Wong, "#StaceyTaughtUs"; Brea, *Unrest*; Samuels, "On the Hospital"; Wendell, "Notes from Bed"; Lazard, "Carolyn Lazard"; McArthur, "Edition One and Two."

3. Hedva, "Sick Woman Theory"; Morales, *Kindling*; Piepzna-Samarasinha, *Care Work*; Samuels, "On the Hospital"; Sins Invalid, *Skin, Tooth, and Bone*; Wendell, "Notes from Bed."

4. Macías-Rojas, *From Deportation* and "Immigration and the War"; Richie, Brown, and Shah, "Reciprocal Politics."

5. Hedva, "Sick Woman Theory"; Morales, *Kindling*; Piepzna-Samarasinha, *Care Work*; Sins Invalid, *Skin, Tooth, and Bone* and *Birthing, Dying, Becoming*; Fat Rose, "Stacey Milbern"; Lazard, "Carolyn Lazard"; Piepzna-Samarasinha and Wong, "#StaceyTaughtUs"; Brea, *Unrest*; Samuels, "On the Hospital"; Wendell, "Notes from Bed"; McArthur, "Edition One and Two."

6. Sins Invalid, *Skin, Tooth, and Bone* and *Birthing, Dying, Becoming*.

7. See, for example, Malatino, "Tough Breaks"; Spade, "Solidarity Not Charity."

8. I am asking these questions with a hope to build on works by Johanna Hedva and Victoria Rodríguez-Roldán, as well as Leah Lakshmi Piepzna-Samarasinha and Aurora Levins Morales. See Hedva, "Sick Woman Theory"; Rodríguez-Roldán, "Who Gets to Be"; Piepzna-Samarasinha, *Care Work*; Morales, *Kindling*.

9. Brown, "Neo-Liberalism"; Harvey, *Brief History*.

10. See, for example, Mitchell and Snyder, *Biopolitics of Disability*; Puar, *Right to Maim*.

11. Macías-Rojas, *From Deportation* and "Immigration and War."

12. Piepzna-Samarasinha, *Care Work*, 183.

13. Also, I acknowledge the privilege in flexibility afforded by my current work at a university and other benefits (e.g., health insurance), which is a buffer to my life and survival. I am not sure if *privilege* would be the best word here, though, since they should be basic rights given to all the people no matter what.

14. Malatino, "Tough Breaks"; Spade, "Solidarity Not Charity."

15. Richie, Brown, and Shah, "Reciprocal Politics"; Ben-Moshe, *Decarcerating Disability*; Macías-Rojas, *From Deportation* and "Immigration and War."

16. See, for example, Arendt, *Human Condition*, cited in Hedva, "Sick Woman Theory."

17. Piepzna-Samarasinha, *Care Work*.

18. Morales, *Kindling*.

19. Sins Invalid, *Skin, Tooth, and Bone* and *Birthing, Dying, Becoming*; Fat Rose, "Stacey Milbern"; see also Piepzna-Samarasinha and Wong, "#StaceyTaughtUs"; Wendell, "Notes from Bed"; Samuels, "On the Hospital"; Brea, *Unrest*: Lazard, "Carolyn Lazard"; McArthur, "Edition One and Two."

20. See, for example, Haley, *No Mercy Here*; Molina, "Medicalizing the Mexican"; Chapter 1 of this book.

21. Bailey and Mobley, "Work in the Intersections"; Haley, *No Mercy Here*; Molina, "Medicalizing the Mexican"; Schalk and Kim, "Integrating Race"; Pickens, *Black Madness*; Erevelles, *Disability and Difference*.

22. Iyengar, "Framing Responsibility."

23. Miles, "'Strong Black Women.'"

24. Piepzna-Samarasinha, *Care Work*, 184.

25. Fireweed Collective, "Our Framework."

26. See Samuels, "Six Ways," where Samuels beautifully describes such a mixture and reality with details.

27. Morales, *Kindling*, 77–78.

28. Wendell, "Notes from Bed," 209–210 [emphasis added].

29. Sins Invalid, *Skin, Tooth, and Bone.*

30. Sins Invalid, *Skin, Tooth, and Bone;* "Our existence is our resistance" is printed on a T-shirt that the Disability Visibility Project created as well.

31. See, for example, Baynton, "Disability and the Justification."

32. Hedva, "Sick Woman Theory."

33. Garland-Thomson, "Feminist Disability Studies."

34. Hedva, "Sick Woman Theory," sec. 1, para. 3.

35. Hedva, "Sick Woman Theory," sec. 1, para. 1; sec. 4, para. 3.

36. Hedva, "Sick Woman Theory," sec. 4, para. 3.

37. McRuer, *Crip Theory.*

38. Clare, *Brilliant Imperfection.* A critique is that even the form of self-care has been commercialized and turned into a mechanism to surveil and self-discipline people to fit into capitalist demands. See Jones, "Beyond Self-Care"; Kim and Schalk, "Resistance, Care"; Gibson, "Grounding Movement"; Krip Hop Nation and 5th Battalion ent., *Broken Bodies;* Lewis, "Honoring Arnaldo Rios-Soto"; Moore, Gray-Garcia, and Thrower, "Black and Blue"; Sins Invalid, *Skin, Tooth, and Bone;* Thrower and Moore, *Where Is Hope.*

39. Piepzna-Samarasinha, *Care Work,* 184 (emphasis in original).

40. Piepzna-Samarasinha, *Care Work,* 186–188.

41. Puar, "coda" and *Right to Maim;* Berlant, "Slow Death."

42. Malatino, "Tough Breaks"; Spade, "Solidarity Not Charity."

43. Mbembe, "Necropolitics" and *Necropolitics;* Berlant, "Slow Death"; Gilmore, *Golden Gulag;* Hong, *Death beyond Disavowal;* Ferguson and Hong, "Sexual and Racial Contradictions"; Reeve, "Biopolitics and Bare Life."

44. Weheliye, *Habeas Viscus.*

45. DeLanda, *A New Philosophy.*

46. Piepzna-Samarasinha, *Care Work,* 184.

47. Morales, *Kindling,* 6–9.

48. Hedva, "Sick Woman Theory."

49. Morales, *Kindling,* 6–8 [emphasis added].

50. See, for example, Harvey, *Brief History;* Puar, "coda."

51. Morales, *Kindling.*

52. Morales, *Kindling,* 10–11.

53. Malatino, "Tough Breaks"; Spade, "Solidarity Not Charity."

54. It is also crucial to note that those images of the disability rights movement are overwhelmingly occupied and represented by white U.S. citizens with physical disabilities, and it also deterred many who do not identify similarly to them from disability communities. See Nishida, "Understanding Political Development."

55. See, for example, Dixon et al., "26 Ways"; Malatino, "Tough Breaks"; Spade, "Solidarity Not Charity."

56. See also Sins Invalid, *Skin, Tooth, and Bone.*

57. Hedva, "Sick Woman Theory," sec. 1, para. 7 (emphasis in original).

58. See, for example, Dixon et al., "26 Ways"; Malatino, "Tough Breaks"; Spade, "Solidarity Not Charity."

59. See, for example, Price, *Mad at School;* Wendell, "Notes from Bed."

60. Hedva, "Sick Woman Theory," sec. 5, para. 1 [emphasis added].

61. Hedva, "Sick Woman Theory."

62. Macías-Rojas, *From Deportation* and "Immigration and War."

63. Macías-Rojas, *From Deportation* and "Immigration and War"; Ben-Moshe, Chapman, and Carey, *Disability Incarcerated*.

64. See, for example, Nelson, *Body and Soul*; Park, Jimenez, and Hoekstra, "Decolonizing the US Health System."

65. Disability Justice Culture Club, "All Living"; see also Chapter 4.

66. Hedva, "Sick Woman Theory," sec. 6, para. 2.

67. The term *crip-licious* was first introduced to me by disability studies scholar Lezlie Frye.

POSTSCRIPT

1. In addition to the list of content warnings provided for this book, this chapter includes mentions of ableist care rationing and death.

2. Centers for Disease Control and Prevention, "When You've Been."

3. Price, *Mad at School*; Pickens, *Black Madness*; Samuels, "On the Hospital" and "Six Ways"; Hedva, "Sick Woman Theory"; Morales, *Kindling*; Piepzna-Samarasinha, *Care Work*; Sins Invalid, *Skin, Tooth, and Bone*.

4. Parrey, "Being Disoriented."

5. I am building this way of thinking—that the COVID pandemic and other concurrent violent oppressions are related—from the talk given by Nirmala Erevelles. See Center for 21st Century Studies, "Long 2020." See also African American Policy Forum, *Under the Blacklight*.

6. Stacey Park Milbern and others have engaged in grounded activism and care by embodying disability justice activism principles. See Milbern, "Reflections as Congress Debates"; Piepzna-Samarasinha and Wong, *#StaceyTaughtUs*.

7. Stramondo, "COVID-19 Triage"; Center for Public Representation, "CPR and Partners File Complaint" and "CPR and Partners File Second Complaint"; Shaviro, "Disability Groups File."

8. Lupus Foundation of America. "Hydroxychloroquine" and "Lupus Facts and Statistics."

9. Asch, "Reproduction"; McGuire, *War on Autism*; Stramondo, "COVID-19 triage."

10. Crip Fund, "Crip Fund Is Pooling."

11. Green, "Coronavirus"; Disability Culture Crip and Ally Care Exchange, "About."

12. Here, I am lifting the wisdom shared by writer and disability justice activist Aaron M. Ambrose, who shared a series of Facebook posts with their crip wisdom during the COVID pandemic.

13. Black, "Pod Mapping for Mutual Aid."

14. Hedva, "Sick Woman Theory"; Morales, *Kindling*; Piepzna-Samarasinha, *Care Work*; Berne, "Disability Justice"; Sins Invalid, *Skin, Tooth, and Bone* and *Birthing, Dying, Becoming*; Fat Rose, "Stacey Milbern"; Piepzna-Samarasinha and Wong, "#StaceyTaughtUs"; Brea, *Unrest*; Samuels, "On the Hospital"; Wendell, "Notes from Bed."

15. Dixon et al., "26 Ways to Be."

16. Richie, Brown, and Shah, *Reciprocal Politics*.

17. Here, I am bringing back the notion of "needs as sacred" by Disability Justice Culture Club, whose quote I started this book with. See Disability Justice Cultural Club, "All Living Creatures."

Bibliography

Abbott, Pamela. "Conflict over the Grey Areas: District Nurses and Home Helps Providing Community Care." *Journal of Gender Studies* 3, no. 3 (1994): 299–306.

Abdelhadi, Abla. "Addressing the Criminalization of Disability from a Disability Justice Framework: Centring the Experiences of Disabled Queer Trans Indigenous and People of Colour." *Feminist Wire*, November 21, 2013. https://www.thefeministwire .com/2013/11/addressing-the-criminalization-of-disability-from-a-disability-justice -framework-centring-the-experiences-of-disabled-queer-trans-indigenous-and -people-of-colour/.

Abolition and Disability Justice Coalition. *Abolition and Disability Justice Coalition.* https://abolitionanddisabilityjustice.com/.

Acs, Gregory, and Paloma Loprest. *Leaving Welfare: Employment and Well-being of Families That Left Welfare in the Post-Entitlement Era*. Kalamazoo, MI: W. E. Upjohn Institute for Employment Research, 2004.

Aetna Better Health of New York. *New York Managed Long-Term Care Program Member Handbook.* 2020. https://www.aetnabetterhealth.com/ny/assets/pdf/members/mem ber-materials/handbook/mltc/Final%20ABHNY%20Member%20HB%20expansion .pdf.

African American Policy Forum. *Under the Blacklight: The Intersectional Vulnerabilities That COVID Lays Bare*. Podcast series. https://www.aapf.org/aapfcovid.

Aizura, Aren. "Communizing Care in the Left Hand of Darkness." *Ada: A Journal of Gender, New Media, and Technology* 12 (2017). https://adanewmedia.org/2017/10 /issue12-aizura/.

Ajo, Tanja, Liat Ben-Moshe, and Leon J. Hilton. "Mad Futures: Affect/Theory/Violence." *American Quarterly* 69, no. 2 (2017): 291–302.

Altiraifi, Azza. "Grounding Movements in Disability Justice." Webinar, 2020. https:// www.dustinpgibson.com/offerings/groundingmovementsindj.

Arendt, Hannah. *The Human Condition*. Chicago: University of Chicago Press, 1958.

Artiga, Samantha, Jessica Stephens, and Harry Heinman. "Advancing Opportunities, Assessing Challenges: Key Themes from a Roundtable Discussion of Health Care and Health Equity in the South." *Kaiser Family Foundation*, June 19, 2014. https://www .kff.org/racial-equity-and-health-policy/issue-brief/advancing-opportunities -assessing-challenges-key-themes-from-a-roundtable-discussion-of-health-care-and -health-equity-in-the-south/.

Asch, Adrienne. "Reproduction." In Keywords for Disability Studies, edited by Rachel Adams, Benjamin Reiss, and David Serlin, 155–157. New York: New York University Press, 2015.

Ashley, Collin P., and Michelle Billies. "The Effective Capacity of Blackness." *Subjectivity* 10, no. 1 (2017): 63–88.

Bach, Stephen. "International Migration of Health Workers: Labour and Social Issues." Sector Sctivities Programme Working Paper. Geneva: International Labour Office, 2003.

Baggs, Mel. "Holding onto My Humanity." *Cussin' and Discussin'* (blog), August 22, 2017. https://cussinanddiscussin.wordpress.com/2017/08/22/holding-onto-my-hu manity/.

———. "Why We Should Listen to 'Unusual' Voices." *Anderson Cooper Blog 360°*, February 21, 2007. http://www.cnn.com/CNN/Programs/anderson.cooper.360/blog/2007 /02/why-we-should-listen-to-unusual-voices.html.

Bailey, Moya, and Izetta A. Mobley. "Work in the Intersections: A Black Feminist Disability Framework." *Gender and Society* 33, no. 1 (2018): 19–40.

Baines, Donna. "Staying with People Who Slap Us Around: Gender, Juggling Responsibilities and Violence in Paid (and Unpaid) Care Work." *Gender, Work and Organization* 13, no. 2 (2006): 129–151.

Baker, Mike. "Seeing 'Black Lives Matter' Written in Chalk, One City Declares It a Crime." *New York Times*, July 16, 2020. https://www.nytimes.com/2020/07/16/us /sidewalk-chalk-police-selah-washington.html.

Banks, Nina. "Black Women's Labor Market History Reveals Deep-Seated Race and Gender Discrimination." Economic Policy Institute, February 19, 2019. https://www .epi.org/blog/black-womens-labor-market-history-reveals-deep-seated-race-and -gender-discrimination/.

Baynton, Douglas. "Disability and the Justification of Inequality in American History." In *The New Disability History: American Perspectives*, edited by Paul K. Longmore and Lauri Umansky, 33–57. New York: New York University Press, 2001.

Ben-Moshe, Liat. *Decarcerating Disability: Deinstitutionalization in Prison Abolition*. Minneapolis: University of Minnesota Press, 2020.

Ben-Moshe, Liat, Chris Chapman, and Allison C. Carey, eds. *Disability Incarcerated: Imprisonment and Disability in the United States and Canada*. New York: Palgrave Macmillan, 2014.

Berkin, Carol. *Revolutionary Mothers: Women in the Struggle for America's Independence*. New York: Knopf, 2005.

Berlant, Lauren. "Slow Death (Sovereignty, Obesity, Lateral Agency)." *Critical Inquiry* 33, no. 4 (2007): 754–780.

Berne, Patty. "Disability Justice—a Working Draft." *Sins Invalid* (blog), June 9, 2015. https://www.sinsinvalid.org/blog/disability-justice-a-working-draft-by-patty -berne.

Bernhardt, Annette, Siobhan McGrath, and James DeFilippis. *Unregulated Work in the Global City: Employment and Labor Law Violation in New York City.* New York: Brennan Center for Justice, 2007.

Bernstein, Nina. "Advocates Say Managed-Care Plans Shun the Most Disabled Medicaid Users." *New York Times,* May 1, 2013. https://www.nytimes.com/2013/05/01/nyre gion/advocates-say-ny-managed-care-plans-shun-the-most-disabled-seniors.html.

———. "Lives Upended by Disrupted Cuts in Home-Health Care for Disabled Patients." *New York Times,* July 20, 2016. https://www.nytimes.com/2016/07/21/nyregion /insurance-groups-in-new-york-improperly-cut-home-care-hours.html.

———. "Medicaid Home Care Cuts Are Unjust, Lawsuit Says." *New York Times,* July 15, 2014. https://www.nytimes.com/2014/07/16/nyregion/legal-group-sues-over-cuts-to -assistance-in-medicaid-home-care-services-.html.

———. "Medicaid Shift Fuels Rush for Profitable Clients." *New York Times,* May 8, 2014. https://www.nytimes.com/2014/05/09/nyregion/medicaid-shift-fuels-rush-for-prof itable-clients.html.

———. "Pitfalls Seen in a Turn to Privately Run Long-Term Care." *New York Times,* March 17, 2014. https://www.nytimes.com/2014/03/07/nyregion/pitfalls-seen-in -tennessees-turn-to-privately-run-long-term-care.html.

Black, Rebel Sidney. "Pod Mapping for Mutual Aid." 2020. http://www.pdxdisabilityjus tice.org/pod-mapping.pdf.

Blackman, Lisa. "Embodying Affect: Voice-Hearing, Telepathy, Suggestion and Model-ling the Nonconscious." *Body and Society* 16, no. 1 (2010): 163–192.

Boris, Eileen, and Jennifer Klein. *Caring for America: Home Health Workers in the Shadow of the Welfare State.* Oxford, UK: Oxford University Press, 2015.

Bouie, Jamelle. "Mississippi's Race to the Bottom." *Slate,* October 20, 2014. http://www .slate.com/articles/news_and_politics/politics/2014/10/mississippi_the_affordable _care_act_and_racism_the_state_s_failures_are.html.

Braun, Virginia, and Victoria Clarke. "Using Thematic Analysis in Psychology." *Qualita-tive Research in Psychology* 3, no. 2 (2006): 77–101.

Brea, Jennifer, dir. *Unrest.* Glendale, CA: Shella Films, 2017.

Brown, Lydia X. Z. "I Am Not Afraid." *Autistic Hoya* (blog), June 18, 2013. https://www .autistichoya.com/2013/06/i-am-not-afraid.html.

———. "Like Festering Wounds: Ableism, White Supremacy, and the Prison-Industrial Complex." Paper presented at the Western Massachusetts Disability Studies Confer-ence, Northampton, MA, February 2016.

Brown, Lydia X. Z., E. Ashkenazy, and Morénike Giwa Onaiwu, ed. *All the Weight of Our Dreams: On Living Racialized Autism.* Lincoln, NE: DragonBee Press, 2017.

Brown, Wendy. "Neo-Liberalism and the End of Liberal Democracy." *Theory and Event* 7, no. 1 (2003). https://doi.org/10.1353/tae.2003.0020.

Butler, Judith. *Precarious Life: The Powers of Mourning and Violence.* London: Verso Books, 2004.

Cacho, Lisa M. *Social Death: Racialized Rightlessness and the Criminalization of the Unprotected.* New York: New York University Press, 2012.

Cambiando Vidas. "Cambiando Vidas—Changing Lives." https://www.accessliving.org /get-involved/join-a-community-organizing-group/cambiando-vidas/.

Caring Across Generations. "About." https://caringacross.org/about/.

Center for 21st Century Studies. "The Long 2020: Nirmala Erevelles, Bernard Perley, Tom Rademacher." Webinar, April 16, 2021.

Center for Public Representation. "CPR and Partners File Complaint Regarding Illegal Disability Discrimination in Treatment Rationing during COVID-19 Pandemic." Center for Public Representation, March 23, 2020. https://www.centerforpublicrep .org/news/cpr-and-partners-file-complaint-regarding-illegal-disability-discrimina tion-in-treatment-rationing-during-covid-19-pandemic/.

———. "CPR and Partners File Second Complaint Regarding Illegal Disability Discrimination in Treatment Rationing during COVID-19 Pandemic." Center for Public Representation, March 24, 2020. https://www.centerforpublicrep.org/news/cpr-and-part ners-file-second-complaint-regarding-illegal-disability-discrimination-in-treat ment-rationing-during-covid-19-pandemic/.

Centers for Disease Control and Prevention. "When You've Been Fully Vaccinated." May 16, 2021. https://www.cdc.gov/coronavirus/2019-ncov/vaccines/fully-vaccinated .html.

Centers for Medicare and Medicaid Services. "Eligibility." n.d. https://www.medicaid .gov/medicaid/eligibility/index.html.

———. "Managed Care." n.d. http://www.medicaid.gov/Medicaid-CHIP-Program-In formation/By-Topics/DeliverySystems/Managed-Care/Managed-Care.html.

———. "National Health Expenditure Projections 2019–2028." 2020. https://www.cms .gov/Research-Statistics-Data-and-Systems/Statistics-Trends-and-Reports/National HealthExpendData/NationalHealthAccountsProjected.

———. "Section 1115 Demonstrations." n.d. http://www.medicaid.gov/Medicaid-CHIP -Program-Information/By-Topics/Waivers/1115/Section-1115-Demonstrations. html.

Chandler, Eliza. "Cripping Community: New Meanings of Disability and Community." *Nomorepotlucks*, 2012.

Chang, Grace. *Disposable Domestics: Immigrant Women Workers in the Global Economy.* Chicago: Haymarket Books, 2016.

Chen, Mel. *Animacies: Biopolitics, Racial Mattering, and Queer Affect.* Durham, NC: Duke University Press, 2012.

Choy, Catherine C. *Empire of Care: Nursing and Migration in Filipino American History.* Durham, NC: Duke University Press, 2003.

Clare, Eli. *Brilliant Imperfection: Grappling with Cure.* Durham, NC: Duke University Press, 2017.

Clough, Patricia T. "The Affective Turn: Political Economy, Biomedia and Bodies." *Theory, Culture and Society* 25, no. 1 (2008): 1–22.

Cohen, Cathy, and Sarah J. Jackson, "Ask a Feminist: A Conversation with Cathy J. Cohen on Black Lives Matter, Feminism, and Contemporary Activism." *Signs: Journal of Women in Culture and Society* 41, no. 4 (2016): 775–792.

Cowing, Jess L. "Occupied Land Is an Access Issue: Interventions in Feminist Disability Studies and Narratives of Indigenous Activism." *Journal of Feminist Scholarship* 17, Fall (2020): 9–25.

Cranford, Cathy J. *Home Care Fault Lines: Understanding Tensions and Creative Alliances.* Ithaca, NY: Cornell University Press, 2020.

Creating Collective Access. *Creating Collective Access.* https://creatingcollectiveaccess .wordpress.com/.

Crip Fund. "Crip Fund Is Pooling . . ." *Crip Fund.* https://cripfund.wordpress.com/.

Cuomo, Andrew. *Governor Cuomo Issues Executive Order Creating Medicaid Redesign Team.* 2011. http://www.governor.ny.gov/press/01052011medicaid.

Curti, Giorgio H., and Christopher M. Moreno. "Institutional Borders, Revolutionary Imaginings and the Becoming-Adult of the Child." *Children's Geographies* 8, no. 4 (2010): 413–427.

Daly, Mary, and Guy Standing. "Introduction." In *Care Work: The Quest for Security*, edited by Mary Daly, 1–12. Geneva: International Labour Organization, 2001.

Dandy Shots. "Loree's Care Collective." January 25, 2016. https://www.youtube.com /watch?v=i3rX8MAHULk.

Daniel, Matt. "Who Died during Hurricane Sandy, and Why?" *EarthlySky*, 2012. https:// earthsky.org/earth/who-died-during-hurricane-sandy-and-why.

da Silva, Denise F. "No-Bodies: Law, Raciality and Violence." *Griffith Law Review* 18, no. 2 (2014): 212–236.

DeLanda, Manuel. *A New Philosophy of Society Assemblage Theory and Social Complexity*. London: Continuum, 2006.

Deleuze, Gilles. *Expressionism in Philosophy: Spinoza*. Translated by Martin Joughin. New York: Zone Books, 1990.

———. "Postscript on Control Societies." In *Negotiations*, 177–182. Translated by Martin Joughin. New York: Columbia University Press, 1995.

———. *Spinoza: Practical Philosophy*. Translated by Robert Hurley. San Francisco: City Lights, 1988.

Deleuze, Gilles, and Félix Guattari. *Anti-Oedipus: Capitalism and Schizophrenia*. Translated by Robert Hurley. New York: Penguin, 2009.

———. *A Thousand Plateaus: Capitalism and Schizophrenia*. Translated by Brian Massumi. Minneapolis: University of Minnesota Press, 1987.

DiNapoli, Thomas P. *Medicaid in New York: The Continuing Challenge to Improve Care and Control Costs*. March 2015. https://www.osc.state.ny.us/files/reports/special-top ics/pdf/health-medicaid-2015.pdf.

Disability Culture Crip and Ally Care Exchange. "About." https://www.facebook.com /DisabilityCultureCACE/about/.

Disability Justice Culture Club. "All Living Creatures Have Needs." November 4, 2019. https://www.facebook.com/disabilityjusticecultureclub/posts/147532293278738.

Dixon, Ejeris, Piper Anderson, Kay U. Barrett, Ro Garrido, Emi Kane, Bhabvana Nancherla, Deesha Narichania, Sabelo Narasimhan, Amir Rabiyah, and Meejin Richart. "26 Ways to Be in the Struggle, beyond the Streets." Accessible version adapted by Alejandra Ospina and Akemi Nishida. Disability Visibility Project, June 6, 2020. https://disabilityvisibilityproject.com/2020/06/06/26-ways-to-be-in-the-struggle -beyond-the-streets-june-2020-update/.

Dodson, Lisa, and Wendy Luttrell. "Untenable Choices: Taking Care of Low-Income Families." *Contexts: Understanding People and Their Social World* 10, no. 1 (2011): 39–42.

Donovan, Rebecca. "Home Care Work: A Legacy of Slavery in U.S. Health Care." *Affilia* 2, no. 3 (1987): 33–44.

Driskill, Qwo-Li. "Anti-Colonial Disability Arts & Activism." Arts Everywhere Festival. Presentation at Art Gallery of Guelph, Guelph, ON, January 27, 2019. https://vimeo .com/346876230.

Duarte, Fernando David Márquez. "Black Earth Rising and Queer Sono: A Critical Decolonial Analysis." *Open Philosophy* 5, no. 1 (2021): 118–135.

Duffy, Mignon. *Making Care Count: A Century of Gender, Race, and Paid Care Work*. New Brunswick, NJ: Rutgers University Press, 2011.

Duguay, Jennie. "Repeat after Me: Care Collectives and the Practice of Community Based Care." *The Peak* (blog), May 21, 2017. http://peakmag.net/disability-justice/repeat-after-me/.

Dunbar-Ortiz, Roxanne. *An Indigenous People's History of the United States.* Boston: Beacon Press, 2014.

Durano, Mariana. "Women in International Trade and Migration: Examining the Globalized Provision of Care Services." In *Gender and Development Discussion Paper Series, No. 16,* organized by Economic and Social Commission for Asia and the Pacific, 2005.

Ehrenreich, Barbara, and Arlie R. Hochschild, eds. *Global Woman: Nannies, Maids, and Sex Workers in the New Economy.* New York: Macmillan, 2004.

Elflein, John. "Total Medicaid Expenditure 1966–2019." *Statista,* 2020. https://www.statista.com/statistics/245348/total-medicaid-expenditure-since-1966/.

Erdos, Emily. "Hurricane Sandy and the Inequalities of Resilience in New York." *American Prospect: Ideas, Politics, and Power,* 2018. https://prospect.org/infrastructure/hurricane-sandy-inequalities-resilience-new-york/.

Erevelles, Nirmala. *Disability and Difference in Global Contexts: Enabling a Transformative Body Politic.* New York: Palgrave, 2011.

Espiritu, Yén L. *Home Bound: Filipino American Lives across Cultures, Communities, and Countries.* Berkeley: University of California Press, 2003.

Fabricant, Michael, and Michelle Fine. *The Changing Politics of Education.* Boulder, CO: Paradigm, 2013.

Fat Rose. "Stacey Milbern: California Care Rationing Coalition May 6 Press Conference." May 12, 2020. https://www.youtube.com/watch?v=Oy3WgvCZEjg.

——. "What Is Fat Rose?" *Fat Rose.* https://fatrose.org/vision/.

Ferguson, Roderick A. *One-Dimensional Queer.* Cambridge, UK: Polity Press, 2019.

Ferguson, Roderick A., and Grace K. Hong. "The Sexual and Racial Contradictions of Neoliberalism." *Journal of Homosexuality* 59, no. 7 (2012): 1057–1064.

Fine, Michael D. *A Caring Society? Care and the Dilemmas of Human Service in the Twenty-First Century.* London: Palgrave Macmillan, 2007.

Fineman, Martha A. *The Autonomy Myth: A Theory of Dependency.* New York: New Press, 2004.

Fireweed Collective. "Our Framework." *Fireweed Collective.* https://fireweedcollective.org/.

Fisher, Lucy T., and Miliann Kang. "Reinventing Dirty Work: Immigrant Women in Nursing Homes." In *Immigrant Women Workers in the Neoliberal Age,* edited by Nilda Flores-González, Anna R. Guevarra, Maura Toro-Morn, and Grace Chang, 164–185. Champaign: University of Illinois Press, 2013.

Flanders, Laura. "Can 'Caring across Generations' Change the World?" *The Nation,* 2012. http://www.thenation.com/article/167354/can-caring-across-generations-change-world#.

Fleischer, Doris Z., and Frieda Zames. *The Disability Rights Movement: From Charity to Confrontation.* Philadelphia: Temple University Press, 2001.

Flores-González, Nilda, Anna R. Guevarra, Maura Toro-Morn, and Grace Chang, eds. *Immigrant Women Workers in the Neoliberal Age.* Champaign: University of Illinois Press, 2013.

Folbre, Nancy, ed. *For Love and Money: Care Provision in the United States.* New York: Russell Sage Foundation, 2012.

———. "Nursebots to the Rescue? Immigration, Automation, and Care." *Globalizations* 3, no. 3 (2006): 349–360.

Foucault, Michael. *The Birth of Biopolitics (Lectures at the Collège de France 1978–1979).* Translated by Graham Burchell. New York: Palgrave Macmillan, 2008.

———. *Society Must Be Defended: Lectures at the Collège de France 1975–1976.* Translated by David Macey. New York: Picador, 2003.

Fox, Nick J. *The Body.* Cambridge, UK: Polity Press, 2012.

Fox, Nick J., and Pam Alldred. "The Sexuality-Assemblage: Desire, Affect, Anti-Humanism." *Sociological Review* 61, no. 4 (2013): 769–789.

Francisco-Menchavez, Valerie. *Labor of Care: Filipina Migrants and Transnational Families in a Digital Age.* Champaign: University of Illinois Press, 2018.

Fritsch, Kelly. "Gradations of Debility and Capacity: Biocapitalism and the Neoliberalization of Disability Relations." *Canadian Journal of Disability Studies* 4, no. 2 (2015): 1–48.

———. "Intimate Assemblages: Disability, Intercorporeality, and the Labour of Attendant Care." *Critical Disability Discourse* 2 (2010): 1–14.

———. "Resisting Easy Answers: An Interview with Eli Clare." *Upping the Anti: A Journal of Theory and Action* 9 (2009): 45–59.

Garland-Thomson, Rosemarie. "Feminist Disability Studies." *Signs: Journal of Women in Culture and Society* 30, no. 2 (2005): 1557–1587.

Genzlinger, Neil. "Mel Baggs, Blogger on Autism and Disability, Dies at 39." *New York Times,* April 28, 2020. https://www.nytimes.com/2020/04/28/health/mel-baggs-dead .html.

Gibson, Barbara E., Franco A. Carnevale, and Gillian King. "'This Is My Way': Reimagining Disability, In/Dependence and Interconnectedness and Assistive Technologies." *Disability and Rehabilitation* 34, no. 22 (2012): 1894–1899.

Gibson, Dustin P. "Grounding Movements in Disability Justice." Webinar, 2020. https:// www.dustinpgibson.com/offerings/groundingmovementsindj.

Gillett, James. *A Grassroots History of the HIV/AIDS Epidemic in North America.* Spokane, WA: Marquette Books, 2011.

Gilmore, Ruth W. *Golden Gulag: Prisons, Surplus, Crisis, and Opposition in Globalizing California.* Berkeley: University of California Press, 2007.

Giroux, Henry A. *Neoliberalism's War on Higher Education.* Chicago: Haymarket Books, 2014.

———. "Reading Hurricane Katrina: Race, Class, and the Biopolitics of Disposability." *College Literature* 33, no. 3 (2006): 171–196.

Glazer, Greer. "Nurse Immigration." *Online Journal of Issues in Nursing* 9, no. 1 (2004): 15.

Glenn, Evelyn N. *Forced to Care: Coercion and Caregiving in America.* Cambridge, MA: Harvard University Press, 2010.

Goodley, Dan, Rebecca Lawthom, and Katherine R. Cole. "Dis/Ability and Austerity: Beyond Work and Slow Death." *Disability and Society* 29, no. 6 (2014): 980–984.

———. "Posthuman Disability Studies." *Subjectivity* 7 (2014): 342–361.

Goodley, Dan, and Mark Rapley. "How Do You Understand Learning Difficulties: Towards a Social Theory of 'Impairment.'" *Mental Retardation* 39, no. 3 (2001): 229–232.

Gordon, Linda. *Pitied but Not Entitled: Single Mothers and the History of Welfare.* New York: Free Press, 1994.

Gorman, Rachel. "Quagmires of Affect: Madness, Labor, Whiteness, and Ideological Disavowal." *American Quarterly* 69, no. 2 (2017): 309–313.

Gossett, Reina, Eric A. Stanley, and Johanna Burton. "Known Unknowns: An Instruction to Trap Door." In *Trap Door: Trans Culture Production and the Politics of Visibility*, edited by Reina Gossett, Eric A. Stanley, and Johanna Burton, xv–xxvi. Cambridge, MA: MIT Press, 2017.

Grech, Shaun. "Disability, Poverty and Development: Critical Reflections on the Majority World Debate." *Disability and Society* 24, no. 6 (2009): 771–784.

Green, Matthew. "Coronavirus: How These Disabled Activists Are Taking Matters into Their Own (Sanitized) Hands." KQED *News*, March 17, 2020. https://www.kqed.org /news/11806414/coronavirus-how-these-disabled-activists-are-taking-matters-into -their-own-sanitized-hands.

Gregg, Melissa, and Gregory J. Seigworth. "An Inventory of Shimmers." In *The Affect Theory Reader*, edited by Melissa Gregg and Gregory J. Seigworth, 1–28. Durham, NC: Duke University Press, 2010.

Guevarra, Anna R. *Marketing Dreams, Manufacturing Heroes: The Transnational Labor Brokering of Filipino Workers*. New Brunswick, NJ: Rutgers University Press, 2010.

Halberstam, Jack. "The Wild Beyond: With and For the Undercommons." In *The Undercommons: Fugitive Planning and Black Study*, by Stephano Harney and Fred Moten, 2–13. Brooklyn, NY: Autonomedia, 2013.

Haley, Sarah. *No Mercy Here: Gender, Punishment, and the Making of Jim Crow Modernity*. Chapel Hill: University of North Carolina Press, 2016.

Hall, Kim Q., ed. *Feminist Disability Studies*. Bloomington: Indiana University Press, 2011.

Haraway, Donna J. *When Species Meet*. Minneapolis: University of Minnesota Press, 2008.

Hardt, Michael, and Antonio Negri. *Empire*. Cambridge, MA: Harvard University Press, 2001.

———. *Multitude: War and Democracy in the Age of Empire*. New York: Penguin, 2004.

Harney, Stephano, and Fred Moten. *The Undercommons: Fugitive Planning and Black Study*. Brooklyn: Autonomedia, 2013.

Harris-Kojetin, Lauren, Manisha Sengupta, Eunice Park-Lee, and Roberto Valverde. *Long-Term Care Services in the United States: 2013 Overview*. Hyattsville, MD: National Center for Health Statistics, 2013.

Harvey, David. *A Brief History of Neoliberalism*. Oxford, UK: Oxford University Press, 2005.

Hayman, Bridget. "Independent Living History." In *Access Living* (blog), May 31, 2019. https://www.accessliving.org/newsroom/blog/independent-living-history/.

Healthcare Education Project. *Managed Long-Term Care and Nursing Homes: Frequently Asked Questions*, 2012. https://healthcareeducationproject.org/wp-content/uploads /2015/05/Managed_Care_FAQ_FINAL.pdf.

Hedva, Johanna. "Sick Woman Theory." *Mask Magazine*, 2016. http://www.maskmaga zine.com/not-again/struggle/sick-woman-theory.

———. "sick woman theory: an interview." Interview by Brianna Albers. *Monstering Magazine*, 2020. https://monsteringmag.com/magazine/sick-woman-theory-an-interview.

Henriques, Julian. "The Vibrations of Affect and Their Propagation on a Night Out on Kingston's Dancehall Scene." *Body and Society* 16, no. 1 (2010): 57–89.

Henschel, Haley. "Judge Stripped of Disability Cases, Not Job." *Milwaukee Journal Sentinel*, September 5, 2016. https://www.jsonline.com/story/news/politics/2016/09/05/judge-stripped-disability-cases-not-job/89774320/.

Hinton, Elizabeth, Robin Rudowitz, Lina Stolyar, and Natalie Singer. "10 Things to Know about Medicaid Managed Care." *Kaiser Family Foundation*, December 16, 2019. https://www.kff.org/medicaid/issue-brief/10-things-to-know-about-medicaid-managed-care/.

Hochschild, Arlie R. "Behind Every Great Caregiver: The Emotional Labour in Health Care." In *Emotional and Interpersonal Dimensions of Health Services: Enriching the Art of Care with the Science of Care*, edited by Laurette Dubé, Guylaine Ferland, and D. S. Moskowitz, 67–72. Montreal: McGill-Queen's University Press, 2004.

———. "Global Care Chains and Emotional Surplus Value." In *On the Edge. Living with Global Capitalism*, edited by Will Hutton and Anthony Giddens, 130–146. London: Jonathan Cape, 2000.

Hoffman, Amy. *Hospital Time*. Durham, NC: Duke University Press, 1997.

Hogg, Michael A., and Dominic Abrams. "Editorial: Group Processes and Intergroup Relations." *Group Processes and Intergroup Relations* 1, no. 1 (1998): 5–6.

Hong, Grace K. *Death beyond Disavowal: The Impossible Politics of Difference*. Minneapolis: University of Minnesota Press, 2015.

hooks, bell. "Theory as Liberatory Practice." *Yale Journal of Law and Feminism* 4, no. 1 (1991): 1–12.

Hughes, Bill. "Disabled People as Counterfeit Citizens: The Politics of Resentment Past and Present." *Disability and Society* 30, no. 7 (2015): 991–1004.

Hung, Elena, and Katherine Perez. "Trump's New Wall to Keep Out the Disabled." *New York Times*, November 20, 2018. https://www.nytimes.com/2018/11/29/opinion/trumps-disability-public-charge.html.

Internal Revenue Service. "ABLE Accounts: Tax Benefits for People with Disabilities." *Internal Revenue Service*, February 24, 2020. https://www.irs.gov/government-entities/federal-state-local-governments/able-accounts-tax-benefit-for-people-with-disabilities#::text=The%20Achieving%20a%20Better%20Life,pay%20for%20qualified%20disability%20expenses.

Iyengar, Shanto. "Framing Responsibility for Political Issues." *Annals of the American Academy of Political and Social Science* 546 (1996): 59–70.

Jacobs, Douglas. "A Tortured Choice for Immigrants: Your Health or Your Green Card?" *New York Times*, October 12, 2018. https://www.nytimes.com/2018/10/10/opinion/immigration-trump-health-public-charge.html.

Johnson, Antoine S., Elise A. Mitchell, and Ayah Nuriddin. "Syllabus: A History of Anti-Black Racism in Medicine." *Black Perspectives*, August 12, 2020. https://www.aaihs.org/syllabus-a-history-of-anti-black-racism-in-medicine/.

Johnson, Merri L., and Robert McRuer. "Cripistemologies: Introduction." *Journal of Literary and Cultural Disability Studies* 8, no. 2 (2014): 127–148.

Jones, Abeni. "Beyond Self-Care Bubble Baths: A Vision for Community Care." *Autostraddle*, July 20, 2017. https://www.autostraddle.com/on-being-a-burden-whats-missing-from-the-conversation-around-self-care-385525/.

Kafer, Alison. *Feminist, Queer, Crip*. Bloomington: Indiana University Press, 2013.

Kaiser Family Foundation. *Date Note: 5 Charts about Public Opinion on Medicaid*. February 28, 2020. https://www.kff.org/medicaid/poll-finding/data-note-5-charts-about-public-opinion-on-medicaid/.

————. *Five Key Facts about the Delivery and Financing of Long-Term Services and Supports*, 2013. http://kff.org/medicaid/fact-sheet/five-key-facts-about-the-delivery-and-financing-of-long-term-services-and-supports/.

————. *Medicaid and Managed Care*. 2001. http://kaiserfamilyfoundation.files.word press.com/2013/01/medicaid-and-managed-care-fact-sheet.pdf.

————. *Medicaid in the United States*. October, 2019. http://files.kff.org/attachment /fact-sheet-medicaid-state-US.

————. *Medicaid State Fact Sheets*. 2020. https://www.kff.org/interactive/medicaid -state-fact-sheets/.

————. *Status of State Medicaid Expansion Decisions: Interactive Map*. 2020. https:// www.kff.org/medicaid/issue-brief/status-of-state-medicaid-expansion-decisions-in teractive-map/.

Katz, Michael. *In the Shadow of the Poorhouse: A Social History of Welfare in America*. New York: Basic Books, 1986.

————. *Poverty and Policy in American History*. New York: Academic Press, 1983.

————. *The Undeserving Poor: America's Enduring Confrontation with Poverty: Fully Updated and Revised*. London: Oxford University Press, 2013.

Keller, Josh. "Mapping Hurricane Sandy's Deadly Toll." *New York Times*, November 12, 2012. https://archive.nytimes.com/www.nytimes.com/interactive/2012/11/17/nyre gion/hurricane-sandy-map.html.

Kelly, Christine. *Disability Politics and Care: The Challenge of Direct Funding*. Toronto: UBC Press, 2016.

Kim, Eunjung. *Curative Violence: Rehabilitating Disability, Gender and Sexuality in Modern Korea*. Durham, NC: Duke University Press, 2017.

Kim, Jina B., and Sami Schalk. "Resistance, Care, and Activist Scholarship." Paper presented at Symposium on Disability, Intersectionality, and Transnational Feminist Praxis, Mansfield, CT, March 2019.

Kittay, Eva F. *Love's Labor: Essays on Equality, Women, and Dependency*. New York: Routledge, 1999.

Kolářová, Kateřina. "'Grandpa Lives in Paradise Now': Biological Precarity and the Global Economy of Debility," *Feminist Review* 111, no. 1 (2015): 75–87.

Krip Hop Nation and 5th Battalion ent. *Broken Bodies, PBP, Police Brutality Profiling Mixtape*. Compact disc. Krip Hop Nation, 2011.

LaDuke, Winona. *All Our Relations: Native Struggles for Land and Life*. Cambridge, MA: South End Press.

Lara, Ali. "Wine's Time: Duration, Attunement, and Diffraction." *Subjectivity* 10, no. 1 (2017): 104–122.

Lara, Ali, Wen Liu, Collin P. Ashley, Akemi Nishida, Rachel J. Liebert, and Michelle Billies. "Affect and Subjectivity." *Subjectivity* 10, no. 1 (2017): 30–43.

Lazard, Carolyn. *Carolyn Lazard*. http://www.carolynlazard.com/.

Leong, Nancy. "Racial Capitalism." *Harvard Law Review* 126, no. 8 (2013): 2151–2226.

Lewis, Abram J. "Trans History in a Moment of Danger: Organizing within and beyond 'Visibility' in the 1970s." In *Trap Door: Trans Cultural Production and the Politics of Visibility*, edited by Reina Gossett, Eric A. Stanley, and Johanna Burton, 57–90. Cambridge, MA: MIT Press, 2017.

Lewis, Talila A. "Ableism 2020: An Updated Definition." *Talila A. Lewis* (blog), January 25, 2020. https://www.talilalewis.com/blog/ableism-2020-an-updated-definition.

──────. "Honoring Arnaldo Rios-Soto & Charles Kinsey: Archiving Liberation through Disability Solidarity." *Talila A. Lewis* (blog), July 22, 2016. https://www.talilalewis.com/blog/achieving-liberation-through-disability-solidarity.

Liebert, Rachel J. "Beside-the-Mind: An Unsettling, Reparative Reading of Paranoia." *Subjectivity* 10, no. 1 (2017): 123–145.

Lindquist, Johan, Biao Xiang, and Brenda S. A. Yeoh. "Opening the Black Box of Migration Brokers, the Organization of Transnational Mobility and the Changing Political Economy in Asia." *Public Affairs* 85, no. 1 (2012): 7–19.

Lipson, Debra, Maria Dominiak, Michelle Herman Soper, and Brianna Ensslin. *Developing Capitation Rates for Medicaid Managed Long-Term Services and Supports Programs: State Considerations.* 2016. https://www.chcs.org/media/MLTSS-Rate-Setting_Final.pdf.

Liu, Wen. "Toward a Queer Psychology of Affect: Restarting from Shameful Places." *Subjectivity* 10, no. 1 (2017): 44–62.

Livingston, Julie. *Debility and the Moral Imagination of Botswana.* Bloomington: Indiana University Press, 2005.

Longmore Institute. "Disability Visibility Justice with ASL/CC." Webinar, November 20, 2015. https://www.youtube.com/watch?v=qo8oVI7Jb5g.

Lorde, Audre. *Sister Outsider: Essays and Speeches.* New York: Ten Speed Press, 1984.

Lowe, Lisa. *Immigrant Acts.* Durham, NC: Duke University Press, 1997.

Lupus Foundation of America. "Hydroxychloroquine (Plaquenil) and Coronavirus (COVID-19) Questions and Answers." *Lupus Foundation of America* (blog), October 29, 2020. https://www.lupus.org/resources/hydroxychloroquine-plaquenil-coronavirus-covid19-questions-answers#.

──────. "Lupus Facts and Statistics." *Lupus Foundation of America* (blog), October 6, 2016. https://www.lupus.org/resources/lupus-facts-and-statistics#:~:text=Lupus%20is%20two%20to%20three,537%20young%20African%20American%20women.

Lynch, Kathleen, John Baker, and Maureen Lyins, with Sara Cantillon, Judy Walsh, Maggie Feeley, Niall Hanlon, and Maeve O'Brien. *Affective Equality: Love, Care and Injustice.* Hampshire, UK: Palgrave Macmillan, 2009.

Macías-Rojas, Patrisia. *From Deportation to Prison: The Politics of Immigration Enforcement in Post-Civil Rights America.* New York: New York University Press, 2016.

──────. "Immigration and the War on Crime: Law and Order Politics and the Illegal Immigration Reform and Immigrant Responsibility Act of 1996." *Journal of Migration and Human Security* 6, no. 1 (2018): 1–25.

Malatino, Hil. *Trans Care.* Minneapolis: University of Minnesota Press, 2020.

Malatino, Hilary. "Tough Breaks: Trans Rage and the Cultivation of Resilience." *Hypatia* 34, no. 1 (2019): 121–140.

Manalansan, Martin F., IV. "Messy Mismeasures: Exploring the Wilderness of Queer Migrant Lives." *South Atlantic Quarterly* 117, no. 3 (2018): 491–506.

──────. "Queering the Chain of Care Paradigm." *Scholar and Feminist Online* 6, no. 3 (2008). http://sfonline.barnard.edu/immigration/manalansan_01.htm.

Massumi, Brian. "The Autonomy of Affect." *Cultural Critique* 31, no. 2 (1995): 83–109.

──────. *Ontopower: War, Powers, and the State of Perception.* Durham, NC: Duke University Press, 2015.

————. "Pleasures of Philosophy." In *A Thousand Plateaus: Capitalism and Schizophre-nia*, by Gilles Deleuze and Félix Guattari. Translated by Brian Massumi, xvi–xv. Minneapolis: University of Minnesota Press, 1987.

————. *Politics of Affect*. Cambridge: Polity Press, 2015.

Mbembe, Achille. "Necropolitics." *Public Culture* 15, no. 1 (2003): 11–40.

————. *Necropolitics: Theory in Forms*. Durham, NC: Duke University Press, 2018.

McArthur, Park. *Edition One and Two Fantasies*. https://www.artland.com/exhibitions /solo-exhibition-48e9b4.

McArthur, Park, and Constantina Zavitsanos. "Other Forms of Conviviality: The Best and Least of Which Is Our Daily Care and the Host of Which Is Our Collaborative Work." *Women and Performance: A Journal of Feminist Theory* 23, no. 1 (2013). https://www.womenandperformance.org/ampersand/ampersand-articles/other -forms-of-conviviality.html.

McCann, Adam. "States with the Most and Least Medicaid Coverage." *WalletHub*, March 23, 2020. https://wallethub.com/edu/states-with-the-most-and-least-medi caid-coverage/71573/#methodology.

McCarthy, Jane R., and Raia Prokhovnik. "Embodied Relationality and Caring after Death." *Body and Society* 20, no. 2 (2014): 18–43.

McGuire, Anna. *War on Autism: On the Cultural Logic of Normative Violence*. Ann Arbor: University of Michigan Press, 2016.

McKenzie, Kwame. "Autonomy and Automatons: Managed Care in the USA." *Psychiatric Bulletin* 22, no. 12 (1998): 765–768.

McRuer, Robert. *Crip Theory: Cultural Signs of Queerness and Disability*. New York: New York University Press, 2006.

————. *Crip Times: Disability, Globalization, and Resistance*. New York: New York Uni-versity Press, 2018.

Medicaid Matters New York and National Academy of Elder Law Attorneys, New York Chapter. *Mis-managed Care: Fair Hearing Decisions on Medicaid Home Care Reduc-tions by Managed Long Term Care Plans*. July 2016. https://www.ilny.org/phoca download/Report-on-Medicaid-Home-Care-Reductions-in-New.pdf.

Meekosha, Helen. "Decolonizing Disability: Thinking and Acting Globally." *Disability and Society* 26, no. 6 (2011): 667–682.

Metzl, Jonathan M. *The Protest Psychosis: How Schizophrenia Became a Black Disease*. Boston: Beacon Press, 2011.

Meyer, Madonna H., ed. *Care Work: Gender Labor and the Welfare State*. New York: Routledge, 2000.

Michener, Jamila. *Fragmented Democracy: Medicaid, Federalism, and Unequal Politics*. Cambridge, UK: Cambridge University Press, 2018.

Milbern, Stacey. "Reflections as Congress Debates Our Future." In *Resistance and Hope: Essays by Disabled People. Crip Wisdom for the People*, edited by Alice Wong, 2018. https://disabilityvisibilityproject.com/resist/.

Milbern, Stacey, and Leah Lakshmi Piepzna-Samarasinha. "Disability Justice Activists Look at 'Ways to Maintain Ableism.'" *Democracy Now!*, June 23, 2010. https://www .youtube.com/watch?v=ONxbe0j0K6s.

Miles, Angel L. "Being Disabled IS A JOB!" Facebook, 2015.

————. "'Strong Black Women': African American Women with Disabilities, Intersect-ing Identities, and Inequality." *Gender and Society* 33, no. 1 (2019): 41–63. https:// journals.sagepub.com/doi/10.1177/0891243218814820.

Million, Dian. "Felt Theory: An Indigenous Feminist Approach to Affect and History." *Wicazo Sa Review* 24, no. 2 (2009): 53–76.

Mingus, Mia. "Access Intimacy, Interdependence and Disability Justice." *Leaving Evidence* (blog), April 12, 2017. https://leavingevidence.wordpress.com/2017/04/12/access-intimacy-interdependence-and-disability-justice/.

———. "Access Intimacy: The Missing Link." *Leaving Evidence* (blog), May 5, 2011. https://leavingevidence.wordpress.com/2011/05/05/access-intimacy-the-missing-link/.

———. "Changing the Framework: Disability Justice." *Leaving Evidence* (blog), February 12, 2011. https://leavingevidence.wordpress.com/2011/02/12/changing-the-framework-disability-justice/.

Minich, Julie A. "Enabling Whom? Critical Disability Studies Now." *Lateral* 5, no. 1 (2016). https://csalateral.org/issue/5-1/forum-alt-humanities-critical-disability-studies-now-minich/

Miserandino, Christine. "The Spoon Theory." *But You Don't Look Sick* (blog). https://butyoudontlooksick.com/articles/written-by-christine/the-spoon-theory/.

Mitchell, David T., and Sharon L. Snyder. *The Biopolitics of Disability: Neoliberalism Ablenationalism, and Peripheral Embodiment.* Ann Arbor: University of Michigan Press, 2015.

Mohanty, Chandra T. *Feminism without Borders: Decolonizing Theory, Practicing Solidarity.* Durham, NC: Duke University Press, 2003.

Mol, Annemarie. *The Logic of Care: Health and the Problem of Patient Choice.* New York: Routledge, 2008.

Molina, Natalia. "Medicalizing the Mexican: Immigration, Race, and Disability in the Early Twentieth-Century United States." *Radical History Review* 94 (2006): 22–37.

Moore, Leroy. "The Tearing Down of Black Disabled Movements, Constantly Starting Over." *Krip Hop Nation.* 2020. https://kriphopnation.com/the-tearing-down-of-black-disabled-movements-constantly-starting-over/.

Moore, Leroy F., Jr., Tiny aka Lisa Gray-Garcia, and Emmitt H. Thrower. "Black and Blue: Policing Disability and Poverty beyond Occupy." In *Occupying Disability: Critical Approaches to Community, Justice, and Decolonizing Disability,* edited by Pamela Block, Devva Kasnitz, Akemi Nishida, and Nick Pollard, 295–318. New York: Springer, 2016.

Morales, Aurora L. "Genealogies of Empowerment." In *Telling to Live: Latina Feminist Testimonios,* edited by Aurora L. Morales, Patricia Zavella, Norma Alarcon, Ruth Behar, Luz del Alba Acevedo, Celia Alvarez, Rina Benmayor, Claea Lomas, Daisy Cocco e Filippis, Gloria Holguin Cuadraz, Liza Fiol-Matta, Yvette Gisele Flores-Orrtiz, Mirtha F. Quintanales, Eliana Rivero, and Caridad Souza, 25–26. Durham, NC: Duke University Press, 2001.

———. *Kindling: Writings on the Body.* Cambridge, MA: Palabrera Press, 2013.

Morris, Jenny. *Independent Lives: Community Care and Disabled People.* Hampshire, UK: Palgrave Macmillan, 1993.

———. "Independent Living and Community Care: A Disempowering Framework." *Disability and Society* 19, no. 5 (2004): 427–442.

Nadasen, Premilla. *Household Workers Unite: The Untold Story of African American Women Who Built a Movement.* Boston: Beacon Press, 2016.

Nadasen, Premilla, Jennifer Mittelstadt, and Marisa Chappell, eds. *Welfare in the United States: A History with Documents, 1935–1996.* New York: Routledge, 2009.

Naidoo, Rajani. "Entrenching International Inequality: The Impact of the Global Com-modification of Higher Education on Developing Countries." In *Structure and Agency in the Neoliberal University*, edited by Joyce E. Canaan and Wesley Shumar, 84–100. New York: Routledge, 2008.

Narayan, Uma. "Colonialism and Its Others: Considerations on Rights and Care Dis-courses." *Hypatia* 10, no. 2 (1995): 133–140.

National Center for Health Statistics. "Table P-11: Type of Health Insurance Coverage for Persons under Age 65 and for Persons Aged 65 and over, by Selected Character-istics: United States, 2018." *National Health Interview Survey*, 2018. https://ftp.cdc .gov/pub/Health_Statistics/NCHS/NHIS/SHS/2018_SHS_Table_P-11.pdf.

National Conference of State Legislatures. *Managed Care, Market Reports and the States*. July 1, 2017. https://www.ncsl.org/research/health/managed-care-and-the -states.aspx.

National Council on Disability. *Chapter 1. An Overview of Medicaid Managed Care*. n.d. https://ncd.gov/policy/chapter-1-overview-medicaid-managed-care.

National Priorities Project. *Federal Spending: Where Does the Money Go*. n.d. https:// www.nationalpriorities.org/budget-basics/federal-budget-101/spending/.

Nedelsky, Jennifer. *Law's Relations: A Relational Theory of Self, Autonomy, and Law*. Oxford, UK: Oxford University Press, 2001.

Nelson, Alondra. *Body and Soul: The Black Panther Party and the Fight against Medical Discrimination*. Minneapolis: University of Minnesota Press, 2013.

New York State Department of Health. *Access* NY *Health Care. Health Insurance Applica-tion for Children, Adults and Families*. 2015. https://www.health.ny.gov/forms/doh -4220.pdf.

———. *Chapter* II *Administrative Rules and Regulations Subchapter R Park 98: Managed Care Organizations*. 2009. https://www.health.ny.gov/health_care/managed_care /pdf/subpart98-1and2.pdf.

———. MCO*'s Certified by New York State Department of Health*. 2012. https://www .health.ny.gov/health_care/managed_care/mcodefs.htm.

———. *Medicaid Enrollees and Expenditures by County*. 2014. https://www.health.ny .gov/statistics/health_care/medicaid/eligible_expenditures/.

———. *Quality Strategy for the New York State Medicaid Managed Care Program*. 2018. https://www.health.ny.gov/health_care/managed_care/quality_strategy.htm#i.

———. *Redesigning New York's Medicaid Program*. 2014. https://www.health.ny.gov /health_care/medicaid/redesign/.

———. *Transitional Cases Service Plan Submission Tracking: November 2012*. 2015. https://www.health.ny.gov/health_care/medicaid/redesign/2012-11_2013-04_transi tional_cases.htm.

Nga, Thach T., and Joshua M. Weiner. "An Overview of Long-Term Services and Sup-ports: Final Report." *U.S. Department of Health and Human Services*. 2018. https:// aspe.hhs.gov/basic-report/overview-long-term-services-and-supports-and-medicaid -final-report.

Nishida, Akemi. "Abuse." In *Disability in American Life: An Encyclopedia of Concepts, Policies, and Controversies*, 2 vols., edited by Tamer Heller, Sarah Parker Harris, Carol Gill, and Robert Gould, 5–8. Santa Barbara, CA: ABC-CLIO.

———. "Relating through Differences: Disability, Affective Relationality, and the U.S. Public Health Care Assemblage." *Subjectivity* 10, no. 1 (2017): 89–103.

———. "Understanding Political Development through an Intersectionality Framework: Life Stories of Disability Activists." *Disability Studies Quarterly* 36, no. 2 (2016).

Nishida, Akemi, and Joan M. Ostrove. "Power as Control/Power as Resistance and Vision: Disability and Gender in Psychology (and Beyond)." In *The Palgrave Handbook of Psychology, Power, and Gender*, edited by E. Zurbriggen and R. Capdevila. New York: Palgrave, forthcoming.

Oliver, Michael. *The Politics of Disablement.* London: Macmillan Education, 1990.

Olson, Laura K. *The Politics of Medicaid.* New York: Columbia University Press, 2010.

Ong, Paul, and Tania Azores. "The Migration and Incorporation of Filipino Nurses." In *The New Asian Immigration in Los Angeles and Global Restructuring*, edited by Paul Ong, Edna Bonacich, and Lucie Cheng, 164–195. Philadelphia: Temple University Press, 1994.

Organized Communities Against Deportations. "Campaigns." *Organized Communities Against Deportations*, n.d. https://www.organizedcommunities.org/campaigns.

O'Toole, Corbett J. *Fading Scars: My Queer Disability History.* Fort Worth, TX: Autonomous Press, 2015.

Paradise, Julia. "Medicaid Moving Forward." *Kaiser Family Foundation.* 2014. http://kff .org/medicaid/fact-sheet/the-medicaid-program-at-a-glance-update/.

Park, Lisa S.-H., Anthony Jimenez, and Erin Hoekstra. "Decolonizing the US Health System: Undocumented and Disabled after ACA." *Health Tomorrow: Interdisciplinarity and Internationality* 5 (2018): 24–54.

Parreñas, Rhacel. *Servants of Globalization: Migration and Domestic Work*, 2nd ed. Stanford, CA: Stanford University Press, 2015.

Parrey, Ryan C. "Being Disoriented: Uncertain Encounters with Disability." Disability Studies Quarterly 36, no. 2 (2016). https://dsq-sds.org/article/view/4555/4299.

Patterson, James T. *America's Struggle against Poverty 1900–1980.* Cambridge, MA: Harvard University Press, 1981.

Patton, Michael Q. *Qualitative Research and Methods*, 4th ed. Thousand Oaks, CA: SAGE Publications, 2015.

Pham, Xoai. "Principles of Pride: We Owe Our Lives to Trans Elders like Ceyenne Doroshow." *Autostraddle,* June 30, 2020. https://www.autostraddle.com/principles-of -pride-we-owe-our-lives-to-trans-elders-like-ceyenne-doroshow/.

PHI. "FACTS 5: Home Care Aides at a Glance." PHI, 2014. http://phinational.org/fact -sheets/facts-5-home-care-aides-glance.

———. "Projected Growth of Direct-Care Workers over Age 55, 2012–2022." PHI, 2014. http://phinational.org/policy/resources/chart-gallery.

———. "Workforce Data Center." PHI, 2017. https://phinational.org/resource/facts-5 -home-care-aides-at-a-glance/.

———. "Workforce Data Center." PHI, 2020. https://phinational.org/policy-research /workforce-data-center/#tab=National+Data&natvar=Health+Insurance.

Phillips, John W. P. "Agencement/Assemblage." *Theory, Culture and Society* 23, no. 2/3 (2006): 108–109.

Pickens, Therí A. *Black Madness:: Mad Blackness.* Durham, NC: Duke University Press, 2019.

Piepzna-Samarasinha, Leah L. *Care Work: Dreaming Disability Justice.* Vancouver: Arsenal Pulp Press, 2018.

Piepzna-Samarasinha, Leah L., and Alice Wong, eds. #StaceyTaughtUs Syllabus: Work by Stacey Park Milbern. 2020. https://disabilityvisibilityproject.com/2020/05/23/staceytaughtus-syllabus-work-by-stacey-milbern-park/.

Pimpare, Stephen. A People's History of Poverty in America. New York: New Press, 2008.

Polson, Diana. "The Caring Precariat: Home Health Care Work in New York City." PhD dissertation, Graduate Center, City University of New York, 2013.

Polson, Diana, James DeFilippis, and Annette Bernhardt. "Working without Laws in New York City." Challenge 54, no. 2 (2011): 80–108.

Poo, Ai-Jen with Ariane Conrad. The Age of Dignity: Preparing for the Elder Boom in a Changing America. New York: New Press, 2015.

Powers, Lauri, E., and Mary Oschwald. Violence and Abuse against People with Disabilities: Experiences, Barriers, and Prevention Strategies. N.d. https://www.temple.edu/instituteondisabilities/programs/justice/docs/bibliographyScans/Powers_Oschwald.pdf.

Price, Margaret. "The Bodymind Problem and the Possibilities of Pain." Hypatia 30, no. 1 (2014): 278–284.

———. "Defining Mental Disability." In The Disability Studies Reader, 4th ed., edited by Lennard J. Davis, 298–307. New York: Routledge, 2013.

———. Mad at School: Rhetoric of Mental Disability and Academic Life. Ann Arbor: University of Michigan Press, 2011.

Puar, Jasbir K. "CODA: The Cost of Getting Better: Suicide, Sensation, Switchpoints." GLQ: A Journal of Lesbian and Gay Studies 18, no. 1 (2012): 149–158.

———. "'I Would Rather Be a Cyborg Than a Goddess': Becoming-Intersectional in Assemblage Theory." Philosophia 2, no. 1 (2012): 49–66.

———. The Right to Maim: Debility, Capacity, Disability. Durham, NC: Duke University Press, 2017.

Puig de la Bellacasa, Maria. Matter of Care: Speculative Ethics in More Than Human Worlds. Minneapolis: University of Minnesota Press, 2017.

Quadagno, Jill. "The Transformation of Medicaid from Poor Law Legacy to Middle-Class Entitlement?" In Medicare and Medicaid at 50: America's Entitlement Programs in the Age of Affordable Care, edited by Alan B. Cohen, David C. Colby, Keith A. Wailoo, and Julian E. Zelizer, 77–94. Oxford, UK: Oxford University Press, 2015.

Reclaim Ugly. "Mission and Values." Reclaim Ugly, n.d. https://reclaimugly.org/about-us/.

Reeve, Donna. "Biopolitics and Bare Life: Does the Impaired Body Provide Contemporary Examples of Homo Sacer?" In Arguing about Disability: Philosophical Perspectives, edited by K. Kristianse, S. Vehmas, and T. Shakespeare, 203–218. New York: Routledge, 2009.

Rehabilitation Research and Training Center on Disability Statistics and Demographics. The Annual Disability Statistics Compendium Section 10: Medicaid and Medicare, n.d. http://disabilitycompendium.org/compendium-statistics/medicaid-and-medicare.

Richie, Beth E., Brown, Lydia X. Z., and Shah, Silky. "The Reciprocal Politics of Bed Space Activism: From Confinement to Radical Care." Webinar, April 9, 2021.

Robinson, Cedric J. Black Marxism: The Making of the Black Radical Tradition. Chapel Hill: University of North Carolina Press, 2000.

Rodríguez-Roldán, Victoria. "Who Gets to Be the Activist." In Resistance and Hope: Essays by Disabled People. Crip Wisdom for the People, edited by Alice Wong, 2018. https://disabilityvisibilityproject.com/resist/.

Roulstone, Alan. "Personal Independence Payments, Welfare Reform and the Shrinking Disability Category." *Disability and Society* 30, no. 5 (2015): 673–688.

Ruddick, Susan. "The Politics of Affect: Spinoza in the Work of Negri and Deleuze." *Theory, Culture and Society* 27, no. 4 (2010): 21–45.

Rudowitz, Robin, Kendal Orgera, and Elizabeth Hinton. "Medicaid Financing: The Basics." *Kaiser Family Foundation*, 2019. https://www.kff.org/medicaid/issue-brief /medicaid-financing-the-basics/view/print/.

Rupp, Kalman, Gerald F. Riley. "State Medicaid Eligibility and Enrollment Policies and rates of Medicaid Participation among Disabled Supplemental Security Income Recipients." *Social Security Bulletin* 76, no. 3 (2016). https://www.ssa.gov/policy/docs /ssb/v76n3/v76n3p17.html

Samuels, Ellen. "On the Hospital." *Rogue Agent: A Journal for Work That Inhabits the Body 51*, 2019. http://www.rogueagentjournal.com/esamuels.

———. "Six Ways of Looking at Crip Time." *Disability Studies Quarterly* 37, no. 3 (2017). https://dsq-sds.org/article/view/5824/4684.

Sandahl, Carrie. "Queering the Crip or Cripping the Queer? Intersections of Queer and Crip Identities in Solo Autobiographical Performance." GLQ: *A Journal of Lesbian and Gay Studies* 9, no. 1–2 (2003): 25–56.

Scales, Kezia. "It's Time to Care: A Detailed Profile of America's Direct Care Workforce." PHI, 2020. https://phinational.org/wp-content/uploads/2020/01/Its-Time-to-Care -2020-PHI.pdf.

Schalk, Sami. *Bodyminds Reimagined: (Dis)Ability, Race, and Gender in Black Women's Speculative Fiction*. Durham, NC: Duke University Press, 2018.

Schalk, Sami, and Jina B. Kim. "Integrating Race, Transforming Feminist Disability Studies." *Signs: Journal of Women in Culture and Society* 46, no. 1 (2020): 31–55.

Schweik, Susan. "Lomax's Matrix: Disability, Solidarity, and the Black Power of 504." *Disability Studies Quarterly* 31, no. 1 (2011). https://dsq-sds.org/article/view/1371.

Sequenzia, Amy, and Elizabeth J. Grace, eds. *Typed Words Loud Voices*. Fort Worth, TX: Autonomous Press, 2015.

Shakespeare, Tom. *Help*. Birmingham: British Association of Social Workers, 2000.

———. "The Social Relations of Care." In *Rethinking Social Policy*, edited by G. Lewis, S. Gewirtz, and J. Clarke, 52–65. New York: SAGE Publications, 2000.

Sharpe, Christina. *In the Wake: On Blackness and Being*. Durham, NC: Duke University Press, 2016.

Shaviro, Joseph. "COVID-19 Infections and Deaths Are Higher among Those with Intellectual Disabilities." NPR, June 9, 2020. https://www.npr.org/2020/06/09/872401607 /covid-19-infections-and-deaths-are-higher-among-those-with-intellectual -disabili.

———. "Disability Groups File Federal Complaint about COVID-19 Care Rationing Plans." NPR, March 23, 2020. https://www.npr.org/transcripts/820303309.

Shaviro, Steven. The "Bitter Necessity" of Debt: Neoliberal Finance and the Society of Control, 2010. http://www.shaviro.com/Othertexts/Debt.pdf.

Shildrick, Margrit. "'Why Should Our Bodies End at the Skin?': Embodiment, Boundaries, and Somatechnics." *Hypatia* 30, no. 1 (2015): 13–29.

Shildrick, Margrit, and Janet Price. "Deleuzian Connections and Queer Corporealities: Shrinking Global Disability." *Rhizomes* 11, no. 12 (2006).

Silentmiaow. "In My Language." January 14, 2007. https://www.youtube.com/watch?v =JnylM1hI2jc.

Sins Invalid. *Birthing, Dying, Becoming Crip Wisdom*. Performance, OCD Theater, San Francisco, October 14-15, 2016.
———. *Skin, Tooth, and Bone: The Basis of Movement Is Our People*, 2nd ed. Sins Invalid, 2019.
Skloot, Rebecca. *The Immortal Life of Henrietta Lacks*. New York: Crown, 2010.
Skowronski, Jeanine. "A State-by-State Guide to Medicaid: Do I Qualify?" *Policygenious*, 2018. https://www.policygenius.com/blog/a-state-by-state-guide-to-medicaid/.
Slife, Brent D. "Taking Practice Seriously: Toward a Relational Ontology." *Journal of Theoretical and Philosophical Psychology* 24, no. 2 (2004): 157–178.
Smith, Leah. "The Institutional Bias." *Center for Disability Rights*, n.d. http://cdrnys.org/blog/disability-dialogue/the-disability-dialogue-the-institutional-bias/.
Social Security Administration. *Supplemental Security Income (ssi)*, n.d. https://www.ssa.gov/pubs/EN-05-11000.pdf.
Soldatic, Karen. *Disability and Neoliberal State Formations*. New York: Routledge, 2019.
———. "The Transnational Sphere of Justice: Disability Praxis and the Politics of Impairment." *Disability and Society* 28, no. 6 (2013): 744–755.
Soldatic, Karen, and Shaun Grech. "Transnationalising Disability Studies: Rights, Justice and Impairment." *Disability Studies Quarterly* 34, no. 2 (2014).
Soldatic, Karen, and Helen Meekosha. "The Place of Disgust: Disability, Class and Gender in Spaces of Workfare." *Societies* 2, no. 3 (2012): 139–156.
Spade, Dean. *Mutual Aid: Building Solidarity during This Crisis (and the Next)*. London: Verso Books, 2020.
———. "Solidarity Not Charity: Mutual Aid for Mobilization and Survival." *Social Text* 38, no. 1 (2020): 131–151.
Spinoza, Baruch. *Ethics*. Translated by Edwin Curley. New York: Penguin Classics, 2005.
Stoljar, Natalie. "Informed Consent and Relational Conceptions of Autonomy." *Journal of Medicine and Philosophy* 36, no. 4 (2011): 375–384.
Stoll, Laurie Cooper. "Fat Is a Social Justice Issue, Too." *Humanity and Society* 43, no. 4 (2019): 421–441.
Stramondo, Joseph. "COVID-19 Triage and Disability: What NOT to Do." *Bioethics.net*, March 30, 2020. http://www.bioethics.net/2020/03/covid-19-triage-and-disability-what-not-to-do/.
Sweeney, Elizabeth. "Young, Hot, Queer and Crip: Sexing Up Disability Is a Way of Life for Loree Erickson." Xtra, September 9, 2009. https://xtramagazine.com/culture/young-hot-queer-crip-12141.
Thomas, Carol. *Sociologies of Disability and Illness: Contested Ideas in Disability Studies and Medical Sociology*. London: Macmillan International Higher Education, 2007.
Thrower, Emmitt H., and Leroy Moore Jr. "Where Is Hope: The Art of Murder." New York: Wabi Sabi Productions, 2015.
Timmons, Niamh. "Towards a Trans Feminist Disability Studies." *Journal of Feminist Scholarship* 17 (Fall 2020): 46–63.
Trattner, Walter I. *From Poor Law to Welfare State: A History of Social Welfare in America.*, 6th ed. New York: Free Press, 1999.
Trnka, Susanna, and Catherine Trundle. *Competing Responsibilities: The Ethics and Politics of Contemporary Life*. Durham, NC: Duke University Press, 2017.
Tronto, Joan C. *Caring Democracy: Markets, Equality, and Justice*. New York: New York University Press, 2013.

———. *Moral Boundary: A Political Argument for an Ethic of Care.* New York: Routledge, 1993.

———. "There Is an Alternative: Homines Curans and the Limits of Neoliberalism." *International Journal of Care and Caring* 1, no. 1 (2017): 27–43.

U.S. Bureau of Labor Statistics. *Labor Force Characteristics of Foreign-Born Workers Summary,* 2020. https://www.bls.gov/news.release/forbrn.nr0.htm/labor-force-char acteristics-of-foreign-born-workers-summary#::text=See%20table%201.)-,The%20 share%20of%20the%20U.S.%20civilian%20labor%20force%20that%20was,from%20 62.3%20percent%20in%202018.

U.S. Census Bureau. *Annual Services Report Data,* 2010. http://www.census.gov/ser vices/sas_data.html.

———. *Nearly 1 in 5 People Have a Disability in the U.S.: Census Bureau Reports,* 2012. https://www.census.gov/newsroom/releases/archives/miscellaneous/cb12-134.html.

U.S. Department of Health and Human Services. *2017 Poverty Guidelines,* 2017. https:// aspe.hhs.gov/2017-poverty-guidelines.

———. *What Is the Difference between Medicare and Medicaid?,* n.d. https://www.hhs .gov/answers/medicare-and-medicaid/what-is-the-difference-between-medicare -medicaid/index.html.

U.S. Department of Labor. *Fact Sheet: Application of the Fair Labor Standards Act to Domestic Service, Final Rule,* 2013. https://www.dol.gov/agencies/whd/fact-sheets /flsa-domestic-service.

Vasey, Sean. *The Rough Guide to Managing Personal Assistants.* London: National Centre for Independent Living, 2001.

Venn, Couze. "Individuation, Relationality, Affect: Rethinking the Human in Relation to the Living." *Body and Society* 16, no. 1 (2010): 129–161.

Verlinden, Jasper J. "On Affect Theory's Hidden Histories: Toward a Technological Genealogy." *American Quarterly* 69, no. 2 (2017): 321–326.

Vermont Center for Independent Living. *The Independent Living Movement and Disability Rights,* n.a. https://www.vcil.org/resources/pas-toolkit/the-independent-living -movement-and-disability-rights.

Vora, Kalindi. *Life Support: Biocapital and the New History of Outsourced Labor.* Minneapolis: University of Minnesota Press, 2015.

Ware, Syrus M. "Disabled: Not a Burden, Not Disposable." Webinar, 2020. https:// transgenderlawcenter.org/resources/covid19/disabled-not-a-burden.

Washington, Harriet A. *Medical Apartheid: The Dark History of Medical Experimentation on Black Americans from Colonial Times to the Present.* New York: Anchor Books, 2008.

Watermeyer, Brian. *Toward a Contextual Psychology of Disablism.* New York: Routledge, 2012.

Watson, Nick, Linda McKie, Bill Hughes, Debra Hopkins, and Sue Gregory. "(Inter) Dependence, Needs and Care: The Potential for Disability and Feminist Theorists to Develop an Emancipator Model." *Sociology* 38, no. 2 (2004): 331–350.

Wearing, Sadie, Yasmin Gunaratnam, and Irene Gedalof. "Frailty and Debility." *Feminist Review* 111, no. 1 (2015): 1–9.

Weheliye, Alexander G. *Habeas Viscus: Racializing Assemblages, Biopolitics, and Black Feminist Theories of the Human.* Durham, NC: Duke University Press, 2014.

Wendell, Susan. "Notes from Bed: Learning from Chronic Illness." In *Dissonant Disabilities: Women with Chronic Illnesses Explore Their Lives,* edited by Diane Driedger and Michelle Owen, 209–217. Toronto: Canadian Scholars' Press, 2008.

Wiley, Maya. "After Sandy: New York's 'Perfect Storm' of Inequality in Wealth and Housing." *The Guardian*, October 28, 2013. https://www.theguardian.com/commen tisfree/2013/oct/28/sandy-new-york-storm-inequality.

Wong, Alice. "My Medicaid, My Life." *New York Times*, May 3, 2017. https://www.ny times.com/2017/05/03/opinion/my-medicaid-my-life.html.

Wright, Beatrice A. *Physical Disability—A Psychosocial Approach*, 2nd ed. New York: HarperCollins, 1983.

Wynter, Sylvia. "Unsettling the Coloniality of Being/Power/Truth/Freedom: Towards the Human, after Man, Its Overrepresentation—An Argument." CR: *The New Centennial Review* 3, no. 3 (2003): 257–337.

Wynter, Sylvia, and Katherine McKittrick. "Unparalleled Catastrophe for Our Species? Or, to Give Humanness as Different Future: Conversations." In *Sylvia Wynter: On Being Human as Praxis*, edited by Katherine McKittrick, 9–89. Durham, NC: Duke University Press, 2015.

Yeates, Nicola. "Global Care Chains: A State-of-the-Art Review and Future Directions in Care Transnationalization Research." *Global Network* 12, no. 2 (2012): 135–154.

Zola, Irving K. "Bringing Our Bodies and Ourselves Back In: Reflections on a Past, Present, and Future 'Medical Sociology.'" *Journal of Health and Social Behavior* 32, March (1991): 1–16.

Index

Abbott, Pamela, 81
Ableism, 1, 11–13, 86, 103, 126, 139, 145,
    158, 182, 195n113; abuse and, 6; affect
    theory and, 25; dependency used to
    justify, 8; encompassing sanism, aud-
    ism, and healthism, 31; experienced by
    care workers, 12–13; independence and,
    132–133; interdependency and, 151;
    intersecting identities and, 69; intersec-
    tion with other violence, 164; label of
    disability and, 27; long-term care and,
    16, 71; medical industrial complex and,
    158; messy dependency and, 131–133;
    neoliberalism as incubator for, 17, 101;
    pity or fear in, 23; productivity and, 141;
    social justice and, 146; social oppressions
    and, 28–31
"Access Intimacy, Interdependence and
    Disability Justice," 126
Achieving a Better Life Experience (ABLE)
    Act, 207n39
Affective bodymind, 119–121
Affective collectivity, 103–107, 210n6;
    affective bodymind and, 119–121,
    213n40; bed activism and, 170; beyond
    slow death and cerebral connectivity,
    107–109; co-capacitation and undercom-

mons, 122–123; co-capacitative force of,
    123; defined, 105–106; first encounter,
    109–113; recursive encounters, 113–116,
    213n41; shared vulnerability, 116–119;
    significance of, 104–105; undercommons
    and, 124–125
Affective labor industry, 80–81
Affective relationality, 106
Affect theory, 22–26
Agencement, 50
Aid to Families with Dependent Children,
    64
Altiraifi, Azza, 28
Americans with Disabilities Act, 23
Anzaldúa, Gloria, 164, 173
Assistance, defined, 11
Audism, 31, 195n113

Baggs, Mel, 131
Becoming *versus* being, 26
Bed activism, 8, 35–36, 178–180; defined,
    159–160; discussions of, 160; growth
    of, 163; neoliberalism and, 161–162,
    171–172; neplantla place of opening, 169;
    ontological resistance, 166–172; protests
    and, 160–161, 176–177; pulse of col-
    lectivity, 172–174; Sick Woman Theory,

Akemi Nishida is Assistant Professor of Disability and Human Development and Gender and Women's Studies at the University of Illinois Chicago. She is the coeditor of *Occupying Disability: Critical Approaches to Community, Justice, and Decolonizing Disability*.